# DERMATOLOGY
## *for the* PRIMARY CARE PROVIDER

# DERMATOLOGY
## *for the* PRIMARY CARE PROVIDER

**Reid A. Waldman, MD**
University of Connecticut Health Center
Department of Dermatology

**Jane M. Grant-Kels, MD, FAAD**
University of Connecticut Health Center
Department of Dermatology

ELSEVIER

Elsevier
1600 John F. Kennedy Blvd.
Ste 1800
Philadelphia, PA 19103-2899

DERMATOLOGY FOR THE PRIMARY CARE PROVIDER, FIRST EDITION ISBN: 9780323712361

---

**Notice**

Practitioners and researchers must always rely on their own experience and knowledge in evaluating and using any information, methods, compounds, or experiments described herein. Because of rapid advances in the medical sciences, in particular, independent verification of diagnoses and drug dosages should be made. To the fullest extent of the law, no responsibility is assumed by Elsevier, authors, editors, or contributors for any injury and/or damage to persons or property as a matter of products liability, negligence or otherwise, or from any use or operation of any methods, products, instructions, or ideas contained in the material herein.

---

**Library of Congress Control Number: 2021935844**

*Content Strategist:* Charlotta Kryhl
*Content Development Specialist:* Erika Ninsin
*Publishing Services Manager:* Shereen Jameel
*Project Manager:* Aparna Venkatachalam
*Design Direction:* Ryan Cook

Printed in India

Last digit is the print number: 9 8 7 6 5 4 3 2 1

Working together
to grow libraries in
developing countries

www.elsevier.com • www.bookaid.org

*Dedicated to my personal hero, my father, Steven D. Waldman, MD.*

*To Barry, the love of my life and best friend, and to our children (Charlie, Lori, Joanna, and Luke) and grandchildren (Grant, Landon, Chase, and Carson Kels and Charlotte Albright), who fill our lives with joy and wonder.*

# LIST OF CONTRIBUTORS

**Rana Abdat, MD**
Resident Physician
Department of Dermatology
Tufts Medical Center
Boston, Massachussetts

**Casey Abrahams, BA**
Medical Student
The Warren Alpert Medical School of Brown University
Providence, Rhode Island

**Tatiana Abrantes, BS**
Medical Student
The Warren Alpert Medical School of Brown University
Providence, Rhode Island

**Jonas Adalsteinsson, MD**
Resident Physician
Department of Dermatology
University of Connecticut Health Center
Farmington, Connecticut

**Douglas A. Albreski, DPM**
Assistant Professor of Dermatology
Department of Dermatology
University of Connecticut Health Center
Farmington, Connecticut

**Erisa Alia, MD**
Department of Dermatology
University of Connecticut Health Center
Farmington, Connecticut
Dermatology Resident
MedStar Washington Hospital Center
Georgetown University Hospital
Washington, D.C.

**Savannah M. Alvarado, MD**
Department of Dermatology
University of Connecticut
Farmington, Connecticut

**Kathryn Bentivegna, MPH**
Medical Student
University of Connecticut Health Center
Farmington, Connecticut

**Gregory Cavanagh, BS**
Medical Student
The Warren Alpert Medical School of Brown University
Providence, Rhode Island

**Afton Chavez, MD, FAAD,**
Dermatologist/Mohs Surgery Fellow
Beth Israel Lahey Health
Burlington, Massachusetts

**Michelle W. Cheng, MD**
Resident Physician
Division of Dermatology, Department of Medicine
David Geffen School of Medicine at UCLA
Los Angeles, California

**Taylor Cole, BS**
Medical Student
David Geffen School of Medicine at UCLA
Los Angeles, California

**Elizabeth Dupuy, MD**
Pediatric Dermatology Fellow
Children's Hospital Los Angeles
Los Angeles, California

**Hao Feng, MD, MHS**
Assistant Professor of Dermatology
Director of Laser Surgery and Cosmetic Dermatology
Department of Dermatology
University of Connecticut
Farmington, Connecticut

**Katalin Ferenczi, MD, FAAD**
Associate Professor
Department of Dermatology
University of Connecticut Health Center
Farmington, Connecticut

**Lynne J. Goldberg, MD**
Jag Bhawan Professor of Dermatology and Pathology
and Laboratory Medicine
Boston University School of Medicine
Boston, Massachusetts

**Ayman Grada, MD, MS**
Dermatologist, Wound Specialist
Department of Dermatology
Boston University School of Medicine
Boston, Massachusetts

**Christian Gronbeck, MD**
Resident Physician
University of Connecticut Health Center
Farmington, Connecticut

**Neelesh Jain, MD**
Resident Physician
Department of Dermatology
University of Connecticut Health Center
Farmington, Connecticut

**Preeti Jhorar, MD**
Clinical Instructor
Division of Dermatology, Department of Medicine,
David Geffen School of Medicine at UCLA
Los Angeles, California

**Christina Jiang**
University of Connecticut School of Medicine
Farmington, Connecticut

**Layla Kazemi, BA**
Medical Student
The Warren Alpert Medical School of Brown University
Providence, Rhode Island

**Andrew Kelsey, MD**
Assistant Professor
Department of Dermatology
University of Connecticut
Farmington, Connecticut

**Philip E. Kerr, MD, FAAD**
Chair, Department of Dermatology
Associate Professor of Dermatology and
Dermatopathology
University of Connecticut Health Center
Farmington, Connecticut

**Aziz Khan, MD**
Assistant Professor of Medicine
University of Connecticut School of Medicine
Farmington, Connecticut

**Nikita Lakdawala, MD**
Clinical Assistant Professor of Dermatology
The Ronald O. Perelman Department of Dermatology
NYU Langone Health
New York, New York

**Gloria Lin, MD**
Chief Resident
Department of Dermatology
University of Connecticut Health Center
Farmington, Connecticut

**Regina Liu, BA**
Medical Student
David Geffen School of Medicine at UCLA
Los Angeles, California

**Sarah Lonowski, MD, MBA**
Resident Physician
Division of Dermatology, Department of Medicine,
David Geffen School of Medicine at UCLA
Los Angeles, California

**Jun Lu, MD**
Associate Professor
Director, Clinical Trial Unit
Department of Dermatology
University of Connecticut
Farmington, Connecticut

**Mohammed Malik**
Medical Student
University of Connecticut School of Medicine
Farmington, Connecticut

**Sonal Muzumdar, MD**
Resident Physician
Department of Dermatology
University of Connecticut
Farmington, Connecticut

**Tania Phillips, MD FRCPC**
Professor of Dermatology
Boston University School of Medicine
Boston, Massachusetts

**Payal C. Shah**
Medical Student
NYU Langone School of Medicine
New York, New York

**Jeff Shornick, MD**
Associate Professor (Retired)
Department of Dermatology
Dartmouth Medical School
Hanover, New Hampshire

**Shivani Sinha, MS**
Frank H. Netter MD School of Medicine
Quinnipiac University
North Haven, Connecticut

**Brett Sloan, MD, FAAD**
Professor of Dermatology
University of Connecticut
Farmington, Connecticut

**Campbell L. Stewart, MD, FAAD**
Assistant Professor
Department of Dermatology
University of Connecticut Health Center
Farmington, Connecticut

**Victoria Stoj, MD, MPH**
Department of Dermatology
University of Connecticut
Farmington, Connecticut

**Logan Thomas, MD**
Resident Physician
Division of Dermatology, Department of Medicine,
David Geffen School of Medicine at UCLA
Los Angeles, California

**Amy R. Vandiver, MD, PhD**
Dermatology Resident
Division of Dermatology, Department of Medicine
University of California at Los Angeles
Los Angeles, California

**Diane L. Whitaker-Worth, MD, FAAD**
Associate Professor
Department of Dermatology
UConn Health
Farmington, Connecticut

# TABLE OF CONTENTS

*All sections not specified were authored by Reid A. Waldman and Jane M. Grant-Kels

# DERMATOLOGY
## *for the* PRIMARY CARE PROVIDER

# Red and Purple Lesions That Look Like a Rash or Dermatitis

# 1

# Scalp Dermatitis

*Reid A. Waldman and Jane M. Grant-Kels*

## CHAPTER OUTLINE

# SCALP PSORIASIS

## Clinical Features

Scalp psoriasis is characterized by the presence of well-demarcated erythematous plaques with overlying white scale of variable thickness affecting the occipital scalp more commonly than the remainder of the scalp.

- The scalp may be the only area of the body affected by plaque psoriasis.
- More commonly, scalp psoriasis occurs concomitantly with psoriasis elsewhere.
- The main differential diagnosis for isolated scalp psoriasis is seborrheic dermatitis.
  - In cases where scalp psoriasis and seborrheic dermatitis cannot be readily distinguished from one another, the rash is referred to as "sebopsoriasis."
- Psoriasis can be differentiated from seborrheic dermatitis based on:
  - The location of scalp involvement—Isolated occipital scalp involvement in subtler cases of scalp psoriasis versus encroachment onto the forehead and temples in seborrheic dermatitis;
  - The presence of characteristic skin lesions elsewhere—The elbows, gluteal cleft, knees, nails, palms, soles, and trunk for psoriasis or the nasolabial folds, glabella, or chest for seborrheic dermatitis;
  - Plaque and scale appearance—Psoriasis has more sharply circumscribed, redder-looking plaques and whiter-looking scale, whereas seborrheic dermatitis has thinner, pinker-looking plaques and greasier-looking scale;
  - Degree of treatment responsiveness—Classically psoriasis is less treatment responsive than seborrheic dermatitis;
  - Family history and past medical history of psoriasis.
- Differentiation of psoriasis from seborrheic dermatitis is important because:
  - Antifungals are a mainstay of treatment in seborrheic dermatitis, but they are much less effective in psoriasis.
  - Refractory cases of psoriasis benefit from the use of phototherapy or systemic therapy, whereas these are not recommended in seborrheic dermatitis.
  - Psoriasis has comorbidities such as psoriatic arthritis and the metabolic syndrome that require prompt recognition and management, whereas seborrheic dermatitis does not.
- Uncontrolled, severe scalp psoriasis can present with a pityriasis amiantacea-like appearance where a patient's hair is engulfed by scale; however, scalp psoriasis in and of itself does not result in alopecia. The presence of scaly alopecic plaques should prompt investigation for other causes of an itchy scalp rash, including tinea capitis.
- Scalp psoriasis often coexists with ear canal psoriasis, which is typically very pruritic and involves its own separate management. Nevertheless, ear involvement with pruritus can also be seen in seborrheic dermatitis and therefore is not always helpful to differentiate the two diseases.

## Work-Up

- A total-body skin examination should be performed to identify other areas of the body affected by psoriasis. Patients frequently do not realize that their scalp rash is related to their body rash.
- All patients with psoriasis require screening for psoriatic arthritis (PsA) at every single visit because a delay in diagnosis of PsA can result in irreparable joint damage.
- Patients with longstanding psoriasis that has suddenly worsened and patients with acute-onset psoriasis should have their medication list reviewed for possible exacerbating triggers (see Chapter 3).
- Routine evaluation for possible systemic triggers of psoriasis (e.g., HIV, streptococcal pharyngitis) is not indicated in the absence of clinical suspicion.
- Routine histologic confirmation is not indicated except in atypical-appearing cases or in cases that fail to respond to treatment as expected.
- Examination of hairs with potassium hydroxide (KOH) and/or submitted for culture should be considered to rule out tinea capitis if possible.

## Initial Steps in Management
### General Management Comments

- Noncompliance with topical therapies is common among patients with scalp dermatoses because of the poor cosmesis of these products.
- There is no cure for psoriasis. Patients will have flare-ups if they discontinue therapy. The goal of therapy is symptom management. It is important to convey this to patients. The course is usually chronic, with a history of waxing and waning.

- Class I, II, and III topical corticosteroids are the mainstay of treatment for scalp psoriasis and are clinically superior and better tolerated than topical vitamin D analogue monotherapy.
- In cases refractory to Class I topical corticosteroids, combination topical corticosteroid vitamin D analogue products can be considered because they have demonstrated superiority over topical corticosteroid monotherapy.
  - Combination products are frequently prohibitively expensive and often require prior authorization by insurance companies.
- Topical vitamin D analogue monotherapy can be used in mild cases where patients prefer to avoid topical steroid use.
- Nowhere is topical medication vehicle more important than on the scalp. Compliance is highly affected by vehicle type. Suitable vehicles for the scalp (in order of suitability) include solution, spray, foam, oil, lotion, and shampoo. Often, insurance formularies dictate which vehicle type is available to the patient. In cases where multiple vehicle types are available, deference to patient preference is reasonable.
- If shampoos are going to be prescribed, then patients must be counseled that these must be left in contact with the scalp for around 15 minutes before rinsing. In the authors' experience, compliance with scalp shampoos is variable.
- If scalp oils are going to be prescribed, then occluding the oil under a shower cap can be considered because scalp oils are frequently very messy. Importantly, children should never be encouraged to use oils under shower cap occlusion because of the risk of shower cap-induced asphyxiation. Additionally, scalp oils should not be used in patients with peanut allergies because the oil vehicle is peanut oil.

## Recommended Initial Regimen

- Clobetasol propionate 0.05% scalp solution, spray, or foam (depending on patient preference and insurance formulary) daily until clear followed by PRN use. Care should be taken to avoid exposure of facial skin to this medication. Patients should be counseled about signs of steroid-related atrophy; however, realistically, this almost never occurs on the scalp.

- A nonexhaustive list of alternatives to clobetasol propionate include in decreasing order of potency: halobetasol propionate 0.05% lotion or foam, betamethasone dipropionate 0.05% lotion or spray, fluocinonide 0.05% topical solution, betamethasone valerate 0.12% foam, fluocinolone 0.025% oil or solution.

What to do if there is a partial but inadequate response after a 4-week trial of potent topical corticosteroid monotherapy:
- Either switch to a combination topical corticosteroid vitamin D analogue product (e.g., betamethasone dipropionate-calcipotriene 0.005%-0.064% scalp solution daily) or add a topical vitamin D analogue product (e.g., calcipotriene 0.005% scalp solution) to the existing corticosteroid regimen.
- Almost all patients who are compliant with therapy should become clear or almost clear with combination therapy.
- In the experience of the authors, compliance is superior for combination products; however, they are often not covered by insurance without prior authorization.

What to do if the response continues to be inadequate:
- Reconsider the diagnosis. If you are not confident in the diagnosis of psoriasis, it is reasonable to consider a punch biopsy of an affected area at this time. Punch biopsies on the scalp are technically more difficult than punch biopsies elsewhere and should only be performed by experienced practitioners. Additionally, the pathology requisition form for a punch biopsy from the scalp must specify that the biopsy is from the scalp because horizontal sectioning is often performed.
- Because scarring alopecia can result from some inflammatory scalp dermatoses, referral to a dermatologist is indicated at this point in time unless one is not available.
- If you are confident that the patient has psoriasis and it is refractory to a combination topical corticosteroid–vitamin D analogue product, then next steps in therapy include intralesional corticosteroid injections, phototherapy (including narrowband ultraviolet B [UVB] and even localized psoralen and ultraviolet A [PUVA] and xenon chloride laser), oral immunosuppressive medications (e.g., methotrexate), acitretin, and biologic medications (reserved for severe scalp psoriasis or for patients with psoriasis elsewhere).

## Other Treatment Options

- Topical coal tar preparations, salicylic acid, glycolic acid, and anthralin are all reported treatments for scalp psoriasis. Data supporting the use of these agents are much weaker than data supporting the use of topical corticosteroids and vitamin D analogues. These agents should only be considered as adjuncts to combination topical corticosteroid vitamin D analogue therapy in patients who fail combination therapy and who are uninterested in phototherapy or systemic therapy for treatment of their psoriasis. The authors' preferential use of these treatments is listed in order of decreasing preference as follows: glycolic acid > salicylic acid > coal tar > anthralin.

# WARNING SIGNS/COMMON PITFALLS

- Patients with psoriasis should be screened at regular intervals for psoriatic arthritis. If any clinical suspicion for psoriatic arthritis exists, then the patient should be referred urgently to a rheumatologist. There are validated screening tools that can easily be implemented in the clinical setting.
- Occasionally, discoid lupus erythematosus can mimic scalp psoriasis. Discoid lupus erythematosus can be differentiated from psoriasis based on its focal, annular nature; the more violaceous hue of its plaques; and its different scale quality; however, this is not always obvious. Promptly recognizing and treating discoid lupus is essential because it is a form of scarring alopecia that causes irreversible hair loss. It is also occasionally associated with systemic lupus erythematosus (around 5% of the time for scalp-only disease).
- Tinea capitis must be excluded if suspected with KOH examination or cultures.
- Never treat scalp psoriasis with systemic corticosteroids. This will almost always trigger a flare once corticosteroids are tapered. This is a chronic disease that requires chronic management.

## Counseling

Psoriasis is a rash that results from your genetics (family history) and immune system causing inflammation in your skin. Psoriasis is a chronic disease that tends to wax and wane. It is incurable, meaning that it lasts for years. Treatments for psoriasis are directed at decreasing inflammation in the skin. The goal of treating psoriasis is to manage symptoms.

Importantly, some people with psoriasis also develop a condition called psoriatic arthritis where they experience painful swelling of the joints and stiffness in the joints when they wake up in the morning that lasts for hours. If you think you may have psoriatic arthritis, it is important that you let us know because psoriatic arthritis can irreversibly damage your joints if it is not treated.

Some patients with psoriasis are at risk for metabolic syndrome (diabetes, obesity, cardiovascular disease, etc.). Therefore weight control and exercise are important to include in your daily routine.

I have prescribed you a topical corticosteroid. You should apply this to your scalp every day while you have the rash. When no rash is present, you do not need to use this medication. It is okay to resume use of the medication when the rash comes back. The major side effect of this medication is that it can thin the skin and cause the blood vessels in the skin to dilate and become visible. This typically does not occur on the scalp but may occur if you use the medication more frequently than instructed or if you apply this medicine to other places on your body, such as your face.

# SEBORRHEIC DERMATITIS—SCALP

## Clinical Features

Seborrheic dermatitis is characterized by the presence of poorly circumscribed, thin, pink plaques with an overlying greasy-looking scale that appear on the seborrheic areas of the body. Seborrheic dermatitis is on a continuum with dandruff because both impact seborrheic areas of the body. Dandruff, however, is limited to the scalp and presents with pruritus and scaling but not erythema. Seborrheic dermatitis can impact other seborrheic areas in addition to the scalp and demonstrates itching, scaling, and evidence of inflammation.

- In adults, seborrheic dermatitis most commonly involves the scalp and is the most common cause of scalp itch.
  - Seborrheic dermatitis may also affect other so-called seborrheic areas, such as the eyebrows, glabella, nasolabial folds, retroauricular area, and chest.
- When seborrheic dermatitis affects the scalp of an infant, it is called "cradle cap."
  - Infantile seborrheic dermatitis also commonly affects the diaper area, axillae, and retroauricular area.

- Uncontrolled, severe seborrheic dermatitis can present with a pityriasis amiantacea-like appearance where a patient's hair is engulfed by scale; however, seborrheic dermatitis in and of itself does not result in alopecia.
- Seborrheic dermatitis commonly develops in immunosuppressed individuals and in individuals with Parkinson disease. In rare cases, severe seborrheic dermatitis can be the presenting sign of HIV.

The etiology of seborrheic dermatitis is multifactorial and is likely because of a normal body yeast called *Malassezia*. If the immune system has a somewhat irregular response to *Malassezia*, it may result in this inflammatory condition. The disease is very common, impacting 1% to 5% of the population and including all races and sexes.

## Differential Diagnosis

- In adults, the main differential diagnosis for seborrheic dermatitis is scalp psoriasis (Fig. 2.8). Rarely, tinea capitis can be mistaken for seborrheic dermatitis (Fig. 2.9).
- Seborrheic dermatitis can be differentiated from scalp psoriasis based on the following characteristics:
  - The location of scalp involvement—Plaques of seborrheic dermatitis are ill defined and can affect anywhere in the scalp. Psoriasis plaques often develop near the hairline in the frontotemporal scalp and may extend onto the forehead and temples. In contradistinction, milder cases of scalp psoriasis are localized to the occipital scalp.
  - Presence of characteristic skin lesions elsewhere— As previously mentioned, seborrheic dermatitis often also affects other seborrheic areas, whereas psoriatic plaques most frequently develop on extensor surfaces.
  - Plaque and scale appearance—Plaques of seborrheic dermatitis are thin, ill defined, and pink and have a greasy-looking scale, whereas psoriatic plaques are thicker, well circumscribed, and covered in white, micaceous scales.
  - Response to antifungals—Seborrheic dermatitis responds to azole antifungals within 4 weeks of treatment; psoriasis, meanwhile, will not typically respond as rapidly to antifungals and even when it does, it tends to recur and to be more resistant.

Tinea capitis can be distinguished from seborrheic dermatitis because tinea capitis usually presents as a solitary, discrete plaque, has overlying alopecia, and predominantly has peripheral scaling rather than diffuse scaling. If there is concern that the patient may have tinea capitis, a KOH examination and fungal culture can distinguish tinea capitis from seborrheic dermatitis.

## Testing and Work-Up

- In both adults and infants, a total-body skin examination, with a focused examination of seborrheic areas (such as the eyebrows, beard, nasolabial folds, retroauricular area, and central chest) should be performed to identify all areas of the body that may be affected by seborrheic dermatitis.
- Adults who present with subacute onset severe seborrheic dermatitis affecting the face and chest should be screened for HIV unless another obvious trigger for development of seborrheic dermatitis has been identified (e.g., organ transplant immunosuppression, Parkinson disease; Fig. 2.10).
- Seborrheic dermatitis is generally a clinical diagnosis; rarely is a biopsy required to make a diagnosis of seborrheic dermatitis.

## How To Manage Seborrheic Dermatitis

Management of seborrheic dermatitis is divided into two phases: (1) an intensive initial treatment phase, which is followed by a (2) less intensive maintenance phase. There is no cure for seborrheic dermatitis. The course is chronic with waxing and waning. Failure to emphasize the importance of using a maintenance therapy virtually guarantees disease recurrence and patient dissatisfaction.

- After an initial period of treatment responsiveness, some patients can become treatment resistant and require a change in therapy. This most frequently is seen in patients receiving antifungals.
- In elderly patients, especially institutionalized elderly patients who require assistance when bathing, a common cause of treatment failure is that these patients are only showered once or twice weekly. Daily bathing is both a treatment for seborrheic dermatitis and is required for medicated shampoos to be effective. Tailoring therapy based on patient bathing habits is essential to success.
- In all infants with cradle cap and in adults with substantial scaling, emollients (e.g., plain petroleum jelly or mineral oil) are necessary for loosening scale. Gentle debridement with a hairbrush is also helpful.

- Treatment options are divided into antifungal and antiinflammatory approaches:
  - Antifungals
    - Azoles (e.g., ketoconazole, clotrimazole, etc.) – The initial treatment of all adults with seborrheic dermatitis should include a topical azole. For scalp disease, shampoos are most commonly prescribed. Ketoconazole is the only prescription azole shampoo available in the United States. It is generally used 2 to 3 times a week. On alternate days, other medicated shampoos are recommended that contain selenium, zinc, salicylic acid, etc. Other azole shampoos (miconazole and climbazole) are available over the counter but do not have the same degree of clinical efficacy as ketoconazole.
    - Ciclopirox—Ciclopirox is a reasonable second-line antifungal. Although it is equally as effective as topical azoles, it is more likely to cause scalp irritation and is typically more expensive. In patients who are bathed infrequently, ciclopirox shampoo is preferential to ketoconazole because it requires less frequent applications (1–2 times a week has been demonstrated to be effective).
    - Selenium sulfide (active ingredient in Selsun Blue)
    - Zinc pyrithione (active ingredient in Head and Shoulders)
  - Antiinflammatory drugs
- Topical corticosteroids—These are equally as effective and possibly more effective than antifungals, but they are more likely to cause cutaneous adverse effects and more likely to cause early disease rebound after discontinuation. Topical corticosteroids should be added in cases that do not respond appropriately to topical antifungals and should be used preferentially in patients with scalp disease who are bathed infrequently. These drugs should be used with caution in cases of cradle cap. Topical steroid scalp preparations can be prescribed as solutions, foams, and even shampoos.
- Topical calcineurin inhibitors—These are equally effective to antifungals and topical corticosteroids. Topical calcineurin inhibitors are only commercially available as ointments and creams, making them less cosmetically acceptable for scalp dermatitis. There is no topical calcineurin inhibitor formulation that is designed for scalp disease.

- Crisaborole—There is limited experience with crisaborole at this point. It is only available as an ointment and therefore is not ideal for scalp disease; it is also often not cosmetically desirable for facial diseases.
- Promiseb—There is not one specific active ingredient in Promiseb. It is a combination of antiinflammatory agents. It is often very expensive but can be considered in refractory cases.

## Recommended Initial Treatment Regimen in Adults

- Initial treatment phase (first 4 weeks of treatment)—Ketoconazole 2% shampoo 2 to 3 times weekly for 4 weeks. The shampoo should be kept in contact with the scalp for 5 to 15 minutes before rinsing. On all other days of the week, over-the-counter (OTC) antifungal shampoos containing either zinc pyrithione or selenium sulfide should be used. Salicylic acid shampoos (such as T-Sal) are also helpful for debridement.
- Maintenance phase (after initial treatment phase)—Ketoconazole 2% shampoo once weekly indefinitely. The shampoo should be kept in contact with the scalp for 5 to 15 minutes before rinsing. On all other days of the week, OTC antifungal shampoos containing either zinc pyrithione or selenium sulfide should be used.
- Patients with severe scaling should also be encouraged to apply mineral oil or another emollient to their scalp nightly. In adults, a shower cap can be used to keep the oil from creating a mess on the patient's bedding. In the morning, a comb can be used to gently debride the now-loosened scale before shampooing.
- Derma-Smooth/FS (fluocinolone acetonide in a peanut oil base) can be prescribed for overnight application. Most patients with a known peanut allergy tolerate this topical therapeutic. Skin testing has shown no immediate (15-min) or delayed (72-h) skin test reactivity, suggesting that refined peanut oil–containing oils are safe to use, even in patients with a history of sensitivity to peanuts. Even the use of this product in atopic children with a history of peanut allergy was found to be safe.

What to do if there is a partial but inadequate response after a 4-week trial of topical azole monotherapy:
- Steroid solutions and foams can be applied to the scalp to reduce inflammation. This should only be

done as needed in the acute phase to avoid secondary side effects from the topical steroids because the scalp skin is highly vascularized and not particularly thick, making it susceptible both to absorption of medications systemically and local atrophy.

- Add or switch to a topical corticosteroid (e.g., clobetasol dipropionate 0.05% solution nightly or fluocinonide acetate 0.05% solution nightly). In cases with severe scaling, fluocinolone acetonide 0.01% scalp oil with or without shower cap occlusion nightly is preferred because the fluocinolone scalp oil serves both as an antiinflammatory and emollient. A much milder topical steroid, topical 1% hydrocortisone scalp solution, is also available over the counter; patients should be warned to use even this mild topical steroid only intermittently.

What to do if response to azole monotherapy wanes over time:

- Initial treatment phase (first 4 weeks of treatment)— Switch to ciclopirox 1% shampoo twice weekly for 4 weeks. The shampoo should be kept in contact with the scalp for 5 to 15 minutes before rinsing. On all other days of the week, OTC antifungal shampoos containing either zinc pyrithione or selenium sulfide should be used.
- Maintenance phase (after initial treatment phase)— Ciclopirox 1% shampoo once weekly indefinitely. The shampoo should be kept in contact with the scalp for 5 to 15 minutes before rinsing. On all other days of the week, OTC antifungal shampoos containing either zinc pyrithione or selenium sulfide should be used.

What to do if the response continues to be inadequate:

- Reconsider the diagnosis. If you are not confident in the diagnosis, it is reasonable to consider a punch biopsy of an affected area at this time. Punch biopsies on the scalp are technically more difficult than punch biopsies elsewhere because of the vascularity of the scalp, resulting in bleeding and the need to place the biopsy at the same angle as the growing hair. Therefore these biopsies should only be performed by experienced practitioners. Additionally, the pathology requisition form for a punch biopsy from the scalp must specify that the biopsy is from the scalp because horizontal sectioning is often performed.
- If you are concerned that the patient may have tinea capitis, a fungal culture or KOH preparation is a reasonable next step.

- Because scarring alopecia can result from some inflammatory scalp dermatoses, referral to a dermatologist is indicated at this point in a timely fashion to avoid unnecessary permanent hair loss.
- It is very rare for scalp seborrheic dermatitis to be refractory to a combination of topical corticosteroids and topical antifungals if the patient is compliant with therapy. If you are confident that the patient has seborrheic dermatitis and it is refractory to a combination of topical corticosteroids and topical antifungals, then evaluation for immunosuppression (e.g., HIV) should be performed. Obtaining a history of the patient's bathing habits is also essential for dictating therapy moving forward. A short course of oral azole antifungals can also be considered (e.g., fluconazole 200 mg PO once weekly for 2 weeks).

## Other Treatment Options

- Other aforementioned treatment options for scalp disease are not frequently employed for seborrheic dermatitis because they are not manufactured in vehicles that are conducive for application to the scalp. Coal tar shampoos have historically been used for treating scalp seborrheic dermatitis, but data supporting their use are limited. Patients with blond or white hair should be warned about the possibility of discoloration of their hair from staining by the tar. As previously mentioned, short-course oral azole antifungals can be considered in severe cases, but they are rarely necessary.

## Recommended Initial Treatment Regimen for Cradle Cap

- Daily hair washing with baby shampoo preceded by application of plain white petroleum jelly (Vaseline) to the scalp once daily. The Vaseline should stay on the scalp for about an hour to help soften the scales before shampooing. Once-daily gentle scale debridement with a soft brush or comb can also be considered.
- Other emollients such as mineral oil, baby oil, or olive oil can be used as alternatives to plain white petroleum jelly if preferred.

What to do if there is a partial but inadequate response after a 4-week trial of topical emollients:

- Given the harmless nature of this condition, no additional treatment is required unless parents are significantly bothered by the condition. In most instances, switching emollients is effective. In cases where this is ineffective or additional therapy is desired, either hydrocortisone 1% cream or ketoconazole 2% cream can be applied once daily for 1 to 2 weeks.

## WARNING SIGNS/COMMON PITFALLS

### In Adults

- See previous commentary about considering a patient's bathing habits when treating seborrheic dermatitis because infrequent bathing and infrequent shampooing are a common cause of treatment failure and nonadherence to medicated shampoos.
- See previous commentary about the importance of incorporating a maintenance treatment into the treatment regimen for seborrheic dermatitis.

### In Children

- Never use a shower cap for medication occlusion in children because this can lead to suffocation and death of the child.
- Atypical-appearing cases, especially those with crusted lesions on the scalp and the diaper area, should be evaluated by a dermatologist because of the remote possibility of a malignancy called Langerhans cell histiocytosis mimicking seborrheic dermatitis (Fig. 1.1). This consideration requires a punch biopsy to help establish the diagnosis.

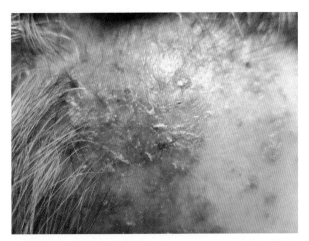

**Fig. 1.1 Langerhans Cell Histiocytosis in An Adult Male.** Note the crusted papules and erosions that help distinguish this condition from seborrheic dermatitis. (From the UConn Department of Dermatology Grand Rounds Collection.)

## Patient Information
### For Adults

You have a rash called seborrheic dermatitis. It is a severe form of dandruff that can involve the scalp but also the face and chest. It is a chronic, recurrent, waxing and waning type of rash, which means that there is no cure. Most importantly, it is a self-limited type of rash, which means that it will not cause you internal harm. This rash is the result of inflammation caused by your immune system. The exact reason that you have developed this rash is unknown. Some experts think that it develops because your immune system overreacts to fats made by a yeast called *Malassezia* that lives on your skin; however, other experts do not think this is the case. Because this is a normal skin yeast, this is not a form of infection and is not contagious.

I have prescribed you an antifungal (yeast) shampoo. You should use this shampoo 3 times per week for 4 weeks. When you wash your hair with this shampoo, it is important that you let the shampoo remain on your scalp for at least 5 minutes before rinsing it out. In 4 weeks, you can decrease the frequency with which you use this shampoo to once per week. It is important that you continue to use this shampoo every week; if you do not, it is likely that the rash will come back. On the days that you do not use the antifungal shampoo, I recommend that you use an OTC shampoo containing either selenium sulfide or zinc pyrithione because these products also have antifungal properties. Examples of brands that contain these ingredients include Selsun Blue and Head & Shoulders. If one of these shampoos that you have been using chronically loses effectiveness, switch to another type of shampoo; always use at least two different types of shampoos during the week to reduce this possibility.

### For Children With Cradle Cap

Your child has a rash called seborrheic dermatitis. This is often referred to colloquially by the name "cradle cap." This rash is not dangerous and will go away with time. It is unknown why infants get this rash.

I recommend that you apply either plain Vaseline or mineral oil to your child's scalp at least an hour before shampooing to soften and loosen the scale. After that, wash your child's hair every day with a baby shampoo. Once daily, you can also gently brush your child's scalp with a comb or soft brush to try to remove the scale. Remember to be gentle! Once your baby has improved, you can eliminate the use of the Vaseline or mineral oil.

Nevertheless, continue shampooing every day or at least every other day.

# LICHEN PLANOPILARIS

## Clinical Features

Lichen planopilaris (LPP) is a variant of lichen planus that affects hair-bearing skin and is a type of scarring hair loss (i.e., primary cicatricial alopecia) that may present as an itchy scalp rash.
- LPP (Fig. 1.2) presents with patchy hair loss with perifollicular erythema and scaling.
  - Affected areas are typically itchy or burn.
    - LPP occurs more commonly in women than in men, in Caucasians than in other groups, and in people in their 50s or 60s than in other age groups.
    - Clinically, LPP is divided into three subtypes, based on distribution of involvement, that may demonstrate overlap:
  - Classic LPP—LPP involving the frontal and parietal scalp;

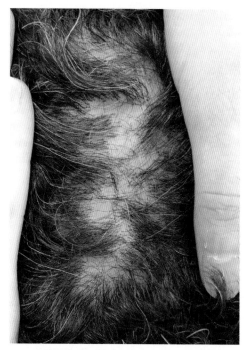

**Fig. 1.2 Lichen Pilanopilaris.** Note the purple perifollicular scale surrounding the burnt-out and scarred areas. (Courtesy Justin Finch, MD.)

- Frontal fibrosing alopecia—Considered by some to be a variant of LPP that exclusively involves the frontal scalp (often presents as hairline regression) and the eyebrows;
- Graham-Little-Piccardi-Lassueur Syndrome—Rare triad of scalp LPP, nonscarring alopecia of the axillae and pubic hair, and an eruption of follicular papules all over the body.
  - In a minority of cases, LPP coexists with lichen planus on non–hair-bearing skin or on the mucosa.
  - Although there are specific clinical findings that are more common in different subtypes of LPP, all types of LPP can present with the following:
    - Eyebrow loss;
    - Other non-scalp hair loss, including hair loss in the beard area and the extremities;
    - Flesh-colored facial papules (which likely represent involvement of the vellus hairs on the face).
  - Early LPP is often misdiagnosed as androgenetic alopecia occurring in combination with seborrheic dermatitis.
    - Early LPP can be differentiated from androgenetic alopecia based on the following:
      - LPP presents with discrete patches of alopecia.
      - LPP presents with perifollicular erythema and scaling, although this may be subtle.
      - LPP causes scarring and therefore follicular ostia will not be identifiable in areas of scarring.
- Other common mimickers of LPP include the other primary cicatricial alopecias (Figs. 1.3 and 1.4; e.g., central centrifugal cicatricial alopecia, chronic cutaneous lupus erythematosus).

## Work-Up

- In all cases of LPP, a total-body skin and mucosal examination should be performed and a targeted history should be obtained to evaluate for disease activity elsewhere (e.g., in the extremities, groin, axillae).
- In cases where a diagnosis of LPP cannot be rendered on clinical grounds alone, a punch biopsy is required to confirm the diagnosis. A biopsy should be obtained from an active area of inflammation, not from a scarred area.

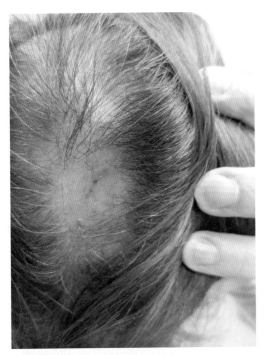

**Fig. 1.3 End-Stage Cicatricial Alopecia.** Note the absence of hair follicles in the scarred areas. Hair regrowth within those areas is not possible. (From the UConn Department of Dermatology Grand Rounds Collection.)

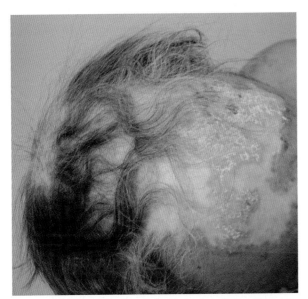

**Fig. 1.4 Discoid Lupus Erythematosus Affecting the Scalp.** Note the surrounding inflammatory border. (From the UConn Department of Dermatology Grand Rounds Collection.)

- Thyroid function tests should be ordered for all patients with LPP because around 10% of patients with LPP have hypothyroidism.

## Initial Steps in Management

All patients with presumed primary cicatricial alopecia, including LPP, should be referred urgently to a dermatologist who is comfortable treating scarring alopecia because the scarring that results from these conditions is permanent but can be curtailed with appropriate management.

There is no cure for LPP and the scarring that it causes is not reversible. The goal of therapy is to stop active inflammation and prevent disease progression. A secondary goal of therapy is to hasten hair regrowth in nonscarred areas; however, this should not be emphasized until the inflammatory component of the disease is under control. It is important to convey this to patients.

Most patients with LPP require the combination of ultra-potent topical corticosteroids with an oral immunosuppressive agent (e.g., mycophenolate mofetil, cyclosporine, methotrexate) or an antimalarial (e.g., hydroxychloroquine) to obtain complete remission of their disease. These medications should be started and monitored by a dermatologist.

## Recommended Initial Regimen

- Clobetasol propionate 0.05% scalp solution, spray, or foam (depending on patient preference and insurance formulary) daily or twice daily. Patients should be counseled that daily use is mandatory and that this can safely be continued for months. On average, it takes almost a year of continuous therapy to obtain complete remission of LPP, and it may take months of continuous use to notice any clinically significant benefit. Before obtaining complete remission, no topical steroid drug holiday should occur.
  - Patients should be counseled that topical steroids do not hasten hair regrowth and that their hair will grow, if scarring has yet to take place, at its normal growth rate once the inflammation has been stopped.
- A nonexhaustive list of alternatives to clobetasol propionate include in decreasing order of potency: halobetasol priopionate 0.05% lotion or foam, betamethasone dipropionate 0.05% lotion or spray, fluocinonide 0.05% topical solution, betamethasone valerate 0.12% foam, fluocinolone 0.025% oil or solution.

What to do if there is extensive inflammation or if there is going to be a delay in access to a dermatology appointment:

- As previously mentioned, the majority of patients require either an oral immunosuppressant or an antimalarial to obtain control of their LPP; however, in cases where there is going to be a delay in the initiation of one of these agents, oral corticosteroids can be used. Initiation of oral corticosteroids is not a replacement, however, for requesting an urgent dermatology referral so that a steroid-sparing oral medication can be initiated.
- If you are going to start oral corticosteroids, they should be started as follows in most cases: Prednisone 1 mg/kg PO every morning with a plan to down-titrate the dose by 10% per week to the lowest dose possible that still maintains satisfactory disease control.
  - It is important to consider the significant systemic toxicities of long-term high-dose corticosteroids before starting treatment.
    - Most patients need a baseline dual-energy X-ray absorptiometry (DEXA) scan and qualify for osteoporosis prophylaxis.
    - Some patients qualify for pneumocystis pneumonia prophylaxis.
  - Patients who are titrated off oral corticosteroids without the substitution of an appropriate steroid-sparing agent are at a high risk for disease relapse.
  - Short-course steroids (e.g., a 5-day dose pack) are not helpful and may trigger severe disease rebound.

### Warning Signs/Common Pitfalls

This disease causes irreversible scarring hair loss and therefore requires aggressive management to prevent progression. Once scarring has occurred, there is nothing that can be done to reverse it. If you are suspicious that a patient may have LPP or another primary cicatricial alopecia, refer the patient urgently to an experienced dermatologist.

Patients with LPP often have coexistent androgenetic alopecia. The presence of androgenetic alopecia does not rule out LPP or any other primary cicatricial alopecia nor does it make these diagnoses less likely.

Do not place a stop date on the use of ultrapotent topical corticosteroids out of fear of local corticosteroid-induced adverse effects because these adverse effects are unlikely to develop on the scalp and long-term therapy is necessary to achieve clinical benefit.

## COUNSELING

You have an uncommon type of hair loss called lichen planopilaris, or LPP for short. This type of hair loss is caused by inflammation in your hair follicles. It is unknown why people develop LPP; however, it is a chronic condition, which means that it lasts for a long time and is currently incurable.

If left untreated, LPP can cause permanent scarring and hair loss. Permanently scarred areas will never regrow hair. This is why it is important to treat LPP early and to continue treatment until the condition has burned out, which may take years. The goal of treating your condition is to reduce the inflammation, prevent additional scarring from occurring, and allow hair regrowth to occur in nonscarred areas.

You have been prescribed an ultrapotent topical corticosteroid. It is important that you use this medication every day. It is important that you do not stop this medication without consulting your doctor first. It may take months of daily use for you to notice improvement. If you stop your medication, your disease may come back. You should not put this medication on your face or other areas of your body not specifically mentioned by your doctor. It can cause thinning of the skin and visible blood vessel formation.

Many patients will also need an oral medication in addition to this topical medication to get satisfactory control of their disease. It is important that you see a dermatologist to determine whether you are a patient that might benefit from a pill for this condition.

## HEAD LICE

### Clinical Features

- Head lice infestation (pediculosis capitis) is a not infrequent cause of itchy scalp rash that more commonly occurs in children than adults.
  - The itch related to a head lice infestation is caused by sensitization to head louse saliva; therefore itch usually does not develop until weeks after an initial infestation.

- Head lice are not a vector for any infectious disease; however, infestation with head lice is stigmatized and frequently symptomatic.
- Head lice infestation primarily spreads person-to-person from direct head-to-head contact, but it can less frequently spread indirectly from sharing objects that have come into contact with an infested scalp (e.g., a hat, comb, pillowcase, movie seats).
- The primary differential diagnoses for head lice are dandruff (seborrheic dermatitis), hair casts (so-called "pseudonits"), and the presence of foreign debris (commonly hairspray and hair gel residue). In the authors' experience, many patients are misdiagnosed with head lice by non–healthcare personnel but do not have lice.
  - Head lice can be distinguished from the other items on the differential by identification of an actual louse.
  - Nits are distinguished from hair casts ("pseudonits") because nits are firmly adherent to hair shafts; hair casts easily slide on the hair shaft.
  - Foreign debris can be distinguished from the other items on the differential because it will be removed from the scalp during a wet comb examination.

## Work-Up

The initial work-up for head lice involves an examination of the scalp hair to identify the presence of lice and/or nits. If needed, a wet comb examination should be undertaken.

- To perform a wet comb examination, water, conditioner, or mineral oil is applied to the scalp hair. Using a louse comb, all of the patient's hair is combed through in the hopes of identifying adult head lice, nymphs, eggs, and/or nits.
- Head lice diagnosis includes the finding of any of the following:
  - Adult head lice: 2 to 3 mm, 6-legged, mobile, and tan-white in color.
  - Nymphs: Immature head lice that are smaller than adult lice and go through three separate stages of development before maturing into adult lice.
  - Eggs: Hair colored, barely large enough to see, and residing within 4 mm of the scalp for temperature regulation.
  - Nits: Empty eggs (i.e., eggs from which nymphs have already hatched) that are whitish in color;

nits can still be identified after successful treatment of lice because they are not alive and are adherent to the hair.

- A diagnosis of active head lice is made based on the identification of a live louse or nymph on a patient's scalp.
- Lice can only move by crawling and do not jump from head to head; however, static electricity can reportedly propel a louse up to 1 meter, which is why the scalp hair examination is best performed on wet hair.

Close contacts and family members should also be inspected for head lice; however, schoolwide lice checks are not recommended because they have been shown to be ineffective at slowing the spread of head lice.

## Initial Steps in Management
### General Management Comments

The authors recommend reading the American Academy of Pediatrics' recommendations for the management of head lice (published in 2015) from which the recommendations herein are adapted.

There are age restrictions for most treatments for head lice. It is important to ensure that the treatment prescribed is safe to use in young children (<4 years of age) to avoid harm to the patient. Some of these treatments have been reported to cause death in infants (<6 months).

Local resistance patterns, if available, should be reviewed before determining the appropriate treatment for a patient because resistance patterns to certain agents vary geographically.

## Recommended Initial Regimen

Patients who have not received an appropriate trial of OTC therapy should be started on one of the following because they are far less expensive than prescription head lice treatments and are reasonably effective:

- The entirety of the scalp and hair should be lathered with permethrin 1% lotion (brand name Nix). This should be left on for 10 minutes and then rinsed out. This should be repeated in 9 days.
- Pyrethrin with piperonyl butoxide (brand name Rid) is available in both shampoo and mousse forms. Either form is suitable and should be applied to the entirety of the scalp and the hair, left for 10 minutes, and then rinsed out. This should be repeated in 9 days.

Individuals who are allergic to chrysanthemums should not receive pyrethrin-containing products because these allergens cross-react.

- Malathion 0.5% lotion (brand name Ovide) should be applied to the entirety of the scalp and hair and then rinsed out 8 to 12 hours later. The decision to repeat treatment 7 to 9 days later depends on whether active lice infection presents after initial treatment. This product's vehicle is highly flammable. There is a report of a smoker's hair catching fire the morning after applying this product.

Patients who have failed an OTC topical agent can undergo treatment with one of the following prescription products:

- Benzyl alcohol 5% is an asphyxiant; appropriate application of benzyl alcohol involves soaking the entirety of the scalp and hair with the product. The product can be rinsed out after 10 minutes and should be repeated 9 days after initial application. This product is strictly prohibited in neonates because it has been known to cause asphyxiation and death.
- Spinosad 0.9% suspension also requires careful application with a goal of saturating the entire scalp and hair with the suspension. This product should also be rinsed out after 10 minutes and can be repeated in 1 week if active infection is still present. This product is also strictly prohibited in neonates because it contains benzyl alcohol.
- Ivermectin 0.5% lotion is applied to the entirety of the scalp and hair and rinsed out after 10 minutes. Only one application is required.

In persistent nonresponders or in mass treatment settings where patient compliance is in doubt (e.g., homeless shelters, institutions), the following oral therapy can be considered:

- Oral ivermectin 200 ug/kg with the plan to repeat in 10 days is a viable oral option for lice.

What can be done for the children of parents who say that they prefer a "natural" approach to management?

- Galderma, the makers of Cetaphil, demonstrated that weekly applications of Cetaphil cleanser to the entirety of the scalp left in overnight before rinsing for 3 weeks may be an effective treatment for lice. Instructions for this treatment are available on their website. If such an approach is employed, the patient should be brought back to evaluate for successful treatment of the infestation.

## Other Treatment Options

- Lindane, essential oils, smothering agents (e.g., mayonnaise), and manual removal are not recommended for the treatment of head lice.

## Regarding School Attendance

- Schoolchildren should not be dismissed from school for head lice; it is likely that a child diagnosed with head lice has had head lice for weeks before diagnosis. Children with head lice should be discouraged from having head-to-head contact with other children and from sharing fomites (such as hats) with other children.
- "No nit" policies are inappropriate because nits may be present for days to weeks after successful treatment of the infestation. Children should be treated with OTC products (see management recommendations) and be allowed to return to school the following morning.
- In the absence of a schoolwide epidemic, parents of noninfested children do not need to be contacted about the presence of a case of head lice at a school.

## Warning Signs/Common Pitfalls

All topical treatments for lice are prone to user-dependent error. Becoming comfortable with how to apply these therapies and taking time to counsel patients about appropriate application of these therapies can cut down on treatment failures.

Patients should be bought back 14 days after completing treatment to ensure that the treatment was successful.

Identification of nits alone is not diagnostic of active infection because nits can remain for weeks after successful treatment of head lice. Similarly, the persistence of nits after treatment is not a sign of treatment of failure.

Washing and drying bedding, clothing (especially hats), and combs and brushes with high heat is helpful for preventing reinfection and the spread of infection among individuals who share close quarters with an infested patient.

## Counseling

You (or your child) has head lice. This is a type of infestation that is spread from person to person primarily by head-to-head contact. Less commonly, head lice can spread from the sharing of objects, such as a comb or a hat. Head lice will not give you infections.

Please obtain OTC Nix lotion. A pharmacist can help you find this if you are having trouble locating it. You should apply it to all of your hair from the scalp to the ends and rub it into your scalp. After 10 minutes, you can rinse it out. Regardless of whether you still think you have lice, you should repeat this treatment in 9 days because sometimes the lice eggs are not killed by the initial treatment.

We should see you back in 3 weeks to make sure that you have successfully treated the head lice because sometimes this initial treatment is ineffective.

You can go back to school or work immediately after your initial treatment application. The presence of nits (empty lice eggs) on your scalp is not a reason for you to be kept home from school or work because they are not alive and cannot be spread to anyone else.

Hats, scarves, other clothing, and bedding must be washed in hot water to prevent reinfestation. Soaking combs and brushes in hot water for 10 minutes is also recommended.

# ALLERGIC CONTACT DERMATITIS OF THE SCALP

## Clinical Features

Allergic contact dermatitis (ACD) of the scalp is relatively uncommon because the skin on this site is covered by terminal hairs that usually protect it from allergens. The most common causes of scalp ACD include topically applied medications and hair dye.

ACD of the scalp almost never presents as a rash affecting the entire scalp and instead typically presents in one of two ways:
- Geographic pattern—Characterized by geometric plaques (e.g., a bandlike pattern underlying a headband) of eczematous dermatitis on the scalp.
  - Typically caused by accessories such as nickel hair pins, headbands, and hats. Less frequently, it is caused by curling irons.
  - Wig glues and fixatives for hair extensions are other causes.
- Hairline pattern—Characterized by eczematous dermatitis abutting the hairline but not extending into the scalp.
  - Typically caused by scalp-applied allergens that encroach onto the hairline. Classic examples include hair dye, hair gel, and perming solutions.

- Scalp-applied allergens (e.g., shampoos) can also present with a rinse-off pattern with ACD of the cheeks, jawline, and neck. This will be discussed in additional detail in Chapter 3.

The main differential diagnoses for scalp ACD are seborrheic dermatitis and scalp psoriasis:
- Seborrheic dermatitis is often misdiagnosed as ACD because it frequently extends onto the hairline and in severe cases, can be dark red. They both can also be pruritic.
  - Acute ACD can be distinguished from seborrheic dermatitis because acute ACD often presents with vesicles, edema, and weeping, whereas the most prominent feature of seborrheic dermatitis is its characteristic greasy scaling.
  - Subacute ACD can be distinguished from seborrheic dermatitis because of ACD's lack of the typical seborrheic dermatitis greasy scale and ill-defined eczematous patterns from areas exposed to the allergic contactant.
- Scalp psoriasis is often misdiagnosed as ACD because it can occur focally on the occipital scalp or nape of the neck/posterior scalp area and the lesions are often well circumscribed, giving the appearance that something may have come into contact with the affected area. Unlike ACD, scalp psoriasis often has bountiful, micaceous (silvery) scale.

## Work-Up

Patients with suspected ACD in whom the offending agent is either not obviously identified or cannot be easily removed should be referred to a dermatologist who performs patch testing.
- Importantly, patch testing is distinct from prick testing, a type of allergy testing that is performed in many allergist offices; these two tests cannot be used interchangeably.
  - Patch testing is testing for a type IV hypersensitivity reaction, the type of reaction responsible for ACD, whereas prick testing is testing for a type 1 hypersensitivity reaction.
- Blood tests for allergies (i.e., lymphocyte transfer tests) are also not an acceptable substitution for patch testing.

Blindly eliminating or switching products is generally not efficacious because many products within the same class share allergens (e.g., most dark-colored hair dyes contain paraphenylenediamine).

Patients presenting with suspected acute ACD should be questioned about recent exposure to the following:

- Hair dyes
- Perming solutions
- Hair extensions/wig glue
- Topical medications (especially minoxidil)
- New scalp accessories
- Scalp products
  - Although shampoos and hair products can cause scalp ACD, they are less frequent offenders than the aforementioned causes and do not frequently cause acute reactions. When shampoos are the cause of ACD, the most common culprit is the fragrance.

## Initial Steps in Management

The initial management of scalp ACD involves dividing cases into acute ACD (e.g., intense scalp rash with or without facial swelling after hair dye exposure) vs. subacute/chronic ACD (e.g., an eczematous, itchy, usually hairline rash often associated with the use of a hair product or gel).

In all cases where a trigger is easily identifiable, trigger removal should be emphasized.

In acute cases, consider the following:

- A 20-day oral prednisone taper as follows: 40 mg daily for 5 days, 30 mg daily for 5 days, 20 mg daily for 5 days, and 10 mg daily for 5 days. The entire dose is to be taken in the morning.
- This dosing should be adjusted based on the patient's weight. For example, for adult men and larger women, we recommend 60 mg for 5 days, 40 mg for 5 days, 20 mg for 5 days, and then 10 mg for 5 days.
  - Shorter tapers (e.g., 5-day dose packs) typically result in flaring after cessation (rebound effect).
  - Exercise caution when prescribing systemic corticosteroids in patients with diabetes mellitus, poorly controlled hypertension, glaucoma, heart failure, and recent stroke.
- Adjuvant topical corticosteroids should also be employed to help hasten the response and prevent a flare after steroid tapering.
  - For hair-bearing scalp, consider clobetasol dipropionate 0.05% solution nightly or fluocinonide acetate 0.05% solution nightly.
  - For hairline areas, consider hydrocortisone 2.5% cream twice daily or triamcinolone 0.025% cream twice daily. Triamcinolone is fluorinated so it

should only be used for a few days if the rash extends onto facial skin.

In subacute cases on the hairline, consider the following:

- Hydrocortisone 2.5% cream twice daily (or a similar strength topical steroid) twice daily until resolution followed by PRN for flares.
- Topical tacrolimus, pimecrolimus, and crisaborole can also be considered either as an initial therapy or as a steroid-sparing agent for maintenance of response; however, use of these agents may be cost prohibitive.

In subacute cases on the hair-bearing scalp, consider the following:

- Clobetasol dipropionate 0.05% solution nightly (or a similar strength topical steroid) nightly until resolution followed by PRN for flares.

What to do if treatment response is inadequate:

- Reconsider the diagnosis, given the relative rarity of scalp ACD.
- Refer the patient for patch testing because allergen removal is the definitive management for this condition.

## Warning Signs/Common Pitfalls

Patients frequently attribute new rashes to suspected allergies or new products; they can be very emphatic that they have ACD because they understandably want an explanation for their rash. In the case of scalp rashes, ACD is rarely the etiology and patient suspicion should not be used in place of clinical judgment.

As aforementioned, lymphocyte transfer tests (i.e., blood tests for allergies) and prick testing are not appropriate testing for ACD.

Whole scalp rash is almost never ACD.

Geographic patterned rashes in the scalp are almost always ACD.

## COUNSELING

Your scalp rash is caused by an allergy to a product, chemical, or medicine that your scalp is coming into contact with. This type of rash is called allergic contact dermatitis. Identifying what you are allergic to is the most important part of treating this rash. The scalp is very resistant to allergies, which is why you may only have a rash in some areas or only on your hairline. If you have a product that you think may be causing your rash, it is important that you discuss this with your doctor and discontinue its use until your doctor has ruled it out or in as the cause. Switching products without identifying what ingredient in the product you are allergic to is often not helpful for your type of rash. Many products share similar ingredients and sometimes these ingredients are called by different names on the labels depending on who manufactures the product.

Some people with your type of rash benefit from specialized allergen testing, referred to as "patch testing." Patch testing is performed in a dermatologist's office. Generally, after a consultation, potential allergens will be tested. No needles are involved and it is completely painless. Many of the allergens (often dozens) will be applied to your back in discs or chambers and secured with paper tape. The patches are typically applied on a Monday and removed on a Wednesday. During this time, you cannot shower or exercise strenuously because this may cause the patches to come off and interfere with testing. Sponge bathing of other parts of your body is allowed. The site of testing will need to be examined the day of removal of the patches, 2 days later, and often 7 to 10 days after application. Although this testing is frequently very helpful, it is important to understand that sometimes this testing identifies allergies that are not the cause of your immediate problem and sometimes the testing fails to identify the allergens that are. The skin of the back is the ideal site for testing, but it is much thicker and different than skin of the scalp, face, or neck, which is the area affected by your rash.

## TINEA CAPITIS

### Clinical Features

Tinea capitis is a fungal infection of the hair shafts caused by dermatophyte molds. It occurs most frequently in children, followed by adults, and then infants, and it is more frequent in Blacks and immunosuppressed individuals.

Tinea capitis typically presents as patchy hair loss (alopecia) with variable scaling and erythema; however, diagnosis is frequently delayed because of the varied clinical presentations. There are six distinct clinical subtypes that are subdivided into noninflammatory and inflammatory variants. Appropriate subtype identification can theoretically assist with choosing between terbinafine and griseofulvin because some subtypes are more strongly associated with endothrix and vice versa.

- Noninflammatory
  - Grey patch—This presents as patchy alopecia with grey scale in the alopecic areas and minimal inflammation.
  - Black dot—It is similar in appearance to grey patch except that this subtype displays the characteristic broken-off "black dot" hairs for which this subtype is named.
  - Diffuse scale—This subtype is distinct from the other noninflammatory subtypes and easiest to overlook because it is not associated with alopecia. This subtype presents with diffuse grey scale covering the scalp and clinically is difficult to distinguish from seborrheic dermatitis.
- Inflammatory—These subtypes are typically more treatment refractory and require longer treatment courses.
  - Diffuse pustular—This appears similar to grey patch except that it is more inflamed, studded with pustules, and frequently associated with painful lymphadenopathy.
  - Kerion—It is frequently initially misdiagnosed as a bacterial infection because it presents with alopecic patches overlying boggy, inflamed, abscess-like masses.
  - Favus—It typically results from the progression of longstanding untreated tinea capitis and presents with thick, yellow, crusted lesions called scutula that are full of hyphae overlying alopecia that is frequently scarring.

### Differential Diagnosis

The differential diagnosis for tinea capitis differs based on the clinical subtype; however, it includes trichotillomania, bacterial infections (including abscesses), seborrheic dermatitis, psoriasis, and various patchy alopecias, including alopecia areata and discoid lupus erythematosus.

- Trichotillomania (Fig. 1.5)—Black dot tinea capitis and trichotillomania are difficult to distinguish clinically because they are both characterized by patchy alopecia with short, broken hairs within the alopecic patch.
  - Unlike trichotillomania, tinea capitis has scale within its alopecic patches and frequently has some degree of perceptible inflammation.

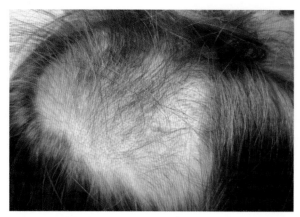

**Fig. 1.5 Trichotillomania.** Note the abnormal pattern and hairs of different length within the affected area. (Courtesy Justin Finch, MD.)

- Bacterial infection—Tinea capitis can be misdiagnosed as a bacterial infection in cases where the patient has painful lymphadenopathy associated with an inflamed scalp rash that is presumed to be bacterial in origin. In most of these cases, the patient has an inflammatory variant of tinea capitis and the pustule formation and/or purulent drainage confuses the clinician.
  - Clinically, differentiating the two can be difficult and may require microbiologic work-up as outlined in the following section (see "Work-Up"); tinea capitis should be suspected in patients who are being treated for bacterial infection of the scalp without improvement.
- Seborrheic dermatitis and psoriasis—Noninflammatory variants of tinea capitis are often misdiagnosed for these conditions, especially in cases of diffuse scale tinea capitis.
  - Diffuse scale tinea capitis can be distinguished from these conditions because it does not have the typically diffuse underlying erythema that hallmarks seborrheic dermatitis and psoriasis.
  - A history of acute onset of the rash is suggestive of tinea over seborrheic dermatitis and psoriasis.
  - The presence of retroauricular scaling and rash on the body are more consistent with psoriasis and seborrheic dermatitis.
- Other patchy alopecias (e.g., alopecia areata, discoid lupus erythematosus)—Tinea capitis, alopecia areata, trichotillomania (as previously discussed),

and discoid lupus erythematosus are the most common causes of patchy alopecia.
- Tinea capitis can be distinguished from alopecia areata because it almost always has scale within its areas of alopecia.
- Plaques of discoid lupus typically have central scarring and may also be present elsewhere on the body, including the conchal bowl.

## Work-Up

In cases where tinea capitis is suspected, clinically treatment should be initiated before confirming the diagnosis with a culture.
- KOH scraping performed by non-experienced personnel is of limited utility. Unless experience and skill are obtained, it is not reliable.
- A Wood's lamp examination can be performed in offices where it is available; however, lack of fluorescence on examination does not rule out tinea capitis because only *Microsporum* species and *T. schoneleinii* fluoresce.
- Culture is recommended, although it is slow (>2 weeks) and can grow contaminants. Several methods are available to obtain culture depending on the patient's age and the tool availability. Although lesional scraping is most commonly performed in dermatologists' offices, the hair plucking and hair clipping methods are frequently easier/more reliable for less experienced practitioners.
  - Lesional scraping—Affected areas of the scalp can be scraped with a glass slide, wet cotton swab, scalpel, or hair brush to obtain scale.
  - Hair pluck—Tweezers can be used to pluck affected hairs.
  - Hair clip—Hairs in affected areas can be trimmed and sent to the laboratory. Hair proximal to the scalp is best.
- In adults, evaluation for immunosuppression, especially in cases of florid tinea, is warranted.

## Initial Steps in Management

The initial management of tinea capitis involves dividing cases into inflammatory and noninflammatory variants.

With inflammatory variants, referral to a specialist is recommended because of the high risk for scarring with the potential for permanent hair loss should improper management ensue; however, treatment should be initiated while the patient is awaiting consultation with a specialist.

For noninflammatory variants, all patients with tinea capitis must be treated with oral antifungals as outlined here:

- Systemic antifungals—Terbinafine and griseofulvin are first-line treatments. We prefer terbinafine because it only requires once daily dosing, has a shorter course, and has fewer adverse effects.
  - Terbinafine—Terbinafine is administered daily for 4 to 6 weeks. No liver function testing is necessary before, during, or after the treatment course. Some authors prefer shorter courses (around 2 weeks); however, the rate of primary failure is higher for shorter courses.
    - Adult dosing
      - 250 mg per day
        - Some adults take medications that have significant CYP interactions with terbinafine (e.g., beta blockers); 126 drugs are known to interact (13 of which are considered major). Therefore a careful review of a patient's medications is mandatory. Additionally, patients should be told to avoid caffeine-containing products and be warned about phototoxicity.
    - Pediatric dosing—weight-based
      - <20 kg: 62.5 mg per day
      - 20 to 40 kg: 125 mg per day
      - >40 kg: 250 mg per day
  - Griseofulvin: 8 to 12 weeks
    - Adult dosing
      - 1 g per day (single or divided dose)
    - Pediatric dosing—weight-based
      - <50 kg: 20 to 25 mg per kg per day (single or divided dose)
      - >50 kg: 1 g per day (single or divided dose)
  - Itraconazole—4 weeks
    - Adult dosing
      - 100 mg per day
      - 428 known drug interactions are known, 169 of which are considered major. This drug should be avoided in patients with a history of congestive heart failure.
    - Pediatric dosing—weight-based
      - 5 mg per kg per day up to 100 mg daily
- Adjuvant topicals—Monotherapy with topical antifungals is not recommended for treatment of tinea

capitis because it is only rarely efficacious; however, using topical antifungals as adjuvants to oral therapy is highly recommended to decrease the transmission of spores. Adjuvants should be continued for the duration of oral therapy and include:
  - Selenium sulfide
  - Ketoconazole shampoo
  - Ciclopirox shampoo

What to do if treatment response is inadequate:
- If a patient does not respond to a full course of one antifungal, switching to another oral antifungal (typically between terbinafine and griseofulvin) is indicated.
  - In cases where the results of fungal culture become available before switching antifungals, they can be used to guide antifungal therapy:
    - Ectothrix—griseofulvin preferred
    - Endothrix—terbinafine preferred

## Warning Signs/Common Pitfalls

Fomites (e.g., hats, hairbrushes) become major reservoirs for dermatophytes in patients with tinea capitis. Cleansing fomites is essential for preventing recurrence.

All close contacts should be evaluated for early signs of tinea capitis. Failure to treat infected contacts is a common cause of recurrence.
- If a patient's fungal culture grows *Trichophyton tonsurans*, then the patient's family/close contacts need to be tested and treated if infected to prevent recurrence.

Initiation of oral antifungals should not be delayed while awaiting fungal culture results.
- Delay in treatment can result in avoidable scarring and permanent hair loss (alopecia) with inflammatory subtypes.

Shorter courses of oral antifungals than are recommended here are frequently used; however, they have a higher rate of primary failure.

Oral corticosteroids have historically been used as adjuncts for treating inflammatory subtypes of tinea capitis. This is no longer recommended because it has not been shown to augment the treatment course or prevent scarring; however, it is associated with a higher rate of adverse events and noncompliance.

## Counseling

You have tinea capitis, which is a fungal infection of your scalp and hair. This infection is very similar to ringworm, although it is more difficult to treat because the fungus has infected the hair itself. This infection is spread from person to person and it can be spread by clothing items (hats) and personal care items (hairbrushes). It is important that all family members and close contacts are evaluated by their doctor for this infection. Additionally, all clothing and personal care items that come into contact with the scalp need to be washed thoroughly with hot water.

We will send a sample collected from your scalp to be tested in a laboratory to find out what specific fungus you have. This is helpful in the unlikely scenario that your infection does not resolve with the antifungal medication we prescribe you today. This testing is very slow and we may not have the results from it for more than a month.

We will have you start an antifungal medication by mouth. It is important that you take this medication every day as directed so that the infection goes away. It may take weeks for you to notice benefit from this medication. In addition, we will recommend a medicated shampoo for you to wash your hair with every day until your therapy is completed and you are cured.

# ACTINIC KERATOSIS

## Clinical Features

Actinic keratoses (Fig. 1.5) are nonobligate precursors to cutaneous squamous cell carcinoma. Scalp actinic keratoses are almost exclusively seen in bald men in whom they are ubiquitous but can also be seen in women with sparse scalp hair, such as in female-patterned hair loss.

- Each individual actinic keratosis has an annual risk of malignant transformation to cutaneous squamous cell carcinoma of around 1%; however, this risk is variable based on the size of the actinic keratosis, the patient's continued sun exposure, and the patient's immunocompetency.
- Actinic keratoses predominantly develop starting in the fifth decade of life and become increasingly prominent in older individuals.
- They occur most frequently in Caucasians, followed by Hispanics and then all other ethnic groups. They occur in men more often than in women and develop predominantly in individuals who have a history of extensive longitudinal sun exposure.

- They are most frequent in immunosuppressed individuals, especially organ transplant recipients.
- Actinic keratosis lesions are characteristically asymptomatic, except for some flaking and a roughness to the touch.
- Pain and bleeding are not characteristic of actinic keratoses and the presence of these symptoms requires the consideration of an alternate diagnosis (e.g., cutaneous malignancy).
- Recent evidence suggests that a painful actinic keratosis has an increased risk for actually representing a squamous cell carcinoma.

Clinically, there are four overlapping subtypes of actinic keratoses. These lesions can occur in isolation but more commonly present as multiple discrete lesions affecting one or more cosmetic units:

*Typical*: These are flat, variably scaled discrete red areas that are characteristically rough to the touch. Sometimes scale is barely perceptible to the naked eye and these lesions are frequently only identifiable by touch.

*Pigmented*: This represents the collision of an actinic keratosis with a solar lentigo (also called a "sun" or "liver" spot). These typically occur in exquisitely photodamaged patients or in darker-skinned patients. They look and feel similar to typical actinic keratoses, but they are tan, brown, or brown-black in appearance.

*Hypertrophic*: These are typically longer-standing actinic keratoses that have developed thickened, compact overlying scale. They look like typical actinic keratoses, but they have a thickened, crust-like scale atop them.

*Cutaneous horn*: As the name suggests, these are actual hornlike projections from the skin. They are classically "taller" than their horizontal width. Not all cutaneous horns are actinic keratoses (25% are squamous cell carcinoma in situ, although 60% can be benign with a wart or seborrheic keratosis at the base). Because you cannot usually determine what is at the base of a cutaneous horn, these lesions invariably need to be biopsied.

## Differential Diagnosis

The differential diagnosis for an actinic keratosis differs based on the subtype; however, a cutaneous malignancy (e.g., squamous cell carcinoma and rarely basal cell carcinoma) is always in the differential for actinic keratoses; therefore lesions that are persistent or recurrent in spite of appropriate management must be biopsied.

Hypertrophic actinic keratoses and cutaneous horns have such characteristic appearances that their differential usually only includes squamous cell carcinoma (+/- in situ), viral wart, and seborrheic keratosis.

- Viral warts are very uncommon on the scalp; therefore this diagnosis should only be made based on histology in lesions biopsied to rule out malignancy.
- Seborrheic keratoses, especially inflamed seborrheic keratoses, can appear almost indistinguishable from hypertrophic actinic keratoses and early squamous cell carcinomas.
  - Nevertheless, in many cases, seborrheic keratoses appear stuck on and are softer to the touch than a hypertrophic actinic keratosis. Hypertrophic actinic keratoses may also have evidences of a typical actinic keratosis lesion surrounding the compact scale.

Typical actinic keratoses may be misdiagnosed as a scalp rash when they are innumerable on the scalp. This situation is not uncommon in light-skinned bald men who have practiced poor photoprotection. In these scenarios, actinic keratoses are typically misdiagnosed as seborrheic dermatitis, xerosis, or another nonspecific inflammatory scalp dermatitis.

- Diffuse actinic keratoses can be distinguished from inflammatory scalp rashes based on their characteristic rough texture. In situations of clinical uncertainty, rubbing one's hand across the scalp without a glove will distinguish actinic keratoses from mimickers.

## Work-Up

Actinic keratoses are a clinical diagnosis. Dermatologists frequently use a dermatoscope (polarized and nonpolarized light with magnification device) to assist with diagnosis; however, learning how to interpret lesions with dermoscopy is not readily available to primary care providers and thus is beyond the scope of this text.

## Initial Steps in Management

All patients with actinic keratoses need a full-body skin examination performed by a trained provider to screen for cutaneous malignancy.

The management of actinic keratoses requires complex decision making based on the nature of an individual actinic keratosis, the patient's overall disease burden, the patient's history of cutaneous malignancy, and the patient's individual preferences. Given the complexity of management and the need for a full-body skin examination by a trained professional, patients with actinic keratoses should be referred to a board-certified dermatologist for evaluation and management.

## Warning Signs/Common Pitfalls

The most feared pitfalls managing actinic keratoses are:

- Misdiagnosing a cutaneous malignancy (e.g. squamous cell carcinoma, basal cell carcinoma, amelanotic melanoma) as an actinic keratosis and delaying definitive management.
- Missing a cutaneous malignancy (including a malignant melanoma) present elsewhere on the body by not performing a thorough full body skin examination.

These pitfalls are best avoided by referring the patient to a specialist when available.

In cases where a primary care provider is responsible for managing actinic keratoses because of a lack of access to a local specialist, avoidance of the following pitfalls is crucial:

- Lesions that are not responding to appropriate therapy (e.g., cryotherapy, topical 5-fluorouracil) should be biopsied to evaluate for malignancy.
- Patients who have more than five actinic keratoses within a cosmetic unit (e.g., on the scalp) should be treated with field therapy (preferably with topical 5-fluorouracil) because their disease burden reflects diffuse actinic damage.

## COUNSELING

You have actinic keratoses, which are precancerous skin lesions. If untreated, these skin lesions have the potential to become a squamous cell carcinoma (pronounced Sk-WAY-miss). Although squamous cell carcinomas are not the same type of skin cancer as melanoma, they do have the potential to spread (metastasize) and therefore we want to prevent them from evolving.

You developed actinic keratoses from chronic sun exposure. The sun damages the skin cells so that they start to turn into cancers. If untreated, the risk of any individual actinic keratosis turning into a squamous cell carcinoma is about 1% per year.

We have referred you to a dermatologist for further treatment and for an examination of your entire skin surface to ensure you have no other serious skin disease and to decrease your risk for developing a skin cancer. Because having been diagnosed with an actinic keratosis means your skin has been exposed to excessive sun exposure throughout your life, you have an increased risk for developing skin cancers, and it is important that the dermatologist examines your entire skin surface, not just the area where you have the actinic keratoses that we found today.

To help decrease your risk for developing additional actinic keratoses, it is very important that you wear a waterproof daily sunscreen with a sun protection factor (SPF) of at least 30 and a broad spectrum label (UVA and UVB). It takes about an ounce or a shot glass full of sunscreen to properly apply the sunscreen to your exposed skin in the warm weather. You should also apply stronger sunscreen with an SPF of at least 50 before going outdoors and should reapply that sunscreen should you spend more than 2 hours outdoors. Despite the label "waterproof," sunscreen should be reapplied after swimming or excessive sweating. Wearing a broad-brimmed sun protective hat that has UPF protection is also essential. Studies have shown that even one summer of appropriate sunscreen use decreases your risk for developing more actinic keratoses.

## DISCOID LUPUS ERYTHEMATOSUS (SEE CHAPTER 2)

# 2

# Face Dermatitis

## CHAPTER OUTLINE

# ATOPIC DERMATITIS—FACE

## Clinical Features

- Atopic dermatitis (AD; often referred to by patients as "eczema") is a chronic inflammatory skin condition characterized by pruritus and pruritic, ill-defined, red, scaly papules and plaques that predominantly affect flexural surfaces (e.g., antecubital fossa, popliteal fossa).
  - The appearance of AD lesions differs based on lesion duration. Chronic lesions are often thickened (i.e., lichenified) from chronic rubbing and excoriated from scratching; acute lesions, on the other hand, can be red and occasionally even weeping.
  - In darker-skinned individuals, long-standing lesions can cause dyspigmentation (either hyperpigmentation or hypopigmentation) that persists after the AD lesion is treated.
- Isolated facial AD is rare except during infancy, in which it is frequently the initial presentation.
  - In infancy, plaques frequently affect the bilateral cheeks which, when the child is able to, they can be observed rubbing.
  - In older children and in adults, facial atopic dermatitis almost always coexists with atopic dermatitis elsewhere on the body.
- In darker-skinned children, facial AD can present as pityriasis alba, which is characterized by scaly, white macules and patches on the face.

- Facial AD frequently becomes secondarily impetiginized (i.e., infected), which presents as acute worsening of eczema with overlying weeping and yellow crusting.
- AD is part of the "atopic triad" with allergic rhinitis and asthma; facial AD may be the heralding sign of this triad in infants.

## Differential Diagnosis

The differential for facial AD includes irritant contact dermatitis (ICD), allergic contact dermatitis (ACD), seborrheic dermatitis, discoid lupus erythematosus, tinea faciei, and psoriasis.

- Facial dermatitis occurring in the presence of AD elsewhere on the body, with or without the presence of clinical signs suggestive of atopy (e.g., nasal crease, allergic shiners), suggests a diagnosis of facial AD.
- Isolated facial dermatitis in adults is unlikely to be AD in the absence of a history of known AD.
- AD often occurs in an overlap state with components of ICD and ACD.
  - Patients with known AD or other facial dermatitis who are treated with topical corticosteroids may also develop steroid-induced rosacea.
  - Topical corticosteroid withdrawal from overuse and discontinuation may mimic an AD flare.
  - Identifying concomitant ACD is important because topical therapy alone is unlikely to be adequate in this setting unless identification of the allergen and avoidance occurs.

- Facial ICD can occur anywhere on the face but most frequently presents in the nasolabial folds and periocular areas because irritants frequently collect into these concave areas.
  - The presence of peeling skin suggests a component of ICD.
  - ICD is common in the winter in arid climates and most frequently occurs in individuals who use harsh facial cleansers and other cosmetics.
    - A subset of facial AD can be seen in acne patients who are using irritating topical therapies (e.g., tretinoin, benzoyl peroxide).
  - AD can be distinguished from ICD in that facial AD frequently coexists with AD present elsewhere. Nevertheless, many patients with facial AD have a component of ICD.
- ACD can be clinically indistinguishable from facial AD; however, a diagnosis of ACD is suggested in adults with no history of AD who develop acute to subacute facial dermatitis.
  - ACD should be suspected in patients with new, persistent facial dermatitis despite treatment with topical corticosteroids.
  - Several distinct patterns of facial ACD are discussed in Chapter 3. Identification of these patterns can help distinguish ACD from AD.
- Seborrheic dermatitis can typically be distinguished from AD because seborrheic dermatitis: 1) predominantly affects seborrheic areas such as the nasolabial folds, eyebrows, scalp, ears, and retroauricular area and 2) typically has greasy-appearing, overlying scale.
- Tinea faciei can typically be distinguished from atopic dermatitis because it is usually unilateral and frequently has central clearing. Additionally, gentle scraping of tinea faciei lesions with a microscope slide will produce large amounts of micaceous scale that can be examined under the microscope with KOH stains, revealing hyphae.
- Discoid lupus can be distinguished from AD because discoid lupus is almost never itchy and is morphologically distinct with rough peripheral scale and central scarring.
- Psoriasis is infrequent on the face and is usually associated with psoriasis elsewhere, such as the scalp, elbows, and knees. The lesions are erythematous with silvery scaling and sharply circumscribed. Unlike with tinea, the KOH scraping would be negative.

## Work-Up

- A total-body skin examination should be performed to look for characteristic skin lesions elsewhere.
- A histopathologic confirmation is almost never necessary.
- Patch testing adults with facial dermatitis is indicated when obvious triggers cannot be identified based on history alone and when topical therapy is inadequate for disease management.

## Initial Steps in Management

- Initial management of atopic dermatitis involves a three-pronged approach:
  - Dry skin care, including:
    - Barrier repair with noncomedogenic (which means it does not cause acne; this is listed on product labels) moisturizing creams at least twice daily.
      - For facial dermatoses, it is frequently helpful to recommend a lighter, more cosmetically acceptable moisturizer for morning application (e.g., Neutrogena Hydro Boost gel cream, CeraVe lotion, Eucerin lotion) and a thicker, more hydrating moisturizer for evening application (e.g., CeraVe moisturizing cream, Eucerin cream).
      - In patients without suspected ACD, morning facial moisturizers should routinely contain a sunscreen (e.g., Neutrogena Hydro Boost City Shield, CeraVe AM, Eucerin Daily Protection).
    - A gentle cleansing of the face with water and with or without a gentle cleanser to remove environmental allergens should be performed twice daily every day (morning and evening). The patient's washed hands should be used rather than a washcloth. Face washing should always be followed immediately by moisturizing.
      - Patients with active dermatitis should be counseled to avoid using exfoliating face washes, such as those containing salicylic acid, glycolic acid, or alpha hydroxy acid.
  - Topical antiinflammatory agents:
    - First-line treatment should include a low-potency topical corticosteroid, such as hydrocortisone 2.5% cream, applied twice daily.
      - Even low-potency topical steroids should be avoided on the eyelids if prolonged use is anticipated.

- Topical steroids around the eyes can precipitate glaucoma in susceptible patients and therefore should be used with caution or avoided and substituted with a noninflammatory steroid, such as a topical tacrolimus product (tacrolimus or Protopic ointment) or a topical pimecrolimus cream (pimecrolimus or Elidel cream).
- On the face, all topical steroids can trigger perioral dermatitis/steroid rosacea.
  - In both of these settings, use a topical calcineurin inhibitor, such as tacrolimus or pimecrolimus, 0.1% twice daily. Note that this treatment is not recommended by the U.S. Food and Drug Administration (FDA) in infants and in children 2 to 15 years of age; instead, tacrolimus 0.03% is FDA endorsed.
  - Another steroid-sparing alternative, crisaborole (commercially available as Eucrisa), is a phosphodiesterase-4 inhibitor and is available as an ointment for the use of AD in patients older than 2 years of age.
- The maintenance of control in patients with relapsing disease that cannot be adequately maintained with dry skin care alone can be performed using topical calcineurin inhibitors, such as topical pimecrolimus 0.1%, twice daily.
  - Some patients require a maintenance application of topical calcineurin inhibitors three times weekly in the absence of active disease to prevent flares.
  - Topical pimecrolimus should not be applied to actively inflamed skin because it can cause a severe burning sensation.
  - Topical tacrolimus and crisaborole only come in ointment form and are often not acceptable cosmetically for daily facial application.
- Trigger avoidance:
  - Questioning patients with facial dermatitis about their daily facial skin care regimen should occur at every visit for facial dermatitis because facial cosmetics and cosmetic removers can worsen AD and cause ICD and ACD.
    - Patients with refractory facial dermatitis often benefit from complete discontinuation of all cosmetics (facial and otherwise) for at

least 4 weeks while actively treating the patient with antiinflammatory topicals. This includes nail polish/acrylic nails that are often found to be the allergic culprit, especially for eyelid or periocular dermatitis.
- Patients with persistent disease despite discontinuation of cosmetics frequently benefit from patch testing.

## Warning Signs/Common Pitfalls

The biggest pitfall when managing AD in any location is failure to promote patient adherence to a dry skin care management regimen. Such a regimen is essential for achieving and maintaining disease control in patients with AD; failure to implement a daily dry skin care regimen ensures treatment failure.

- Patients must specifically be counseled that twice-daily use of their prescription topical antiinflammatory is not a substitute for frequent moisturization.
- Avoidance of harsh soaps and irritating cosmetics/perfumes is essential. Patients need specific product recommendations because the cosmetic aisle in drug stores is otherwise confusing and the internet is full of misinformation on this subject.

Patients with facial dermatitis are frequently noncompliant with therapy if topical medications with poor cosmesis (e.g., ointments) are prescribed.

- If patients are unwilling to use a topical corticosteroid or topical calcineurin inhibitor in the morning because of unacceptable cosmesis, use of a stronger ointment for nightly use only can be considered (e.g., tacrolimus 0.1%, hydrocortisone 2.5% ointment) as long as the patient is counseled extensively about the potential adverse effects of more potent therapies.
- Avoidance of fluorinated topical steroids on the face (topical steroids listed in classes I, II, and III) should be adhered to because these can cause significant adverse effects if used chronically, especially on the thinner skin of the face.
- Noncompliance with moisturizers can occur for similar reasons as noncompliance with therapy.

Failure to identify coexisting dermatoses such as ICD to cosmetics, ACD (including to topical corticosteroids), and/or head and neck dermatitis can interfere with successful management.

- Most patients should be able to achieve disease control with appropriate topical therapies. Coexisting diagnoses should be considered in patients who fail to improve.

## Counseling

You have atopic dermatitis, also known as "eczema." Atopic dermatitis is usually an inherited chronic skin condition (meaning there is no cure) that occurs in people who have skin that does not retain enough water and that does not adequately protect itself against outside allergens. Your skin is sensitive, prone to dryness, and susceptible to becoming itchy and developing rashes.

Individuals with atopic dermatitis develop skin inflammation from within in response to the environment around them. This inflammation makes the skin red and itchy. Importantly, there is no one allergen that causes your skin disease. Additionally, dietary changes have not been reported in the medical literature as curing your disease.

Treating your skin disease requires that you keep your skin healthy by moisturizing it and by avoiding exposure to things that irritate it. To keep your skin healthy, it is important that you wash your face with a gentle cleanser twice daily using your hands instead of a washcloth. After cleansing your face, you should immediately apply a moisturizer. Some people find it helpful to use a different, lighter moisturizing cream (such as a lotion or light cream) in the morning than the one they use at night because the heavy moisturizers (heavy creams or ointments) that are better for keeping the skin hydrated (e.g., CeraVe moisturizing cream or Eucerin Advanced Repair cream) may not be cosmetically suitable for use during the daytime. While your skin is still red and irritated, it is important that you do not apply any cosmetics or fragrances because these can inflame or irritate your skin.

Your doctor has prescribed you a topical mild steroid cream. You should use this cream twice daily only for 7 to 10 days, at which time the redness and irritation should be gone. Alternative steroid-sparing creams may also be prescribed for more chronic or intermittent use.

These prescription creams are not a substitute for your moisturizer and should be used with your moisturizer, not instead of your moisturizer. Once the redness and irritation has resolved, you can stop the prescription cream, although you may need to restart it if the redness

and irritation return. The topical steroid prescribed cream can cause side effects if you use it too frequently or if you use it for too long. This includes possible thinning of the skin, increased visibility of blood vessels in the area of application, discoloration of the skin, and potentially an acnelike rash. Additionally, if this cream is applied around the eye it can cause an increase in eye pressure, which can result in glaucoma, a vision-threatening eye disease. Please tell your doctor if you have a personal or family history of glaucoma.

Atopic dermatitis is cyclical, which means you will have times when your rash is much better and times when it is much worse. Different people flare for different reasons. You should try your best to identify things that are unique triggers for your atopic dermatitis. You will have to work with your doctor over time to find a skin care regimen that is right for you and that keeps your skin disease under control.

# PERIOCULAR AND PERIOTIC PSORIASIS (SEE CH 3, PSORIASIS)

# SEBORRHEIC DERMATITIS—FACE

## Clinical Features

- Seborrheic dermatitis of the face may affect the nasofacial junction, eyebrows, hairline (extending onto the scalp as discussed in Chapter 1), retroauricular area, and, less frequently, the chin.
  - Identifying whether a rash presents with a seborrheic distribution is essential for diagnosing seborrheic dermatitis, especially in subtler cases characterized by barely perceptible pink plaques, pruritus, and mild flaking.
  - Seborrheic distribution is associated with hair-bearing and oily areas of the head, including the scalp, forehead, eyebrows, eyelash line, nasolabial folds, beard area, postauricular area, and submental skin.
- Seborrheic dermatitis is characterized by the development of pink-red thin patches or plaques with overlying greasy, thick scales.
  - Presentation can range from pruritus and a barely perceptible rash to deep red plaques encroaching past the classic seborrheic distribution.
- Isolated facial seborrheic dermatitis is relatively uncommon. In most cases, dandruff or scalp

involvement can be appreciated, regardless of disease severity elsewhere.

## Differential Diagnosis

The differential for facial seborrheic dermatitis includes psoriasis, ICD, acute cutaneous lupus erythematosus, ACD, Darier disease, rosacea, and, rarely, drug reactions.

- Psoriasis is uncommon on the face and, when present, is usually associated with psoriasis elsewhere on the skin. Psoriasis on the scalp, however, is common. Psoriasis usually has silvery scaling and the lesions are well demarcated. The lesions of seborrheic dermatitis are generally not as sharply demarcated and are greasier in appearance with more yellowish scales. It is not uncommon for patients to have both conditions.
- ICD, typically arising from personal care product use or from irritating topical medications for acne (e.g., benzoyl peroxide, tretinoin) mimics seborrheic dermatitis by creating "dermatitis" (manifesting as redness and scaling) at the nasofacial junction (specifically at the alar-facial crease). This so-called "dermatitis" develops because the concavity of the alar-facial crease promotes accumulation of irritating cosmetics and topical medications within the area. This area may develop ICD from topically applied products in the absence of ICD elsewhere.
  - Obtaining a facial skincare regimen history in all patients presenting with a facial rash is a priority and can help differentiate ICD from seborrheic dermatitis.
    - Importantly, seborrheic dermatitis and ICD can occur in an overlap state where underlying seborrheic dermatitis is exacerbated by use of irritating topicals.
  - The presence of rash in nonseborrheic areas, especially concave areas with thin skin such as the periorbital area, suggests a diagnosis of ICD over seborrheic dermatitis; on the other hand, the presence of rash in other classic seborrheic areas (e.g., on the hairline) is suggestive of seborrheic dermatitis.
- Severe seborrheic dermatitis is often misdiagnosed as acute cutaneous lupus because seborrheic dermatitis can mimic a malar rash.
  - Unlike seborrheic dermatitis, which favors the alar-facial crease, acute cutaneous lupus characteristically spares this area because it is sun protected.

- ACD does not typically conform to a typical seborrheic distribution, even though plaques on the cheeks occurring in both diseases may look similar.
- Darier disease can look almost indistinguishable from seborrheic dermatitis; however, disease severity, nail changes, family history of Darier, treatment refractoriness, and the presence of disease elsewhere should all suggest a diagnosis of Darier.
- Rosacea is another cause of red cheeks; however, it typically spares the alar-facial crease and lacks overlying scale; rosacea is also often seen in association with acneiform papules, pustules, and telangiectasia.

## Work-Up

- A total-body skin examination should be performed to look for characteristic skin lesions elsewhere.
- Asking a patient about their daily facial skincare regimen is essential for distinguishing facial seborrheic dermatitis from ICD and for assessing for overlap of the two conditions.
- Adults who present with subacute onset severe seborrheic dermatitis affecting the face and chest should be screened for human immunodeficiency virus (HIV) unless another obvious trigger for development of seborrheic dermatitis is identified (e.g., organ transplant immunosuppression, Parkinson disease).
- Seborrheic dermatitis is generally a clinical diagnosis; rarely is a biopsy required to make a diagnosis of seborrheic dermatitis.

## Initial Steps in Management

There is no cure for seborrheic dermatitis. The course is chronic with waxing and waning. Failure to emphasize the importance of using a maintenance therapy virtually guarantees disease recurrence and patient dissatisfaction.

Treatments for seborrheic dermatitis are primarily divided into topical antifungals and topical antiinflammatory agents.

### Antifungals

- For facial seborrheic dermatitis, topical antifungals formulated either as a shampoo or cream can be used. In cases where a shampoo is used, it must be left in contact with the skin for at least 5 minutes. Application of shampoo to facial skin can be drying and therefore concomitant moisturizer use is necessary.

- Shampoos are preferable in cases with scalp involvement and eyebrow involvement.
- Azoles as creams (e.g., ketoconazole 2%, clotrimazole 1%) can be applied twice daily to affected areas; on the other hand, shampoos (e.g., ketoconazole 2%) are applied two to three times weekly during acute management and once weekly for maintenance. Over-the-counter azole shampoos (e.g., miconazole) are less effective than prescription ketoconazole shampoo.
- Ciclopirox is a reasonable second-line antifungal. It is formulated as both a cream and as a shampoo. Even though it is equally as effective as topical azoles, it is more likely to cause irritation and is typically more expensive. In patients who are bathed infrequently, ciclopirox shampoo is preferential to ketoconazole because less frequent applications (1 to 2 times/week) have been demonstrated to be effective.
- Selenium sulfide (active ingredient in Selsun Blue)
- Zinc pyrithione (active ingredient in Head and Shoulders)
- Salicylic acid (active ingredient in T/Sal Therapeutic shampoo)

## Antiinflammatories

- Topical corticosteroids
  - These are equally as effective and possibly more effective than antifungals, although they are more likely to cause cutaneous adverse effects and early disease rebound after discontinuation.
  - Low-potency topical corticosteroids (e.g., hydrocortisone 2.5% cream twice daily) are more effective then mid-potency and high-potency topical corticosteroids for treatment of seborrheic dermatitis.
  - Mid- and high-potency topical steroids should not be used on the face. Additionally topical steroids around the eyes can precipitate glaucoma and should be avoided.
- Topical calcineurin inhibitors
  - Calcineurin inhibitors are as equally efficacious as topical corticosteroids; nevertheless, they are more expensive and typically require failure of topical corticosteroids before insurance approval.

- Topical pimecrolimus 0.1% cream is recommended for the treatment of facial seborrheic dermatitis because topical tacrolimus 0.1% is only formulated as an ointment, which is typically not cosmetically acceptable to patients.
- Other agents are rarely necessary and lack substantial evidence supporting their use.
  - Crisaborole is only available as an ointment and therefore is not cosmetically desirable for facial disease.
  - There is not one single active pharmaceutical ingredient in Promiseb. It is a combination of antiinflammatory agents. It is often very expensive but can be considered in refractory cases.

## Warning Signs/Common Pitfalls

Consider a patient's bathing habits when treating seborrheic dermatitis because infrequent bathing and infrequent shampooing are a common cause of treatment failure/nonadherence to medicated shampoos.

There is no cure for seborrheic dermatitis; therefore, all patients require maintenance treatment.

For facial seborrheic dermatitis, cream formulations are preferable over ointments because they are typically more cosmetically acceptable.

Failure to identify concomitant personal care product-induced ICD can hinder patient improvement despite appropriate treatment.

Patients with acute onset of severe seborrheic dermatitis should undergo HIV testing.

Patients using antifungal shampoos should alternate daily between different types of shampoos to decrease the likelihood of secondary treatment failure.

## Counseling

You have a rash called "seborrheic dermatitis." It is a severe form of dandruff that can involve the face and also the scalp and chest. This is a chronic, recurrent, waxing and waning type of rash, meaning that there is no cure. Most importantly, it is a self-limited type of rash, meaning that it will not cause you internal harm. This rash is the result of inflammation caused by your immune system. The exact reason that you have developed this rash is unknown. Some experts think that it develops because your immune system overreacts to fats made by a yeast called "*Malassezia*" that lives on your skin; however, other experts do not think this is the case.

Because this is a normal skin yeast, it is not a form of infection and is not contagious.

I have prescribed you an antifungal (yeast) shampoo. You should use this shampoo 3 times per week for 4 weeks. You should apply it to your face and your scalp. You do not need another facewash while using this shampoo. It is important that you let the shampoo remain on your skin for at least 5 minutes before rinsing it out. In 4 weeks, you can decrease the frequency with which you use this shampoo to once per week. It is important that you continue to use this shampoo once every week because if you do not, it is likely that the rash will come back. On the days that you do not use the antifungal shampoo, I recommend that you use an over-the-counter shampoo containing either selenium sulfide or zinc pyrithione because these products also have antifungal properties. Examples of brands that contain these ingredients include Selsun Blue and Head & Shoulders. If one of these shampoos that you have been using chronically loses its effectiveness, switch to another type of shampoo; always use at least two different types of shampoos during the week to reduce this possibility.

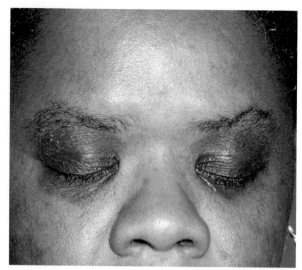

**Fig. 2.1 Periorbital Allergic Contact Dermatitis.** Patient was patch-test positive to gold. Patient wears gold earrings and likely was touching eyelid skin after touching the earrings. (From the UConn Department of Dermatology Grand Rounds Collection.)

## ALLERGIC CONTACT DERMATITIS—FACE

### Clinical Features

Allergic contact dermatitis (ACD) of the face is a delayed hypersensitivity reaction to immunogenic agents, classically soaps, shampoos, hair dyes, cosmetic agents, and nail polish. The face is one of the most common sites for development of ACD.

Common geographic pattern:
- Acute ACD generally presents as pruritic and eczematous plaques, whereas chronic ACD that develops from prolonged allergen exposure classically takes on a lichenified and scaly appearance.
- The rash is normally localized to the specific regions of allergen exposure; however, the overall pattern of facial involvement can be helpful in distinguishing the most likely causal allergen.
  - Involvement of the face that is localized to the lateral neck, preauricular, and temporal regions may be because of allergens applied to the scalp (e.g., hair dyes, shampoos) that rinse off and spread to the face.
  - Lesions that are patchy and develop on the bilateral cheeks may be driven by exposure to cosmetic agents, including moisturizers, fragrances, and sunscreens.
  - Lesions on the upper eyelids (Fig. 2.1) may be the direct result of eye makeup, metal in makeup applicators, or eyelash curlers or may occur indirectly from nail polish exposure when scratching one's eyes.
    - Upper eyelid involvement ("headlight sign") can also be because of airborne contact dermatitis, which classically results from reactivity against specific plants pollens (e.g., ragweed, sunflowers) or occupational exposures (e.g., fiberglass, resins, nickel, wood dust).
      - In these cases, skin involvement may also involve other regions readily exposed to pollen allergens, including the upper chest, neck, and submandibular region.
- The development of ACD on the face involves a sensitization phase of 10 to 14 days after initial exposure.
  - Upon subsequent exposure, dermatitis may appear within 12 to 48 hours.
  - Repeated exposures to the allergen can lead to chronic disease, in which the skin becomes thickened, lichenified, and hyperpigmented.
  - Daily exposure is not required to maintain a reaction.

## Differential Diagnosis

The major differential diagnoses for facial ACD include ICD, AD, seborrheic dermatitis, and phototoxic drug reactions.

- ICD is particularly difficult to distinguish from facial ACD because both follow exposure to a contactant; however, ICD commonly exhibits better demarcation than ACD.
  - Patch testing may be of particular value in these cases; however, ACD/ICD overlap is common and withdrawal of the contactant is a priori in ACD, ICD, and ACD/ICD overlap.
- AD develops in individuals with a personal history of eczema, asthma, or allergic rhinitis at a young age. Isolated facial AD would be unusual. AD typically presents symmetrically in a flexural distribution (antecubital fossae, popliteal fossae, etc.).
- Seborrheic dermatitis can be distinguished from AD because: 1) it typically localizes into a seborrheic distribution (i.e., it affects the nasolabial folds, eyebrows, retroauricular area, and scalp) and 2) it has overlying, greasy-appearing scale.
- A phototoxic drug reaction presents as an exaggerated sunburn in sun-exposed regions, including the face, but patients classically have a history of using specific medications (e.g., tetracyclines, fluoroquinolones, nonsteroidal antiinflammatory drugs [NSAIDs], hydrochlorothiazide).

## Work-Up

Clinical presentation, history, and, in chronic cases, patch testing help establish a diagnosis of facial ACD.

- A total-body skin examination is recommended to identify the presence of a characteristic ACD rash that is localized to the regions previously described.
  - A total-body skin examination is helpful for ruling out other causes of eczematous facial dermatitis, such as AD, because rash elsewhere would be expected in these cases.
- Patient history should be targeted toward identifying a prior history of similar events in addition to evaluating for any new exposures to potential allergens.
  - Classic allergens causing ACD from direct facial contact include cosmetics and lotions with fragrances.
  - Classic facial allergens that impact the face after scalp rinse-off include hair dyes, perming solutions, shampoos, soaps, and topical medications (especially minoxidil).
- The most frequent causes of facial ACD from indirect hand contact are nail polishes and hand lotions.
- Exposure to specific pollens or workplace allergens (e.g., fiberglass, resins, nickel, wood dust) may be suggestive of airborne contact dermatitis.
- A patient history of AD (asthma, hay fever, conjunctivitis) increases the risk for future development of ACD.
- If an offending agent is strongly suspected, it can be useful for the patient to avoid this agent and see if the symptoms resolve or improve.
  - If a particular product is not strongly suspected, however, it is impractical and not recommended to blindly remove potential allergens because many products share similar allergens and this does not frequently lead to identification of the allergen.
  - Instead, in these situations, a "cosmetic holiday," as it is colloquially known, may be recommended to broadly identify the class of allergen exposure.
- For a patient presenting with new-onset facial ACD that is extensive or involves sensitive areas (e.g., the eyelids), it is recommended to refer the patient to a dermatologist for further management and patch testing.
  - Referral to a dermatologist for patch testing can also be pursued if the offending allergen cannot be easily identified or if the patient demonstrates persistent features of ACD.
  - Note that patch testing is different from prick testing, which is an alternative allergy test performed by an allergist.
  - Despite some patients believing that certain foods are causing their ACD, foods are a rare trigger and are more likely to cause a widespread reaction (systemic contact dermatitis) that is not localized to specific skin regions.

## Initial Steps in Management

General management comments:

- The treatment approach for a patient with suspected ACD of the face is targeted toward removing the offending agent (if identified), protecting the skin, and providing treatments to reduce skin inflammation and patient symptoms.

The recommended initial treatment approach for acute ACD of the face involves multiple steps.

- Patients should be informed of common allergen-containing products that can cause ACD of the face.
  - If the trigger is easy to identify, the importance of allergen removal should be emphasized.
  - Patients should be advised to further reference manufacturer sites to identify specific allergens in household items.
- Emollients (e.g., Vaseline, Aquaphor) can be applied to the affected regions to provide a protective barrier against potential allergens.
- To reduce skin inflammation, we recommend the use of moderate-potency topical corticosteroids (fluocinolone acetonide 0.01% cream, triamcinolone acetonide cream 0.1%) twice daily for 2 to 4 weeks on the affected skin areas.
  - Patients with ACD of the hair-bearing scalp may benefit from high-potency corticosteroids (clobetasol propionate 0.05% solution or fluocinonide acetate 0.05% solution) nightly (Chapter 1)
- If immediate reduction in skin inflammation is desired, or if facial involvement is extensive, a 20-day course of oral corticosteroids (e.g., prednisone) is suggested alongside referral to a dermatologist.
  - Dosing should be weight adjusted at a rate of 1 mg/kg.
  - A typical 20-day taper of oral prednisone for an average-weight patient would involve 40 mg daily for 5 days, 30 mg daily for 5 days, 20 mg daily for 5 days, and 10 mg daily for 5 days, with all doses taken in the morning.
  - Shorter, 5- to 7-day doses typically result in rebound flaring after cessation.
  - Systemic comorbidities, such as heart failure, glaucoma, poorly controlled hypertension, and diabetes mellitus should be taken into account when prescribing oral corticosteroids.

What to do if there is a partial but inadequate response after a 4-week trial of topical corticosteroid monotherapy:
- Confirm patient compliance with the treatment regimen and address any compliance barriers.
- Reconsider the diagnosis of ACD or consider other potential allergens.
- Refer patient to a dermatologist for definitive management (patch testing).

## Warning Signs/Common Pitfalls

- Although patients may attribute new rashes to the use of specific products, it is essential to judge the feasibility of these explanations (i.e., if there is a temporal and geographic relationship between product use and rash development).
- Patients with extensive facial involvement or involvement of particularly sensitive areas, such as the eyelids, are unlikely to be adequately treated with topical steroids.
  - In these cases, oral corticosteroids and a referral to a dermatologist for further management are recommended.
- Prick testing is not equivalent to patch testing and is not suitable for identifying allergens causing ACD.

## Counseling

The rash on your cheeks is caused by allergic contact dermatitis, a skin reaction that develops when your immune system reacts to a product, chemical, or medication in your environment. This rash can be bothersome and itchy but is typically not dangerous and can be controlled with medications.

There are a few ways that we manage this rash. First, we want to identify any potential triggers in your day-to-day life. Classic triggers that cause this rash to develop on the face include fragrances, moisturizers, and lotions. You may want to avoid using any skin products that you may have come in contact with recently. If you do not strongly suspect a particular product, however, we do not recommend that you avoid exposing yourself to a number of daily products because this is not usually helpful. In the meantime, we have prescribed you a topical steroid cream to control the rash. You should apply this twice daily on the affected areas of your face for 2 to 4 weeks. Most people tolerate this well over a short period of time, although some say that it causes their blood vessels underneath their skin to become slightly more noticeable. Most patients begin to see their rash resolve within 2 to 4 weeks of consistently using the cream. Some patients also find it helpful to use moisturizers, such as Aquaphor, on their face to protect their skin from further allergen contact.

If your rash continues after these treatments, you may be a candidate for a special type of testing to help us identify the product causing your symptoms. This is called "patch testing," and it is a painless test performed in a dermatologist's office. During this test, many different allergens are placed on your back and secured with tape. They are kept there for 2 days, after which point they are evaluated to determine if you are allergic to any of the agents. This is often helpful in identifying the cause of the rash; however, it can also sometimes identify products that are not causing your immediate problem.

# IRRITANT CONTACT DERMATITIS—FACE

## Clinical Features

Irritant contact dermatitis (ICD) is caused by physical, chemical, or mechanical damage to the skin and it is a common cause of facial dermatitis.

- Facial ICD can be broadly subdivided into three types. All subtypes present with a red, scaling eruption that may become lichenified and result in dyspigmentation if left untreated.
  - Diffuse/spotty—This is the most common subtype of facial ICD. It is characterized by the development of a red and scaly eruption of the cheeks, forehead, and chin. Although the nose can be affected by ICD, it is involved less frequently than other areas because the nose's thick skin and plethora of sebaceous glands are protective against irritants.
    - Diffuse/spotty ICD most commonly develops from personal care products; however, gardeners and lawncare workers may develop this from aerosolized pesticides and other lawncare products; housekeepers may also develop this from aerosolized household cleansing products.
  - Periorbital—This subtype of ICD can present with isolated upper or lower lid dermatitis, or it can present with involvement of both. Upper versus lower lid involvement is caused by different inciting agents (e.g., eye shadow for upper eyelid, eye drops for lower eyelid).
  - Lips—Distinct from perioral dermatitis, a steroid-induced and rosacea-like eruption, lip dermatitis is characterized by cheilitis with or without perioral erythematous plaques. One notable subtype of lip ICD is lip licker dermatitis, a common pediatric dermatosis, where cheilitis and perioral eczematous plaques arise from chronic lip licking. Similarly, infants may have lip/perioral ICD from drooling.
- The biggest cause of both facial ICD and facial ACD is personal care products and their applicators.

Contrary to popular belief, this is true in both men and women.
- Personal care products that are applied to the hair may drip onto the face and neck and cause ICD.
- Isolated facial ICD in the absence of dermatitis elsewhere on the body is very common, especially in cases where facial ICD arises from the application of facial cosmetics.
- Facial ICD is more common in patients with underlying AD because their underlying skin barrier impairment predisposes them to ICD.

## Differential Diagnosis

The differential for facial ICD includes ACD, photodrug reaction, AD, seborrheic dermatitis, rosacea, perioral dermatitis, and angular cheilitis.
- ACD is often clinically indistinguishable from ICD. This is further complicated by the fact that personal care products, the most common cause of facial ICD, are also the most common cause of facial ACD.
  - A combination of the withdrawal of offending agents, repair of the skin barrier, and use of topical antiinflammatories is the treatment of choice for both ACD and ICD.
    - Cases of presumed ICD that fail to respond to treatment or in which an offending agent is not easily identified may benefit from patch testing as outlined in Facial ACD.
- Photodrug reactions can mimic acute, diffuse facial ICD (Fig. 2.2). The sparing of photospared areas (e.g., the nasolabial crease, upper eyelid, and submental area) is supportive of a diagnosis of a photodrug reaction, as is a history of recent initiation of a photosensitizing medication (e.g., doxycycline, hydrochlorothiazide).
- AD can affect the eyelids, face, and flexural neck. This typically occurs in more severe cases and is almost always accompanied by AD elsewhere on the body (e.g., popliteal fossa, antecubital fossa).
  - ICD occurs more commonly in individuals with AD; therefore presence of AD elsewhere on the body does not rule out a diagnosis of facial ICD.
- Seborrheic dermatitis frequently affects the nasolabial folds, eyebrows, hairline, and beard area. Its distribution and overlying greasy scale frequently distinguish it from ICD.
  - ICD also frequently affects the nasolabial fold as irritating cosmetics accumulate within this

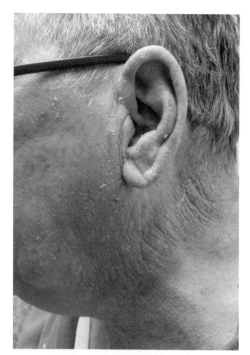

**Fig. 2.2 Chronic Actinic Dermatitis, Lateral Face.** This is thought to be a form of chronic photoallergic dermatitis. (From the UConn Department of Dermatology Grand Rounds Collection.)

concave area. In these cases, ICD may also be identified in the concave periocular area.
- Rosacea may present with redness of the cheeks and nose and superimposed papulopustules; however, it is unlikely to be itchy and is typically associated with telangiectasias.
- Perioral (or periorificial) dermatitis is a misnomer. It is not a true dermatitis. It looks like papulopustular rosacea; however, it concentrates around the mouth and sometimes the eyes and can occur spontaneously or be caused by chronic corticosteroid use. Inhaled corticosteroids are a common, often overlooked culprit. Rarely, topical calcineurin inhibitors can cause perioral dermatitis.
  - Lip ICD can be distinguished from perioral dermatitis because it is a true dermatitis and also frequently coexists with cheilitis.

## Work-Up

All patients with facial ICD need to be asked about their facial skincare regimen, including the use of prescription topical medications and eye drops.

A total-body skin examination should be performed to look for characteristic skin lesions of other diagnoses in the differential.

ICD is generally a clinical diagnosis and rarely is a biopsy required to make the diagnosis.

Patients who fail to improve after the withdrawal of possible offending agents and the use of topical treatment should be offered patch testing.

## Initial Steps in Management

All patients with facial ICD require:
- Withdrawal of the suspected irritant
  - Changing from one brand of personal care product (e.g., mascara) to another does not always improve facial ICD because many products contain similar ingredients.
- For facial dermatoses, it is frequently helpful to recommend lubrication and facial washing twice a day. A lighter, more cosmetically acceptable moisturizer for morning application (e.g., Neutrogena Hydro Boost gel cream, CeraVe lotion, Eucerin lotion) and a thicker, more hydrating moisturizer for evening application (e.g., CeraVe moisturizing cream, Eucerin cream) may enhance patient compliance.
  - In patients without suspected ACD, morning facial moisturizers should routinely contain a sunscreen (e.g., Neutrogena Hydro Boost City Shield, CeraVe AM face, Eucerin daily protection).
  - Patients with significant skin irritation may experience burning with moisturizer application because of preservatives within the moisturizer.
  - Gentle cleansing of the face with water and with or without a gentle cleanser to remove environmental allergens should be performed twice daily every day (morning and evening). The patient's washed hands should be used rather than a washcloth. Face washing should always be followed immediately by moisturizing.
    - Patients with active dermatitis should be counseled to avoid using exfoliating face washes such as those containing salicylic acid, glycolic acid, or alpha hydroxy acid.
    - A topical antiinflammatory
- First-line treatment should include a course of a low-potency topical corticosteroid, such as hydrocortisone 2.5% cream, applied twice daily.
  - Even low-potency topical steroids should be avoided on the eyelids because they can

precipitate glaucoma in susceptible patients and are prone to cause steroid atrophy of this thin skin.

- On the face, all topical steroids can trigger perioral dermatitis/steroid rosacea.
  - In both of these settings, use a topical calcineurin inhibitor, such as pimecrolimus 0.1%, twice daily.
    - Topical pimecrolimus should not be applied to actively inflamed skin because it can cause a severe burning sensation.
- Topical tacrolimus and crisaborole only come in an ointment and are often not cosmetically acceptable for daily facial application.
  - In contradistinction, ointments are usually preferable for irritant cheilitis.

## Warning Signs/Common Pitfalls

The biggest pitfall when managing facial ICD is failure to withdraw the offending irritant. Chronic use of topical corticosteroids is not a substitute for this step of the management process.

- In scenarios where patients are applying multiple personal care products to the affected area(s), withdrawal of all agents should be considered. After resolution of the rash, products can be added back one at a time as tolerated. Initial introduction of a product should be to a limited portion of the skin, such as behind or under the ear, so that if the culprit is identified, a recurrence of a full facial flare is avoided.
- Failure to promote a dry skin care regimen increases the likelihood of ICD relapse after successful treatment.
- Patients must specifically be counseled that twice-daily use of their prescription topical antiinflammatory is not a substitute for frequent moisturization. Patients with facial dermatitis are frequently noncompliant with therapy if topical medications with poor cosmesis (e.g., ointments) are prescribed.
- If patients are unwilling to use a topical corticosteroid or topical calcineurin inhibitor in the morning because of unacceptable cosmesis, use of a stronger ointment for nightly use can be considered (e.g., tacrolimus 0.1%, triamcinolone 0.1%) for a limited duration and as long as the patient is counseled extensively about the potential adverse effects of more potent therapies.
- Noncompliance with moisturizers can occur for similar reasons as stated above.

Failure to identify coexisting dermatoses such as ACD (including to topical corticosteroids), AD, and/ or seborrheic dermatitis can interfere with successful management.

The chronic use of topical corticosteroids on the face, even low-potency topical corticosteroids, can cause skin atrophy, induce an acneiform eruption, what is colloquially known as "red face syndrome," a type of topical steroid addiction in which patients flare after the discontinuation of topicals.

- If red face syndrome is suspected, consider weaning the patient off of topical corticosteroids with diminishing strengths and frequency of use of topical steroids and then a topical calcineurin inhibitor.

## Counseling

You have irritant contact dermatitis (ICD). You developed ICD because your skin is being irritated by something (such as a personal care product) that is coming into contact with it. Our goal is to identify the cause of this irritation and to permanently have you remove/avoid it. If there are multiple potential causes of your rash, then you must try to eliminate all of them until your rash is resolved; you can then add them back one by one as tolerated. Switching brands of products may not be effective because many brands share similar ingredients.

Treating your skin disease requires that you keep your skin healthy by moisturizing it and avoiding exposing it to things that irritate it. To keep your skin healthy, it is important that you wash your face with a gentle cleanser twice daily. After cleaning your face with your hands (rather than a washcloth), you should immediately apply a moisturizer. Some people find it helpful to use a different moisturizer in the morning than they use at night because heavy moisturizers that are better for keeping the skin hydrated (such as CeraVe moisturizing cream) may not be cosmetically suitable for use during the daytime. While your skin is still red and irritated, it is important that you do not apply any cosmetics or fragrances because these can make the skin even more irritated.

Your doctor has prescribed you a cream called "hydrocortisone 2.5%." This cream is a steroid cream. You should use this cream twice daily for a limited time until the redness and irritation is gone. This cream is not a substitute for your moisturizer and should be used with your moisturizer, not instead of your moisturizer. Once the redness and irritation have resolved, you can stop the cream, although you also may restart it when the redness and irritation returns. This cream can cause side effects if you use it too frequently or for too long. This cream can thin the skin, cause blood vessels to be visible in the area of application, discolor the skin, and cause an acnelike rash. Additionally, if this cream is applied around the eye for years, it can cause an increase in eye pressure, which can result in glaucoma, a vision-threatening eye disease.

ETR (See Ch 9, Rosacea)

# ANGULAR CHEILITIS

## Clinical Features

"Angular cheilitis" is an umbrella term for the constellation of conditions that cause irritation, cracking, crusting, and maceration abutting the corners of the mouth (labial commissures). By definition, individuals with angular cheilitis do not have involvement of the entirety of the lips (i.e., diffuse cheilitis).

- Angular cheilitis occurs most frequently in the elderly because of anatomic changes that accompany aging and promote accumulation of saliva in the corners of the mouth.
- Angular cheilitis develops most frequently in individuals with ill-fitting dentures and in those who smoke.

Angular cheilitis has many underlying causes that must be considered when evaluating a patient with this clinical finding. Quite frequently, these different etiologies coexist in the same patient.

- ICD—Almost all cases of angular cheilitis have an underlying component of ICD. This occurs because saliva contains proteases and other enzymes that cause skin breakdown when in prolonged contact with the skin. ICD most commonly causes angular cheilitis in individuals with ill-fitting dentures, smokers, and droolers of any etiology.
  - Clinically, ICD cannot be distinguished from any of the other causes of angular cheilitis and because it almost always occurs in an overlap state with other causes, ICD should always be addressed as a component of management.
- ACD—This is a less common cause of angular cheilitis than ICD; however, the two are virtually clinically indistinguishable. Causes of ACD presenting as

angular cheilitis primarily include metals in dental appliances, flavorings in food and toothpaste, and preservatives and other ingredients in cosmetics. Patients with recurrent angular cheilitis can be patch tested to identify causative contactants.

- Infection—Infection with *Candida sp.*, *Staphylococcus aureus*, and/or *Streptococcus pyogenes* can cause angular cheilitis. The most common infection is a polymicrobial infection caused by *Candida sp.* and bacteria. Although bacterial culture and KOH preparations can be helpful for confirming an infectious cause of angular cheilitis, most patients are treated empirically for a polymicrobial infection. Importantly, patients with confirmed *S. aureus* infection often have *Staph* colonization of their nares and require decolonization to decrease the likelihood of recurrence.
- Nutritional deficiency—Deficiencies of a variety of vitamins and trace elements can cause angular cheilitis. They are thought to account for approximately 20% of cases of angular cheilitis. The most common causative deficiencies are iron deficiency, B vitamin deficiencies, and zinc deficiencies. Work-up for nutritional deficiency should be performed in all patients who are refractory to standard management or who have clear risk factors for nutritional deficiencies.
- Other esoteric causes—These include syphilis, certain medications, and a variety of systemic conditions, such as Sjögren syndrome. A discussion of these less common causes is beyond the scope of this chapter.

## Differential Diagnosis

Angular cheilitis itself is a specific clinical finding; however, the differential for causes of angular cheilitis is quite broad, as previously detailed, and must be considered in all patients presenting with the finding. Differentiating between these causes can be assisted by history and examination of the oral cavity; however, in the majority of cases, work-up after initial treatment failure is necessary to identify the specific cause(s) of an individual's angular cheilitis.

## Work-Up

Work-up is divided into the work-up of patients at initial consultation and the work-up of patients who are refractory to initial management.

## Initial Consultation

- History taking—A history detailing possible irritants, contactants, exacerbating factors, alleviating factors, and dental/orthodontic history should be obtained.
- Oral cavity examination—Examination assessing for thrush, dental appliances, and other contributing clues (e.g., macroglossia, atrophic glossitis) should be performed in all patients.
- Microbial evaluation—If available, bacterial culture and KOH preparation can be helpful for directing therapy. In contradistinction, fungal culture is not typically of any utility given the frequency of asymptomatic colonization with *Candida sp.*

## Refractory Patients

- Laboratory evaluations for underlying diabetes (HgbA1C), HIV, and nutritional deficiencies (CBC, iron and ferritin, Vitamin B2, Vitamin B3, Vitamin B6, Vitamin B9, Vitamin B12, and zinc) should be done.
- Patch testing can be performed in cases where there is sufficient concern for ACD.

## Initial Steps in Management

Angular cheilitis management is divided into initial management, maintenance therapy, and treatment of refractory cases.

### Initial Management

- Patients are frequently initially started on ketoconazole 2% cream twice daily to the affected area for 2 weeks.
- Patients should also be prescribed hydrocortisone 2.5% ointment twice daily as needed to the affected area until clear.
  - Counseling should emphasize that topical antifungal use is obligatory because of the high proportion of cases that are caused by *Candida sp.* and that use of a topical corticosteroid alone is not an appropriate substitute. Additionally, patients should be warned that chronic use of a topical steroid on the face is fraught with potential side effects and is therefore prohibited. Initial time-limited use and then rare intermittent use as needed are the only safe options if using topical steroids in this location.

### Maintenance

- Patients whose skin clears with initial therapy frequently need to continuously apply a barrier cream to the corners of the mouth (e.g., petroleum jelly or Aquaphor) to prevent recurrence of angular cheilitis from additional irritation from saliva.
  - Emphasizing the need for long-term maintenance is critical because most patients develop recurrences over time because their perioral anatomy promotes pooling of saliva in the angles of the mouth.

### Treatment of Refractory Cases

- Patients fail initial management with a topical antifungal and a topical corticosteroid for a variety of reasons, including: 1) the presence of a concomitant bacterial infection; 2) the presence of an underlying nutritional deficiency; 3) the presence of an underlying ACD; and 4) the presence of concomitant oral candidiasis.
- Patients who fail initial therapy should undergo a work-up for systemic causes as previously outlined and should have their therapy plan modified.
  - Patients frequently benefit from the addition of topical mupirocin 2% ointment TID to the existing antifungal regimen, given the commonness of polymicrobial infections causing angular cheilitis.
    - Patients who benefit from the addition of mupirocin or who have *S. aureus* growth on a bacterial culture should have their nares decolonized because it is a frequent cause of disease recurrence. Application of mupirocin ointment into the nares two to three times per day is recommended for nares decolonization.

## Warning Signs/Common Pitfalls

The biggest pitfall when managing angular cheilitis is failure to evaluate for a nonirritant contact dermatitis cause of the condition.

- Importantly, recurrence is not the same as treatment failure and therefore does not necessarily suggest that there is a nonirritant cause to an individual's angular cheilitis.

When prescribing both a topical corticosteroid and a topical antifungal, it is important to emphasize the importance of compliance with the topical antifungal because failure to treat an underlying fungal infection guarantees recurrence as soon as topical therapy is withdrawn.

Given the potential for systemic causes of angular cheilitis, patients should be given short-interval follow-up

(2–4 weeks) appointments to ensure that they are responding appropriately and that they receive appropriate systemic work-up in a timely manner should they not respond.

Denture-wearing patients who have recurrent angular cheilitis should be sent to their dentist for further evaluation.

## Counseling

You have angular cheilitis. Angular cheilitis is inflammation of the skin involving the corners of the mouth. You may have developed this condition for a number of reasons. The most common reason that people develop angular cheilitis is because saliva is pooling in this area of the mouth and irritating the skin. The irritation makes this area especially prone to yeast infections, so we will treat you as if you have a yeast infection as well.

Your doctor has prescribed you an antifungal cream and a topical corticosteroid ointment to treat your condition. It is important that you use the antifungal cream twice daily for at least 2 weeks to treat a possible yeast infection and that you use the topical corticosteroid as frequently as twice daily for 2 weeks or until your rash has cleared. Do not use the topical steroid on this area for more than 2 weeks because it has potential side effects when used chronically on facial skin.

Importantly, angular cheilitis has a tendency to come back. To prevent it from returning, it is important that you apply Vaseline to the corners of your mouth several times a day, or use a Vaseline-based lip balm to protect the corners of your mouth from your saliva.

If your angular cheilitis does not respond to this initial treatment after 2 weeks, it is important that you let your doctor know because there are other less common causes of this rash that you may need to be evaluated for.

## ACTINIC CHEILITIS

### Clinical Features

Actinic cheilitis (Fig. 2.3) is confluent actinic keratoses (AKs) on the lips and is considered to be a premalignant condition. It is more commonly found in lighter-skinned patients and can result from chronic photodamage. Because this has the potential for malignant

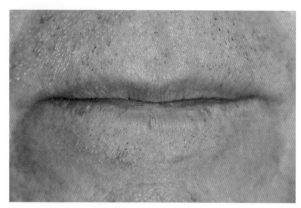

**Fig. 2.3 Actinic Cheilitis.** Note the blurring of the vermilion border. (Courtesy Justin Finch, MD.)

transformation into a squamous cell carcinoma (SCC), treatment or close observation is recommended.

- Patients often relate a history of continued dryness or cracking of the lips (chapped lips) that seems to persist despite moisturization.
- Initial changes may be subtle with only a blurring of the vermilion border; however, the lip will become increasingly scaly, rough, and inflamed. It is more common to see this condition on the lower lip, and erosions and fissures may be appreciated. The upper lip and the corners of the mouth are usually spared because these sites are relatively photo protected.
- Identification of other signs of photodamage on physical examination may help suggest the diagnosis, including poikiloderma of Civatte (mottled erythema on the chest) and cutis rhomboidalis nuchae (thickened leathery skin on the neck with accentuated skin lines forming rhomboidal shapes).

### Differential Diagnosis

The main differential diagnoses for actinic cheilitis are SCC, lip licker's dermatitis, ACD, drug-induced cheilitis, and lichen planus.

- SCC (especially in the earlier in situ stage) can be difficult to distinguish from AKs or actinic cheilitis. An SCC often presents as a thicker, more hyperkeratotic large papule or plaque. Significant tenderness, history of bleeding, ulceration, recurrence, failed treatment of the lesions, or history of immunosuppression should raise clinical suspicion for a malignancy.
- Lip licker's dermatitis is a form of ICD caused by saliva. The patients are often unaware of their lip

licking habit. The lips will appear dry with erythema and fissures, along with a well-demarcated erythematous ring around the lips. This will improve if the patient avoids licking their lips and applies petrolatum as a barrier from the irritant (i.e., saliva).

- ACD occurs because of exposure to allergens. The lips will appear dry, scaly, and erythematous. In this area, common allergens could include ingredients found in lip products and toothpaste. This should improve with avoidance of the allergen.
- Drug-induced cheilitis can be caused by several different medications, including systemic retinoids. It will present similarly to actinic cheilitis with dryness, scaling, and fissures; however, this typically resolves with discontinuation of the medication and can be symptomatically treated with bland emollients. Because oral retinoids are used for skin cancer chemoprophylaxis in high-risk patients, they are frequently necessary to distinguish actinic cheilitis from retinoid-induced cheilitis.
- Lichen planus (Fig. 2.4), an inflammatory dermatosis that can be found inside the oral cavity, can rarely present as isolated lesions on the lips. Wickham striae, which is used to describe the classic white to purple lacy pattern of lichen planus, is typically asymptomatic but can have painful erosions that may be confused with actinic cheilitis. It may respond to topical or systemic immunosuppressive medications, but a referral to a dermatologist is recommended because this may be a challenging diagnosis to make and treat.

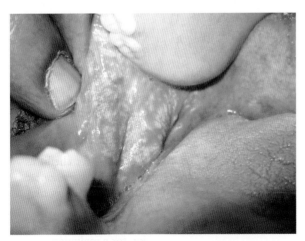

**Fig. 2.4 Oral Lichen Planus.** Notice how these oral lesions appear similar to Wickham striae on the skin. (Courtesy Justin Finch, MD.)

## Work-Up

Patients with suspected actinic cheilitis should be referred to a dermatologist for further evaluation, skin cancer screening, and treatment.

This is usually a clinical diagnosis made by the dermatologist with the aid of physical examination and a dermatoscope (a handheld instrument that uses a transilluminating light source and has magnifying optics of 10X).

- If the diagnosis is unclear, then the dermatologist can perform a skin biopsy for more definitive information.
- If there is any uncertainty in the diagnosis, the patient should be referred to a dermatologist.

## Initial Steps in Management

The most important step in management is prevention of further sun damage. Patients should be counseled regarding the etiology of actinic cheilitis and the fact that sun protection/avoidance are key parts of the strategy.

- Advise against tanning beds and prolonged sun exposure.
- Recommend sun avoidance during peak hours (10 AM–4 PM).
- Even if the patient is outside or in the car for more than 15 minutes, they still require sun protection.
- Recommend physical blocker sunscreens (containing zinc and titanium oxide) with at least SPF 30. To protect the lips, there are lip balms with SPF. Sunscreen needs to be reapplied every 2 hours or more frequently if there is water exposure or excessive sweating. A shot glass full of sunscreen is the amount that is recommended to appropriately cover the entire body. Spray sunscreen is often applied incorrectly because the aerosolized components end up in the air rather than on the skin, so topical formulations are preferred.
- Recommend sun-protective clothing (and built-in sun protection) with wide-brimmed hats to cover the patients' face and ears.

Management of actinic cheilitis involves dividing cases by management plans, which can include localized therapy, field therapy, or, potentially, biopsy. This can vary depending on the size, number, and location of the rashes, as well as the age, comorbidities, and willingness of the patient. Based on the complexity and possible reactions to the treatments, a referral to dermatology is recommended.

## Localized Therapy

- This is beneficial for more discrete lesions and for patients who prefer in-office treatment or are not compliant with daily applications of an at-home cream.
- Cryotherapy can be applied to each lesion with a cryotherapy canister for 10 to 15 seconds for two cycles with a complete thaw in between. There should be an effort to remove any significant scale or crusting over the lesion, so that the liquid nitrogen can be applied to the base.
  - Patients should be counseled that the liquid nitrogen will cause discomfort, erythema, edema, potential blisters, and possible permanent dyspigmentation or a scar.
  - No postcryotherapy wound care is required; however, the patient can apply petrolatum daily to the areas until it has healed. Avoidance of spicy food until the lips heal is recommended.
  - Liquid nitrogen should not be used on melanocytic lesions because treatment of a nevus or melanoma can lead to a delay in diagnosis and inability to diagnose and follow the lesion in question. This highlights the fact that a correct diagnosis is crucial before providing treatment.
  - For those who are not concerned about potential dyspigmentation in the area and who do not want to do treatment at home, cryotherapy should be considered.
- If the entirety of the lip is involved, if cryotherapy is not available, or if the patient elects not to have cryotherapy, then field therapy may be a more optimal solution.

## Field Therapy

- Field therapy is beneficial because it can help to decrease the number of localized treatments that the patients will need in the future by treating the underlying solar damage and even the evolving actinic cheilitis. Sometimes a combination of multiple modalities is used for this condition.
- Chemotherapeutic cream
  - This is better for patients who are compliant and willing to apply a topical cream at home. Although many patients are wary given the expected inflammatory reaction with this medication, they are often pleased by the end results because it improves the photodamage and texture of the lips.

- Topical 5-fluorouracil (5-FU) can be used on the affected areas. Duration may depend on degree of photodamage and tolerability. Patients should be counseled that erythema, discomfort, scaling, crusting, edema, and flu like symptoms are an expected reaction with this medication. Given the variability in response and dosing schedules, this medication is best prescribed by a dermatologist.
- Imiquimod is another topical cream that works by being an immune stimulant. It is available in varied strengths with associated variable schedules and is best prescribed by a dermatologist.
- Ingenol mebutate gel is another topical that dermatologists use. It is known for its quick toxic response after a shorter duration of treatment. Again, this medication is best prescribed by a dermatologist.
- The healing process will take weeks (or, rarely, months) after stopping the cream. It may be helpful to see the patients back 3 to 4 months after using the medication to see if there are any residual areas that require further treatment or biopsy. If crusting persists, consider possible secondary herpes simplex infection or a secondary bacterial infection (impetigo) and work up and treat accordingly.
- The best time to use these creams is in the wintertime because the patient should avoid being outside in the direct sunlight for prolonged periods of time while using these medications.
- Photodynamic therapy (PDT)
  - This is better for patients who are not willing to apply a topical cream at home and would prefer to have an in-office procedure done instead. They need strict sun avoidance for 48 hours after the procedure.
  - A photosensitizing agent (usually aminolevulinic acid) is applied to the affected areas by trained medical staff. The areas are then exposed to a blue light device in the office or the patients are instructed to proceed outside to use sunlight as an activator for the medication.
  - Patients should be counseled on the expected reaction, which includes erythema, edema, crusting, and discomfort.
  - The healing process will take weeks (or, rarely, months) after the procedure. It may be helpful to see the patients back 3 to 4 months afterwards to

see if there are any residual areas that require further treatment or biopsy.

- Electrodessication
  - This is better for patients who are not willing to apply a topical cream at home and would prefer to have an in-office procedure done instead.
  - Electrodessication involves the injection of local anesthesia and then the application of an electrical current, which causes superficial tissue dehydration.
  - Patients should be counseled on the expected reaction, which includes erythema, edema, crusting, and discomfort.
  - Referral to a dermatologist is recommended to evaluate the areas to decide if this is the best treatment modality.
- Chemical peel
  - This is better for patients who are not willing to apply a topical cream at home and would prefer to have an in-office procedure done instead.
  - Patients should be counseled on the expected reaction, which includes erythema, edema, crusting, blistering, and discomfort.
  - Referral to a dermatologist is recommended to evaluate the areas to decide if this is the best treatment modality.
- Laser
  - This is better for patients who are not willing to apply a topical cream at home and would prefer to have an in-office procedure done instead.
  - Several different lasers have been used to treat actinic cheilitis, most notably a $CO_2$ laser.
  - Patients should be counseled on the expected reaction, which includes erythema, edema, crusting, blistering, and discomfort.
  - Referral to a dermatologist is recommended to evaluate the areas to decide if this is the best treatment modality.
- Surgery
  - For severe cases without malignancy, vermilionectomy may be performed.
  - Referral to a dermatologist is recommended to evaluate the areas to decide if this is the best treatment modality.

## Biopsy

- A biopsy should be considered for the following conditions:
  - High clinical suspicion for an SCC
  - Recurrent lesions that failed to respond to previous treatment
  - Larger size or significant hyperkeratosis or ulceration
  - Pain or bleeding
- Given the risk of cutaneous malignancy in the immunosuppressed or immunocompromised population, there should be a lower threshold for potential biopsy if areas do not respond appropriately to treatment.
- If a biopsy is warranted, then referral to a dermatologist is recommended because incorrect sampling can lead to false negatives and a delay in diagnosis.
  What to do if treatment response is inadequate:
- Reconsider the diagnosis and refer to dermatology for further evaluation.

## Warning Signs/Common Pitfalls

- Patients with actinic cheilitis should have periodic skin cancer screenings (at least annually) because this represents cumulative photodamage over their lifetime, putting them at risk for cutaneous malignancies.
- There should be a low threshold for referral to a dermatologist to evaluate the lesions because this condition can mimic other diseases, and there is a wide differential that has to be considered.
- If there is clinical suspicion for a potential SCC, then referral to a dermatologist is recommended, especially on mucosal surfaces and the head and neck in general, where metastases can occur.
- Antiviral prophylaxis against herpes simplex virus (HSV) should be considered when treating actinic cheilitis because this area is at a high risk for developing a herpetic superinfection.

## Counseling

You have precancerous lesions, known as "actinic cheilitis," on your lips that are caused by chronic sun damage. They have the potential to turn into a type of skin cancer called "squamous cell carcinoma," which if left untreated, can be deadly. The most important part of treatment is prevention of further sun damage. You should avoid the sun during peak hours (10 AM–4 PM) and stay away from tanning beds because these can increase your risk for skin cancer. If you are going to be outside or in the car for 15 minutes or more, sun protection is necessary. We recommend physical blocker sunscreens (ones that contain zinc and titanium oxide) with at least SPF 30, along with lip balms with built-in sun protection. The amount of sunscreen required to provide adequate coverage for the face and body amounts to a shot glass full of sunscreen. It needs to be reapplied every 2 hours, or more frequently if there has been water exposure or excessive sweating. Sun-protective clothing can be even more beneficial because this will provide more consistent sun protection and should include a wide-brimmed hat to cover the ears and scalp.

Treatment of actinic cheilitis depends on the number, size, and location of the lesions. Cryotherapy or liquid nitrogen can be used to treat smaller areas but will cause redness, swelling, and some discomfort. Topical chemotherapeutic creams, photodynamic therapy, and other modalities can be prescribed for larger or more diffuse areas but can also cause redness, swelling, and inflammation. In some cases, a biopsy (skin sample) may be necessary to determine a diagnosis. Seeing a dermatologist in the future for evaluation and skin cancer screening will be important.

# ACTINIC KERATOSES

## Clinical Features

Actinic keratoses (AKs) are precancerous lesions that are commonly found in lighter-skinned individuals with significant photodamage. Because they have the potential for malignant transformation into SCC, treatment or close observation is recommended.

- Patients often relate a history of an intermittent rough patch that seems to recur despite exfoliating or moisturizing the area.
- Clinically, they usually present as pink, scaly, or gritty papules on sun-exposed surfaces, such as the scalp, face, ears, neck, upper chest, forearms, dorsal hands, and shins. Nevertheless, the lesions are often subtle and best appreciated through palpation rather than visual examination.
- In males, it is particularly important to examine both the scalp and ears because they lack the photoprotection that longer hair provides for most women.
- In females, the chest and lower extremities become significant areas to examine because they are more likely to wear V-neck shirts, shorts, or skirts.
- There is a pigmented variant that can appear browner in color (rather than pink), but the scaly texture can provide a clue as to the diagnosis.

- An AK variant presents as something called a "cutaneous horn," which literally resembles a column of hyperkeratosis in the shape of a horn. AK can represent one of several potential different diagnoses that present as a cutaneous horn.

## Differential Diagnosis

The main differential diagnoses for AKs are SCC, basal cell carcinoma, seborrheic keratoses, seborrheic dermatitis, and xerosis.

- SCCs (especially in the earlier in situ stage) can be difficult to distinguish from AKs. An SCC often presents as a thicker, more hyperkeratotic larger papule or plaque. Significant tenderness, history of bleeding, recurrence or failed treatment of the lesion, or history of immunosuppression should raise clinical suspicion for a malignancy.
- Basal cell carcinoma usually presents as a pink, pearly papule with or without a central erosion with telangiectasias. Because this is the most common form of skin malignancy, it is often seen in the same population. This growth tends to have less scale and a less gritty texture compared with AKs.
- Seborrheic keratoses commonly coexist among this population and can present in all different shapes, sizes, colors, and textures. These growths often have more of a stuck-on, warty appearance, and patients often confuse them for moles because they most commonly are brownish in color.
- Seborrheic dermatitis, which can manifest as dandruff on the scalp, can appear as pink, scaly patches on the scalp, eyebrows, and nasolabial folds. Some people may confuse these patches with AKs, but they are often more diffuse, less gritty, and greasier in texture and will respond to antifungal creams or shampoos.
- Xerosis is common in older, photodamaged patients because of lack of moisturization, which can make the physical examination more challenging. Although xerosis can appear to be scaly like AKs, it is usually more diffuse and the texture does not appear to be as rough or gritty. The skin lines are more pronounced, with patients complaining of crepey skin. This will improve with gentle skin care and moisturization.

## Work-Up

Patients with suspected AKs should be referred to a dermatologist for further evaluation, skin cancer screening, and treatment.

- AKs are usually a clinical diagnosis made by the dermatologist with the aid of physical examination and dermoscopy (a handheld technology that involves light, magnification, and polarized lenses) to rule out other conditions.
- If the diagnosis is unclear, then the dermatologist can perform a skin biopsy for more definitive information.
- If there is any uncertainty in the diagnosis and there is even the remote possibility of an amelanotic melanoma, the patient should be immediately referred to a dermatologist.

## Initial Steps in Management

The most important step in management is prevention of further sun damage. Patients should be counseled regarding the etiology of the AKs and informed that sun protection and avoidance are key parts of the strategy.

- Advise against tanning beds and prolonged sun exposure.
- Recommend sun avoidance during peak hours (10 AM–4 PM).
- If the patient is outside or in the car for more than 15 minutes, they require sun protection.
- Recommend physical blocker sunscreens (ones that contain zinc and titanium oxide) with at least SPF 30. Sunscreen needs to be reapplied every 2 hours or more frequently if there has been water exposure or excessive sweating. A shot glass full of sunscreen is the amount that is recommended to appropriately cover the entire body. Spray sunscreen is often applied incorrectly and the aerosolized components end up in the air rather than on the skin, so topical formulations are preferred.
- Recommend sun-protective clothing (clothing that has built-in sun protection) with wide-brimmed hats to cover the patients' ears.

Management of AKs includes localized therapy, field therapy, or the need for potential biopsy. This can vary depending on the size, number, and location of the lesions, as well as the age, comorbidities, and willingness of the patient. Based on the complexity and possible reactions to the treatments, a referral to dermatology is recommended.

## Localized Therapy

- Localized therapy is beneficial for solitary, discrete lesions, not for areas that have diffuse actinic or solar damage with numerous evident AKs.

- Cryotherapy can be applied to each lesion with a cryotherapy canister for 10 to 15 seconds for 2 cycles with a complete thaw in between. There should be an effort to remove any significant scale or crusting over the lesion so that the liquid nitrogen can be applied to the base.
  - Patients should be counseled that the liquid nitrogen will cause discomfort, erythema, potential blisters, and possible permanent dyspigmentation or a scar.
  - No postcryotherapy wound care is required; however, the patient can apply petrolatum daily to the areas until it has healed.
  - Liquid nitrogen should not be used on melanocytic lesions because treatment of a nevus or melanoma can lead to a delay in diagnosis and an inability to diagnose and follow the lesion in question. This highlights the fact that a correct diagnosis is crucial before providing treatment.
  - For those who are not concerned about potential dyspigmentation in the area and who do not want to do treatment at home, cryotherapy should be considered.
- If there is significant photodamage or a large number of lesions that need to be treated, field therapy may be more optimal.
- Field therapy
- This is beneficial for multiple or large areas of photodamage. It can help to decrease the number of localized treatments that the patients will need in the future by treating the underlying solar damage and even evolving AKs.
- Chemotherapeutic creams
  - These creams are better for patients who are compliant and willing to apply a topical cream at home. Although many patients are wary given the expected inflammatory reaction with these medications, they are often pleased with the end results because they improve the photodamage and texture of the skin.
  - Apply topical 5-FU to affected areas twice daily for 2 to 6 weeks depending on the location being treated. Patients should be counseled that erythema, discomfort, scaling, crusting, edema, and flu like symptoms are an expected reaction with this medication. For affected areas on the face, the patient may only be able to tolerate 2 to 3 weeks of treatment because of the inflammatory

reaction from the medication. Elsewhere on the body, longer application times are required to get the optimal response.

- Alternatively, topical 5-FU mixed in a 1:1 ratio with calcipotriene (a vitamin D analogue) can be applied to affected areas twice daily for 1 week. Patients should be counseled that erythema, discomfort, scaling, crusting, edema, and flu-like symptoms are an expected reaction with this medication. Because the calcipotriene helps with penetration of the 5-FU, patients often have a more exuberant reaction than with 5-FU alone.
- Imiquimod is another topical cream that works by being an immune stimulant. It is available in varied strengths with associated variable schedules and is best prescribed by a dermatologist.
- Ingenol mebutate gel is another topical that dermatologists use and that is known for its quick toxic response after a shorter duration of treatment. Again, this medication is best prescribed by a dermatologist.
- The healing process will take weeks to months after stopping the cream. It may be helpful to see the patients back 3 to 4 months after using the medication to see if there are any residual areas that require further treatment or biopsy.
- The best time to use these creams is in the wintertime because the patient should avoid being outside in the direct sunlight for prolonged periods of time.
- PDT
  - PDT is better for patients who are not willing to apply a topical cream at home and would prefer to have an in-office procedure done instead. They need to adhere to strict sun avoidance for 48 hours after the procedure.
  - If the lesions are very hyperkeratotic, microdermabrasion may be used before the PDT.
  - A photosensitizing agent (usually aminolevulinic acid) is applied to the affected areas by trained medical staff. The areas are then exposed to a blue light device in the office or the patients are instructed to proceed outside to use sunlight as an activator for the medication.
  - Patients should be counseled on the expected reaction, which includes erythema, edema, crusting, and discomfort.

- The healing process will take weeks (or, rarely, months) after the procedure. It may be helpful to see the patients back 3 to 4 months afterwards to see if there are any residual areas that require further treatment or biopsy.

### Biopsy

- A biopsy should be considered for the following conditions:
  - High clinical suspicion for an SCC
  - A recurrent lesion that has failed to respond to previous treatment
  - Larger size or significant hyperkeratosis
  - Pain or bleeding
  - The remote possibility of an amelanotic melanoma
- Given the risk of cutaneous malignancy in the immunosuppressed or immunocompromised population, there should be a lower threshold for potential biopsy if areas do not respond appropriately to treatment.
- If a biopsy is warranted, then referral to a dermatologist is recommended because incorrect sampling can lead to false negatives and delay in diagnosis.

What to do if treatment response is inadequate:

- Reconsider the diagnosis and refer to dermatology for further evaluation.

### Warning Signs/Common Pitfalls

- Patients with AKs should have periodic skin cancer screenings (at least annually) because AKs represent cumulative photodamage over their lifetime, putting them at risk for cutaneous malignancies.
- There should be a low threshold for referral to a dermatologist to evaluate the lesions because this condition can mimic other diseases, and there is a wide differential that has to be considered.
- If there is clinical suspicion for a potential SCC, then referral to a dermatologist is recommended, especially on the head and neck, where metastases can occur.

### Counseling

You have a precancerous growth, called an "actinic keratosis" (plural: "actinic keratoses"), that is caused by chronic sun damage. It has the potential to turn into a type of skin cancer called "squamous cell carcinoma," which, if left untreated, can be deadly. The most important part of treatment is prevention of further sun damage. You should avoid the sun during peak hours (10 AM–4 PM) and stay away from tanning beds because these can increase your risk for skin cancer. If you are going to be outside or in the car for 15 minutes or more, sun protection is necessary. We recommend physical blocker sunscreens (ones that contain zinc and titanium oxide) with at least SPF 30. The amount of sunscreen required to provide adequate coverage for the face and body amounts to a shot glass full of sunscreen. It needs to be reapplied every 2 hours or more frequently if there has been water exposure or excessive sweating. Sun-protective clothing can be even more beneficial because it will provide more consistent sun protection and should include a wide-brimmed hat to cover the ears and scalp.

Treatment of AKs depends on the number, size, and location of the lesions. Cryotherapy or liquid nitrogen can be used to treat solitary lesions but will cause redness, swelling, and some discomfort. Topical chemotherapeutic creams can be prescribed for larger areas but can also cause redness, swelling, and inflammation. There is also an in-office treatment called "photodynamic therapy," which can be used depending on the situation but will also cause an inflammatory reaction. In some cases, a biopsy (skin sample) may be necessary to determine a diagnosis. Seeing a dermatologist in the future for evaluation and skin cancer screening will be important.

# ACUTE CUTANEOUS LUPUS ERYTHEMATOSUS

- Lupus erythematosus (LE) is a connective tissue disease and autoimmune disorder that can affect one or several organs.
- Circulating autoantibodies and immune complexes are the result of loss of normal immune tolerance and are pathogenic. The clinical features of LE are highly variable. LE nearly always affects the skin to some degree.
- Systemic lupus erythematosus (SLE) may also affect the joints, kidneys, lungs, heart, liver, brain, blood vessels (vasculitis), and blood cells. It may be accompanied by antiphospholipid syndrome.
- LE-specific cutaneous LE (CLE) can be classified as acute, subacute, intermittent, or chronic. Lesions may be localized or generalized. In LE-specific CLE, lesions are often induced by exposure to sunlight.

Ultraviolet B (UVB) irradiation causes keratinocyte necrosis, immune system activation, and antibody formation.
- CLE most often affects young to middle-aged adult women (aged 20–50 years) but children, the elderly, and males may also be affected.
- Acute CLE (ACLE) affects at least 50% of patients with SLE.
- Factors that can exacerbate LE include sun exposure, cigarette smoking, and certain drugs.

## Clinical Features
- ACLE may occur as a manifestation of SLE or independent of SLE.
- ACLE is a manifestation of SLE that may present as a characteristic localized facial eruption (also known as a "malar rash" or "butterfly rash") on the cheeks and bridge of the nose. Atypically, it can affect other sun-exposed areas (Fig. 2.5). The nasolabial folds are spared. Localized ACLE may precede other symptoms of SLE or may be accompanied by other symptoms and signs of acute SLE.
- Involved signs include feeling warm and sometimes a burning sensation after sun exposure.
- Erythema and edema may last hours, days, or weeks and often recur, particularly with sun exposure.
- Postinflammatory hyperpigmentation or hypopigmentation are common in darker-skinned patients.

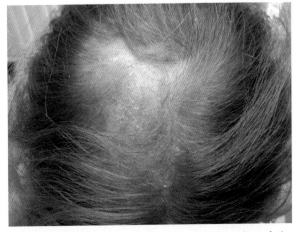

**Fig. 2.5 Ulcerative Oral Lichen Planus.** Ulceration of the gingiva, as shown here, is called "desquamative gingivitis" and can occur in the setting of lichen planus, pemphigus vulgaris, and other diseases.

Other features of ACLE include:

- An erythematous papular rash on the arms, sometimes forming large plaques and spreading widely
- Photosensitivity (a rash on all recently sun-exposed skin)
- Cheilitis and mouth ulcers
- Blisters (bullous SLE) and erosions

## Work-Up

- Cutaneous LE is largely a clinical diagnosis: localized ACLE can be diagnosed by recognition of erythema in the classic malar distribution in a patient with known SLE.
- Patients with cutaneous LE should be evaluated for SLE with a laboratory assessment for the presence of antinuclear antibodies and antibodies to extractable nuclear antigens (double-stranded DNA, Ro, La, Smith).
- Patients should also undergo a comprehensive blood count (CBC), comprehensive metabolic panel (CMP), and urinalysis (UA) to evaluate for systemic involvement.
- If a patient initially presents with CLE, it is recommended to obtain a clinical history with a focus on rheumatologic review of systems.
- Histologic findings are consistent with interface dermatitis and include apoptotic keratinocytes, vacuolization of the basal cell layer of the epidermis, a lymphohistiocytic infiltrate in the superficial dermis, and dermal mucin deposition.

## Initial Steps in Management

- Management of CLE patients includes an emphasis on prevention and controlling flare-ups.
- It also includes counseling on smoking cessation.
- There should be extensive education about avoidance of sun exposure. Mineral-based sunscreens of SPF 30+ should be applied 30 minutes before sun exposure and reapplied every 2 hours. Wide-brimmed hats and sun-protective clothing are also encouraged.
- First-line therapy:
  - Use of topical or topical calcineurin inhibitors.
  - Systemic antimalarial agents, including hydroxychloroquine or chloroquine, with quinacrine added to either of these agents for refractory cases.
  - Depending on the severity of the disease, intralesional or intramuscular corticosteroids and systemic glucocorticoids can be considered.

What to do if initial treatment fails:

- Refer patients with clinical and serologic evidence of LE to a rheumatologist for further evaluation and treatment. Refer patients with red blood cell casts, significant proteinuria (>0.5 g/mL/24h), and a diastolic blood pressure of more than 90 mm Hg to a nephrologist.
- Depending on the severity of systemic and cutaneous involvement, various immunomodulatory therapies should be considered:
  - Methotrexate (oral or subcutaneous)
  - Mycophenolate mofetil
  - Azathioprine
  - Dapsone
  - Intravenous immunoglobulin (IVIG) or belimumab

# DISCOID LUPUS ERYTHEMATOSUS

**Christina Jiang and Jun Lu**

## Clinical Features

- Discoid lupus erythematosus (DLE) is the most common subset of chronic CLE. LE is a polygenic autoimmune disease associated with various human leukocyte antigen (HLA) subtypes, immune signaling, and environmental factors.
- The exact etiology of DLE is not well understood; however, there appears to be contributive environmental factors, including ultraviolet radiation, medications, cigarette smoking, and possibly viruses.
- DLE may occur in association with SLE or in the absence of any systemic disease. DLE occurs as a manifestation of SLE in approximately 20% of patients.
- A complete review of systems should be assessed for serologic and/or hematologic abnormalities, arthralgia or arthritis, pleuritis, pericarditis, neurologic involvement, and renal involvement.
- Morphologically, DLE can present with:
  - Erythematous-violaceous scaly plaques
  - Atrophic scarring
  - Dyspigmentation
  - Follicular hyperkeratosis/plugging
  - Scarring alopecia
- Localized DLE is DLE with only the skin of the head and neck affected (Fig. 2.6). Conchal bowls (Fig. 2.7) and the scalp are common areas of involvement, sometimes with permanent scarring and hair loss.

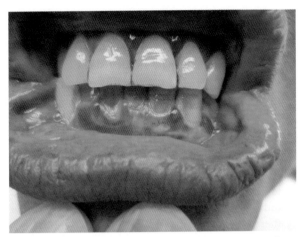

**Fig. 2.6 Acute Cutaneous Lupus, Scalp.** (From the UConn Department of Dermatology Grand Rounds Collection.)

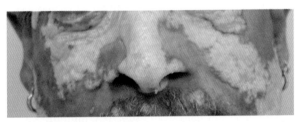

**Fig. 2.7 Discoid Lupus Erythematosus.** This case mimics the malar distribution of acute cutaneous lupus. (From the UConn Department of Dermatology Grand Rounds Collection.)

- Widespread DLE is DLE with an affected area besides just the skin of the head and neck.
  - Differentiation of localized DLE from widespread DLE is important prognostically for determining a patient's risk for SLE.
- Patients may experience mild pruritus or occasional pain with the lesions, but most lesions are asymptomatic.
- DLE is a highly variable disorder. The condition is benign but can result in high morbidity and reduce the patient's quality of life. The disorder has a waxing and waning character. Lesions can result in disfigurement from the scarring or atrophy.

## Differential Diagnosis

Differential diagnoses for DLE include AK, cutaneous SCC, granuloma annulare (GA), AD, seborrheic dermatitis, lichen planus, psoriasis, rosacea, and other subtypes of CLE, including acute or subacute CLE. A punch biopsy will usually exclude these clinical mimickers and establish the correct diagnosis.

## Work-Up

- Screening for SLE is recommended if a patient is diagnosed with DLE.
- The diagnosis of DLE is made based on clinical features, but diagnosis is usually confirmed by skin biopsy.
- Histopathology can demonstrate the following characteristics for DLE:
  - Interface/vacuolar dermatitis
  - Superficial and deep perivascular and periappendageal lymphohistiocytic infiltrate
  - Hyperkeratosis with underlying epidermal thinning
  - Follicular keratin plugs
  - Mucin deposition
  - Basement membrane thickening

## Initial Steps in Management

- Management includes strict sun-protective measures, including sun avoidance, sunscreens of SPF above 30, protective clothing, and wide-brimmed hats.
- Cosmetic measures, such as cover-up makeup or wigs, may be suggested for appropriately selected patients. Makeup used for camouflage includes Covermark and Dermablend.
- Smoking cessation is encouraged.
- Standard first-line therapy includes topical corticosteroids, a topical calcineurin inhibitor, and systemic antimalarials.
  - Topical corticosteroids are selected for the type of lesion under treatment and for the site of involvement. For example, solutions, lotions, oil, or foams are preferred for the scalp, and weaker agents are used on the face.
    - Recommend a twice-daily application of a group 1 or 2 topical corticosteroid, such as clobetasol propionate, for acute flares of DLE.
    - Use a twice-daily application of a low-potency topical steroid (group 6 or 7), such as hydrocortisone 1% or 2.5%, for patients with minimal disease on the face.
    - Use a twice-daily application of a medium- to high-potency topical corticosteroid (groups 2 to 4), such as triamcinolone acetonide 0.1%

cream or fluocinonide 0.05% cream, for trunk, extremity, or scalp disease.

- Improvements with topical corticosteroids are typically noted within days to 2 weeks of the initial therapy.
- Antimalarial therapy has a photoprotective effect and seems to lessen the progression to SLE and to lower the risk for thrombovascular disease.
  - Hydroxychloroquine and chloroquine are currently used; however, the former is preferred because of the lower risk for side effects (retinal toxicity).
  - Adverse effects of antimalarial therapy include gastrointestinal distress, ocular toxicity, and neuromuscular and hematologic abnormalities.
- Intralesional injection of corticosteroids is useful as adjunctive therapy for individual lesions.
  - Dilute concentrations are preferred because of the potential for atrophy related to the amount of corticosteroids injected in any one area.
  - Triamcinolone acetonide in concentrations ranging from 3 to 5 mg/mL is typically used for treatment. Injections are repeated every 3 to 4 weeks until erythema and scale have disappeared.
- If an acute flare of DLE or SCLE fails to improve with high topical corticosteroid application after 2 to 4 weeks, a topical calcineurin inhibitor or intralesional corticosteroid treatment can be attempted.
  - Topical calcineurin inhibitors are pimecrolimus 1% cream and tacrolimus 0.03% or 0.1% ointment. These are favorable for lesions of the face, where topical corticosteroids may induce cutaneous side effects. Disadvantages include the cost and the slow-acting mechanism. Improvement of symptoms can be expected within the first 4 weeks of treatment, and complete clearance of thin patches and plaques may occur within 2 months.
- Topical retinoids and vitamin A analogue have antikeratinizing and antiinflammatory effects and therefore are sometimes used in CLE. Topical retinoids can cause cutaneous irritation and are contraindicated in pregnancy.
- Systemic corticosteroids are typically avoided because the dose and duration of therapy needed to maintain control of cutaneous disease often results in substantial steroid-related adverse effects.

- Systemic immunosuppressives may be considered for refractory cases, including methotrexate, mycophenolate mofetil, and azathioprine, among others.
- Consultation with the following specialists may be helpful:
- Dermatologist for skin lesions
- Rheumatologist for joint involvement or to evaluate for systemic involvement
- Nephrologist for renal involvement
- Ophthalmologist to monitor therapy with hydroxychloroquine or chloroquine. A baseline examination is required within 1 year of starting hydroxychloroquine, then annually after 5 years of cumulative therapy.

### Excision and Laser Therapy

- Excision of burned-out, scarred lesions is possible; however, reactivation of inactive lesions has been reported in some patients.
- Laser therapy (pulsed-dye laser) may be useful for lesions with prominent telangiectasia; however, one must consider the risk for reactivation with this form of therapy. Before using this therapy in patients, a test area should be treated to make certain that the DLE does not flare.

### Long-Term Monitoring

- Follow patients with DLE at regular intervals.
- Response to therapy varies from several weeks to several months.
- At each visit, question the patient about new symptoms that may reflect systemic disease.
- At regular intervals, perhaps annually in otherwise asymptomatic patients, perform routine laboratory studies for assessment, including CBC, renal function tests, complement levels, and UA.

### Counseling

Your rash may or may not be a manifestation of a systemic autoimmune disorder known as "systemic lupus erythematosus." Because of this, we recommend a workup with a rheumatologist. Our goals of management are to stop disease activity to prevent scarring and the development of further lesions. The development of serious systemic disease is possible, although rare.

Although your condition is most consistent with discoid lupus erythematosus, a definitive diagnosis can be attained with a skin biopsy. A skin biopsy is the removal of small sample of affected skin, which is sent to a laboratory to view under the microscope.

Your rash can worsen in the presence of sunlight; therefore we recommend strict sun protection, including sunscreens, wide-brimmed hats, and sun-protective clothing. We recommend applying SPF 30+ sunscreen 30 minutes before going out in the sun and reapplying every 2 hours. Additionally, smoking cigarettes has been associated with worsening of the rash; we encourage smoking cessation to help improve symptoms.

There are multiple treatment options. The initial treatment options include topical corticosteroids for 2 to 3 weeks. If symptoms fail to improve or recur, we can progress to oral medications and immunosuppressant medications.

## OROLABIAL HERPES SIMPLEX

### Clinical Features

Orolabial herpes simplex virus (HSV; also known as "herpes labialis," "cold sores," or "fever blisters") is a common viral infection more often caused by the herpes simplex virus 1 (HSV1) than herpes simplex virus 2 (HSV2).

- It initially presents as crops of vesicles overlying an erythematous base; however, it quickly evolves into eroded or ulcerated papules that may coalesce into plaques with overlying crusting.
- Orolabial HSV most often affects the lips, then the perioral area, then the buccal mucosa, then the gingiva, and finally the oropharynx.
  - HSV almost exclusively affects keratinized mucosa in immunocompetent hosts; however, distribution is less predictable in immunocompromised hosts.
  - The severity of disease is highly variable with initial infections and infections in immunocompromised hosts tending to be most severe.
- Some patients experience systemic prodromal symptoms before each outbreak, which are characterized by malaise with or without a fever.
- Patients frequently complain of localized cutaneous pruritus or, more commonly, pain, burning, soreness, or tingling at the site before the appearance of the visible lesions.
- Frequency of recurrence of orolabial HSV is highly variable with a minority of patients developing more

than 6 recurrences per annum. Recurrences have a tendency to decrease in frequency over time.

- Triggers for recurrences include sunlight, stress, immunosuppression, illness (hence the colloquial names "fever blisters" and "cold sores"), and surgical procedures performed in the vicinity, such as dental work.
  - Patients with eczema may develop a herpes infection within their eczema plaques called "eczema herpeticum," which is characterized by the development of many punched-out ulcerations within established plaques with or without flu like illness. In cases where lesions disseminate to the entire body, eczema herpeticum can be fatal and therefore should be treated as an medical emergency.

### Differential Diagnosis

The differential for orolabial HSV includes aphthous ulcers, erythema multiforme (EM), ulcerative lichen planus (LP), morsicatio buccarum (chronic cheek biting), herpes zoster, cheilitis, and fixed drug eruption (FDE).

- Aphthous ulcers (Fig. 2.8), colloquially known as "canker sores," can be differentiated from orolabial herpes because: 1) they are not preceded by vesicles and 2) they predominantly occur on nonkeratinized mucosa.
- Recurrent EM of the lips is one of the closest mimickers of HSV. It presents with recurrent targetoid lesions with or without bullae that ulcerate and resolve over 2 to 3 weeks. It should be considered in patients with refractory HSV and can be distinguished by its targetoid appearance, the generally larger size of lesions, and histopathologic features. A biopsy of the lip should only be performed by an experienced provider because it is technically difficult.
- Herpes zoster, or reactivation of the varicella-zoster virus, can cause herpetic lesions on the face. It is distinguished from HSV because it presents dermatomally.
- Ulcerative LP is in the differential of a nonhealing herpes lesion on the buccal mucosa. These patients may have classic Wickham striae on the buccal mucosa and may have similar lesions on the genitals as well. These can be differentiated from HSV infection because they are not preceded by a vesicle and they do not resolve as quickly as HSV.

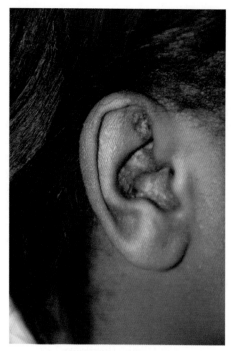

**Fig. 2.8 Discoid Lupus Erythematosus, Conchal Bowl.** This is a classic distribution of discoid lupus erythematosus (DLE). (From the UConn Department of Dermatology Grand Rounds Collection.)

- Morsicatio buccarum, also known as "chronic cheek biting," can be misdiagnosed as HSV because it causes ragged tissue alteration of the buccal mucosa around the bite line, which can mimic a herpes ulceration to the untrained eye. Unlike HSV, these lesions are typically not painful and patients frequently report a history of cheek biting.
- Cheilitis, which has many causes, can result in crusting of the lips, which may be confused for a solitary herpetic lesion. Unlike herpes, which is typically focal or multifocal, cheilitis typically affects the entire lip to some degree.
- FDE can be confused with HSV because it can cause ulceration of the lip; however, it resolves with characteristic hyperpigmentation.

## Work-Up

Diagnosis of orolabial HSV is typically made on clinical grounds alone.
- In cases where the diagnosis is uncertain and HSV is favored, a swab for viral culture or polymerase chain

reaction (PCR, which is more sensitive but also more expensive) can be performed to confirm the diagnosis.
- In cases where the diagnosis is uncertain and HSV is not favored, biopsy can be helpful; however, biopsy should only be performed by someone trained to perform lip and/or oral biopsies because they are technically challenging.
- HSV Ab IgG titers are rarely of any clinical utility and should not be ordered because positive titers can unnecessarily distress patients, despite having limited clinical value.

Patients with severe disease and/or frequent recurrences in the absence of a clear trigger should be evaluated for HIV if clinical suspicion for HIV exists.

## Initial Steps in Management

Acute outbreaks of orolabial herpes should be managed with valacyclovir 2 grams Q12H in 2 doses.
- Resistance to valacyclovir is relatively rare in the immunocompetent population.
- Patients who are resistant to oral treatment can be treated with topical acyclovir; however, it does not decrease the severity or duration of symptoms. It only decreases viral shedding.
- Topical docosanol (Abreva) is of limited clinical utility because it must be applied 5 times per day and its clinical benefit is modest at best.

Severely symptomatic lesions can be managed with adjunctive topical corticosteroids (e.g., hydrocortisone 2.5% ointment for labial involvement or clobetasol propionate 0.05% gel for buccal lesions).

Patients with infrequent flares (less than 6 per year) can be provided with extra valacyclovir to take as previously described at the first sign of a flare (2 grams bid X 1 day).
- Patients who flare more than 6 times per year or who desire suppressive therapy can take 500 mg of valacyclovir daily.
  - Immunosuppressed patients may require higher suppressive doses of valacyclovir.

## Warning Signs/Common Pitfalls

Providers should maintain a strong suspicion for herpes zoster in patients with significant cutaneous head involvement of their herpetic lesions regardless of prior HSV history because facial varicella-zoster virus (VZV) can be vision threatening.

Patients with a history of HSV who undergo perioral or intraoral procedures, including laser resurfacing, should be provided with herpes perioperative prophylaxis to prevent reactivation.

Patients with active orolabial HSV who are around infants should be advised not to kiss the infant because this can transmit the virus to the child.

Patients who develop eczema herpeticum who are febrile and/or have disseminated lesions should be admitted to the hospital for intravenous antiviral therapy.

## Counseling

You have orolabial herpes (also known as "oral herpes"), a type of viral infection within the herpes simplex virus family. Around 80% of American adults are infected with this virus. It is transmitted by saliva and is usually acquired before the age of 20 years old. Importantly, it is infectious, meaning it can be spread from one person to another. This is especially relevant if you are around infants because kissing them when you have an active infection can spread the infection to them. Additionally, performing oral sex while you have an active infection can spread the virus to the genitals of your partner.

There is no cure for orolabial herpes and it frequently comes back. Recurrences are triggered by sunlight, stress, illness, and trauma. You may notice that you feel flu like symptoms or develop a fever before recurrent episodes. Many patients also note local pain, tingling, burning, or pruritus at the site before the appearance of the visible lesions.

Fortunately, there is a treatment for your infection. Your doctor has prescribed you valacyclovir. This medication comes in 1-gram tablets. You should take two of these tablets when you first notice an outbreak and then take two more 12 hours after that. This will shorten the severity and duration of your outbreak and decrease the likelihood that you spread the infection to someone else.

Importantly, if you notice you are having frequent recurrences, you should ask your doctor about treatment to decrease the number of recurrences. Similarly, if you are going to undergo a dental procedure or a procedure affecting the skin around the mouth, you should talk to your doctor about taking an antiviral medication before your procedure to prevent an outbreak.

# HERPES ZOSTER—FACE AND NECK

## Clinical Features

Herpes zoster (HZ), or shingles, is caused by reactivation of VZV, the causative agent of chickenpox. VZV remains dormant in the dorsal root ganglia until reactivation occurs. Not all patients with HZ recall having chickenpox as children.

- The face is the second most common site affected by HZ after the trunk.
  - Facial HZ most commonly occurs from viral reactivation affecting the trigeminal nerve; however, the geniculate ganglion and cervical nerves may also be affected.
- HZ presents with the acute development of painful, tingling, and/or, less commonly, itchy papulovesicles that progress to eroded and crusted papules in a dermatomal distribution.
- HZ is frequently preceded by a 2- to 4-day prodromal period characterized by paresthesia, tingling, pain, and/or, less commonly, itch in the subsequently affected area with or without malaise.
- Acute episodes of herpes zoster frequently last around 2 to 4 weeks.
  - Longer episodes can occur in chronically immunosuppressed individuals.
  - HZ does not have to perfectly respect the midline because dermatomes do not perfectly respect the midline; however, a symmetrical bilateral rash is

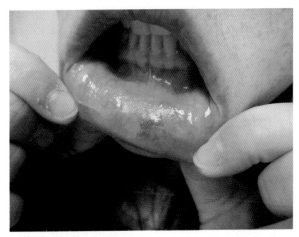

**Fig. 2.9 Aphthous Ulcer.** Note the shallow ulceration involving the soft mucosa. (From the UConn Department of Dermatology Grand Rounds Collection.)

unlikely to be HZ; rarely, bilateral HZ has been reported but mostly in those patients who are more significantly immunosuppressed.
- Some individuals develop a variant called "herpes sine zoster," which is characterized by acute pain, tingling, paresthesia, and/or, less commonly, itch in a dermatomal distribution in the absence of cutaneous findings.
- HZ mostly impacts adults over the age of 50; however, young adults and, rarely, even children can develop HZ.
  - HZ is more common and more severe in immunosuppressed individuals, such as those on chemotherapy, organ transplant patients, those on chronic steroids, those patients with uncontrolled HIV, and patients with advanced lymphoproliferative or hematologic malignancies.
  - Individuals who received the VZV vaccine as children have an almost negligible risk of developing HZ.
There are two more serious subtypes of facial HZ.
- HZ ophthalmicus:
  - HZ of the trigeminal nerve can affect the eye, causing both internal and external (visible on general inspection) ocular complications, which can ultimately culminate in blindness and other ocular morbidity if left untreated.
  - HZ ophthalmicus should be suspected in all patients with trigeminal nerve HZ; however, patients with Hutchinson sign (herpetic lesions on the side, tip, or root of the nose) are at the highest risk for corneal involvement because Hutchinson sign reflects nasociliary nerve involvement (this nerve also innervates the cornea).
    - Clear corneal involvement (e.g., ulceration) may be identifiable on general inspection of some but not all patients with HZ ophthalmicus.
- HZ oticus (also known as "Ramsay Hunt Syndrome"):
  - HZ of the geniculate ganglion, also called "Ramsay Hunt syndrome," classically presents with auricular herpetic lesions (involving the external, middle, or inner ear) with or without ear canal pain, although lesions may be present elsewhere, including on the neck, and may cause facial paralysis.

- HZ oticus can involve the tympanic membrane as well as numerous cranial nerves (CNs; most commonly VII, then VIII, and then all others), resulting in CN palsy.
  - Facial nerve palsy (CN VII) is the most common presentation; however, deafness, tinnitus, and vertigo (CN VIII) are also common.
    - CN palsies can be permanent.
- All patients with HZ may subsequently develop postherpetic neuralgia (PHN). PHN is neuropathic pain at the site of previous herpetic lesions lasting more than 30 days after resolution of the rash. It is the most common complication of acute HZ.
  - It occurs most commonly in the elderly, in immunosuppressed individuals, and in individuals with prolonged episodes of acute HZ.
- Facial HZ can rarely progress to disseminated HZ. This occurs almost exclusively in immunocompromised individuals. Disseminated HZ is characterized by the development of classic papulovesicles diffusely (more than 10 to 12 extradermatomal lesions; if more widespread, it can mimic chickenpox); systemic symptoms can include meningoencephalitis and/or pneumonitis. This variant can be fatal and is almost invariably associated with significant morbidity.
  - Facial HZ is more likely to have neurologic involvement in the absence of disseminated disease (e.g., altered mental status, meningoencephalitis) than other variants of HZ; however, this is still very rare.

## Differential Diagnosis

The differential for facial HZ includes orolabial HSV, ACD, and, rarely, acneiform eruptions such as rosacea.
- Facial HZ can be distinguished from orolabial HSV because it: 1) is unilateral, 2) extends beyond the immediate perioral area throughout a dermatome, and 3) has lesions that are not uniform in size.
- ACD can also present with an acute vesicular facial eruption; however, it is typically: 1) not dermatomal and 2) pruritic, not painful. An inciting contactant can also often be identified.
- Facial HZ is most frequently misdiagnosed as an acneiform eruption in its early stages (e.g., isolated Hutchinson sign) when a patient may only have several isolated lesions. In these cases, pain, including pain in the remainder of the dermatome, suggest a diagnosis of HZ.

## Work-Up

Work-up for Facial HZ involves diagnosis confirmation and identifying complications (e.g., ocular involvement).

### Diagnosis Confirmation

- In typical cases, a diagnosis can be made on clinical grounds alone.
  - In cases where the diagnosis is uncertain and HZ is favored, a swab for viral culture or PCR (which is more sensitive but also more expensive) can be performed to confirm the diagnosis.
  - In cases where the diagnosis is uncertain and HZ is not favored, a punch biopsy can be helpful. A routine hematoxylin and eosin (H&E) stain or a Tzanck smear (which involves scraping the base of a vesicle stained with Giemsa or Wright stain) cannot distinguish HZ from HSV. To do so, immunohistochemistry is required.
- Patients with severe disease and/or frequent recurrences in the absence of a clear trigger should be evaluated for HIV if clinical suspicion for HIV exists.

### Identifying Complications

An evaluation for ocular and neurologic complications, including cranial nerve involvement, is crucial when evaluating patients with facial HZ.

- Ocular evaluation—All patients should be questioned about ocular symptoms and should have a thorough visual inspection done of their eyes.
  - All patients with Hutchinson sign, visible ocular involvement, and/or ocular complaints should be urgently referred to ophthalmology for additional evaluation.
    - Antiviral initiation should not be delayed while awaiting additional evaluation.
  - Otic evaluation—Patients complaining of ear pain should have their ear canals evaluated with an otoscope.
    - All patients with auricular involvement, ear canal involvement, tinnitus, deafness, and/or vertigo should be referred to an otolaryngologist urgently.
  - Neurologic evaluation—A CN examination can help identify impending CN involvement.
    - All altered patients and patients with meningismus should be admitted for intravenous antiviral therapy.

## Initial Steps in Management

Management of acute HZ can be divided into antiviral therapy and pain control.

### Antiviral Therapy

Antivirals shorten the duration of symptoms and decrease the likelihood of postherpetic neuralgia.

- Valacyclovir 1 gram by mouth TID every 7 days is the recommended initial therapy in immunocompetent individuals and works best if given within the first 48 hours of the symptoms or rash.
  - Immunosuppressed patients may require an extended duration of valacyclovir therapy.
  - Valacyclovir-resistant HZ is very rare and almost exclusively occurs in immunosuppressed individuals. It may be considered if HZ persists despite multiple weeks of adequate doses of valacyclovir therapy. If antiviral resistance is expected, a referral to infectious disease is indicated.

### Pain Control

Pain management for HZ can be divided into oral and topical therapies. For the purposes of this chapter, we will focus on a discussion of pain management during acute episodes of HZ.

- Oral therapy:
  - For the vast majority of patients, adequate analgesia can be achieved with the use of scheduled alternating acetaminophen (1 gram Q8H) and ibuprofen (800 mg Q6H).
  - Some patients may require a brief course of opioid analgesics for severe pain. In these cases, opioid prescriptions should be limited to less than 7 days.
  - Systemic steroids, once recommended in the elderly to reduce acute pain and potentially the incidence of postherpetic neuralgia, are now controversial and no longer recommended.
- Topical therapy:
  - Topical corticosteroids—Some experts recommend using topical corticosteroids as a symptomatic adjuvant therapy. The face is a high-risk site for cutaneous atrophy so lower-potency topical corticosteroids should be used than would be used elsewhere on the body.
    - Topical hydrocortisone 2.5% cream/gel/or ointment can be used twice daily for up to 7 days.

- Topical anesthetics
  - Topical lidocaine jelly is frequently prescribed because of its safety; however, its efficacy as an analgesic in this setting is debated.
- Vaccination:
  - Two vaccines are FDA approved for prevention of HZ. The two-dose recombinant zoster vaccine, Shingrix, is the preferred vaccine, according to the Centers for Disease Control and Prevention (CDC) because it is more efficacious.
  - The vaccine is recommended for primary and secondary prevention of HZ in immunocompetent adults over the age of 50. Detailed recommendations can be found on the CDC website.
    - Although the vaccine is recommended for adults on low-dose immunosuppressants, it is not yet recommended for immunocompromised individuals.
- Special scenarios:
  - Ocular involvement
    - Patients with Hutchinson sign and/or ocular involvement require an extended course of 10 days of valacyclovir 1 gram TID.
    - Urgent referral to ophthalmology is critical.
      - All patients should be encouraged to use preservative-free ocular lubricants while awaiting ophthalmology evaluation.
        - Antiviral initiation should not be delayed while awaiting consultation.
  - Ramsay Hunt Syndrome
    - These patients also benefit from extended courses of antivirals as previously described.
    - Some recommend using oral corticosteroids (0.5 mg/kg) for these patients in conjunction with antivirals because it has been shown to improve the likelihood of CN recovery.

## Warning Signs/Common Pitfalls

A high index of suspicion for HZ ophthalmicus and Ramsay Hunt syndrome should be maintained in all patients with facial HZ because of their potential to cause significant morbidity.

Occasionally, patients will present during the prodromal period. If clinical suspicion for impending HZ is high, initiation of valacyclovir should not be delayed because early initiation can decrease the severity of the condition and decrease the likelihood of subsequent postherpetic neuralgia.

Profoundly immunosuppressed patients frequently require prolonged courses of valacyclovir. Failure to improve with 7 days of therapy should be considered to be a treatment failure or a sign of antiviral resistance.

During an acute episode of HZ, contact with children who have not yet received the VZV vaccine should be avoided.

- HZ is infectious for varicella and can be transmitted either by direct contact in immunocompetent hosts or potentially by respiratory secretions in immunocompromised hosts.

Rarely, patients develop neurologic involvement from HZ before the development of disseminated cutaneous lesions. Patients with HZ and acute neurologic symptoms should be hospitalized and urgently undergo lumbar puncture with cerebrospinal fluid (CSF) PCR for VZV.

- All patients in whom disseminated HZ is suspected should be hospitalized.

Shingles occasionally develops in children and pregnant women. The safety of valacyclovir in these populations is less well established.

- In immunocompetent children, antiviral therapy is typically avoided because the episodes are typically mild and self-limited.
- In immunocompromised children, treatment should be directed by a pediatric infectious disease physician.
- In pregnant women, the decision to treat with antivirals is based on disease severity and is at the discretion of the patient's obstetrician.

## Counseling

You have herpes zoster (also known as "shingles"). Shingles is caused by a reactivation of the virus that causes chickenpox. There is no one reason why people develop shingles, although it occasionally develops during periods of stress or illness. Shingles is contagious for chickenpox and it can be transmitted to individuals who have never had chickenpox and that were not vaccinated against chickenpox as children. To decrease the likelihood of spreading the virus, you should cover the affected area with clothing if possible and avoid known contact with those individuals.

Shingles on the face can affect the eye, ear, and nerves of your face. If you develop any visual changes, eye pain, ear pain, hearing difficulties, ringing in your ears, dizziness, or inability to move muscles in your face, you must contact your doctor immediately because this may mean that your shingles is affecting your eyes, ears, or nerves.

Shingles is typically self-limited, which means that it will resolve on its own; however, you have been prescribed valacyclovir to help make the shingles go away faster and to decrease the likelihood that you will develop pain at the area of your shingles from a condition called "postherpetic neuralgia."

Shingles is typically very painful and therefore your doctor has recommended that you take acetaminophen and ibuprofen to help make the pain more manageable. You should alternate between these two medications and take them at set times rather than simply as needed to help manage your pain. You should take 1 gram of acetaminophen every 8 hours alternating with 800 mg of ibuprofen every 6 hours.

You have also been prescribed a prescription steroid cream. You should apply this twice daily for 1 week. Do not apply it to other uninvolved areas because it can thin the skin.

Finally, even though you have shingles, you are still at risk for developing shingles again. To prevent this, you should schedule yourself to receive the shingles vaccine after this acute episode is over. If you previously received the Zostavax, you should still receive the new Shingrix vaccine because these are different vaccines and the Shingrix vaccine is more effective.

# 3

# Body Dermatitis

## CHAPTER OUTLINE

# ATOPIC DERMATITIS—TRUNK AND EXTREMITIES

## Clinical Features

The American Academy of Dermatology (AAD) has developed atopic dermatitis (AD) criteria that are useful in evaluating patients for AD. The three essential criteria (pruritus, typical AD pattern, and chronic/relapsing course) should be used for screening patients with possible AD. If a patient does not display all three of these features, then they are very unlikely to have AD.

- The typical AD pattern is an eruption affecting predominantly flexural surfaces (e.g., flexural neck, antecubital fossa, flexural wrists, popliteal fossa), except during infancy, when it classically affects extensor surfaces and the face.
- Other clinical findings suggestive of AD include xerosis, keratosis pilaris (follicular-based, erythematous or hyperpigmented papules best appreciated on the arms and thighs), hand dermatitis (see Chapter 4), palmar hyperlinearity, ichthyosis (chronic, genetically mediated fish like scaling best appreciated on the lower extremities), and nipple dermatitis.
- Importantly, by definition, all AD is itchy. Patients with a nonpruritic, eczematous-appearing eruption are highly unlikely to have AD.

For most patients, AD flares during the dry, winter months; however, a small subset of patients flare with sweating or light exposure during the summer.

Most adults with AD have had it since childhood, with many patients developing the condition during infancy.

Some children present with a variant of AD called "follicular AD," which is characterized by the development of itchy, follicular-based papules predominantly on the trunk.

- This variant is most common in darker-skinned children and can develop in the absence of typical eczematous plaques.

## Differential Diagnosis

The differential diagnosis for AD is broad and is often confounded by the fact that AD frequently coexists with other conditions, predominantly allergic contact dermatitis (ACD) and irritant contact dermatitis (ICD). The differential diagnosis includes ACD, ICD, asteatotic or dry skin dermatitis, stasis dermatitis, cutaneous T cell lymphoma (CTCL) seborrheic dermatitis, and psoriasis.

- As previously noted, we recommend initially evaluating all patients with possible AD using the AAD's three essential criteria (pruritus, typical AD pattern [Fig. 3.1], and chronic/relapsing course).
  - Using these criteria alone is highly sensitive for detecting AD.

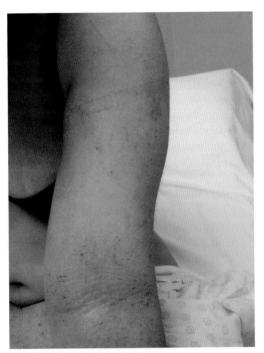

**Fig. 3.1 Atopic Dermatitis.** Notice the flexural distribution and characteristic ill-defined plaques. (From the UConn Grand Rounds Collection.)

- Patients meeting these criteria in whom an alternate diagnosis is still being considered can then be further evaluated for important and associated criteria (see "AAD Criteria", above) using a 3:2:1 approach, where a patient with AD would be expected to display all 3 essential criteria, 2 important criteria, and 1 associated criteria.
- Recognizing the typical AD pattern is essential for differentiating AD from mimickers. Unlike some mimickers, AD is almost always symmetric and AD plaques are ill defined (i.e., do not have distinct borders).
- Patients with AD frequently develop superimposed/concomitant ACD.
  - Concomitant ACD can present either in a clinically obvious manner, such as a new eczematous rash in areas that are not typical for AD, or as AD that is refractory to or worsens with topical therapy, such as in cases where individuals are allergic to components of topical therapy.
  - Individuals with AD are most commonly allergic to fragrances, preservatives, and topical antibiotics. These contactants are frequently present in

both prescription and nonprescription topical treatments for AD and therefore are a frequent cause of treatment failure.
  - AD patients with a new rash in areas that are atypical for AD or that are not responding to conventional therapy should undergo patch testing.
- ICD can be misdiagnosed as AD and can occur concomitantly with AD. Individuals with AD are predisposed to developing ICD because of their underlying skin barrier impairment.
  - ICD on the trunk and extremities most frequently develops from use of personal care products or from cases of obvious occupational exposure (occupational exposure will not be further discussed because it is unlikely to be misdiagnosed as AD).
  - ICD is most commonly a clinical mimicker of trunk and extremity AD when it presents as generalized xerosis and pruritus.
    - This type of ICD can flare existing AD or can exist in the absence of AD, in which case it is characterized by generalized xerosis in the absence of any primary inflammatory skin lesions.
- Stasis dermatitis can be distinguished from AD because it typically presents in individuals older than 50 years of age on the bilateral lower extremities in the absence of rash elsewhere and is often associated with varicosities.
- Psoriasis presents with well-demarcated plaques on extensor surfaces, whereas AD presents with poorly demarcated plaques on flexural surfaces.
- CTCL is the most feared mimicker of AD because it is often very difficult to confirm a diagnosis of CTCL, even histologically, and it can clinically look very similar to AD (Fig. 3.2). CTCL should be considered in patients with atypical-appearing patches and/or plaques, with unusual distribution of disease (e.g., predominant involvement of sun-protected areas, such as the buttocks, inner thighs, and/or breasts), with disease refractory to topical therapy, or with onset of disease in adulthood. Differentiating CTCL from AD is notoriously difficult, and it is prudent to obtain an evaluation from a dermatologist who is experienced in managing CTCL if it is in the differential.

## Work-Up

All patients with presumed AD should be approached systematically using the AAD criteria as previously discussed.

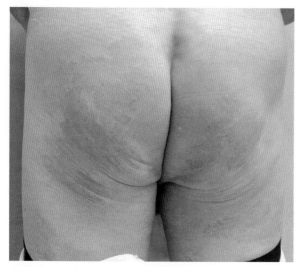

**Fig. 3.2 Cutaneous T Cell Lymphoma.** Notice the bathing suit distribution and atypical appearance of plaques. (From the UConn Grand Rounds Collection.)

A full-body skin examination should be performed in all patients to identify affected areas and to rule out signs of mimickers/concomitant skin conditions.

Histopathologic examination is almost never necessary to confirm a diagnosis of AD; however, it can be important in ruling out mimickers, such as CTCL.

## Initial Steps in Management

Initial management of AD involves a four-pronged approach of dry skin care, topical antiinflammatory agents, trigger avoidance, and itch management.

### Dry Skin Care

Dry skin care involves obtaining a list of all personal care products used and having an understanding of an individual's bathing techniques (e.g., use of a luffa).

- Patients should be counseled that it is okay/encouraged to bathe daily as long as they use appropriate bathing techniques followed by lubrication.
  - Patients should be counseled to use a mild, unscented bar soap, such as Dove White Unscented Bar Soap, CeraVe Hydrating Cleanser Bar, or Cetaphil Gentle Cleansing Bar.
  - Soap should only be routinely applied to the axilla, groin, and overtly dirty areas. A luffa should not be used to apply soap because it may harbor bacteria and is abrasive.

- Hot water should be avoided and showers should not last longer than 10 minutes.
  - Patients should pat dry with a towel rather than rub the towel against their skin.
  - Immediately after bathing, individuals should moisturize.
- Barrier care should be performed by moisturizing at least twice daily (including immediately after showering). Thick moisturizing creams (e.g., Vanicream, CeraVe Moisturizing Cream, Eucerin Advanced Barrier Repair) or ointments (e.g., Vaseline, Aquaphor, Vaniply, Healing Ointment) should be applied to the entire body. Some patients prefer using oils or products containing natural ingredients. Patients should be provided with a list of acceptable moisturizers so that they can identify the products they are willing to use.

### Topical Antiinflammatory Agents

First-line treatment for AD should include a medium-potency topical corticosteroid, such as triamcinolone 0.1% cream, applied twice daily for several weeks (with avoidance of application to facial skin or intertriginous areas to avoid skin thinning).

- Patients who have difficulty complying with twice-daily corticosteroid applications can be offered a slightly more potent topical corticosteroid for once-daily application (e.g., mometasone 0.1% cream)
- Patients should be prescribed 1 gram of cream per day for each percentage of body surface area (BSA) affected.
- Patients who frequently flare in the same locations (e.g., antecubital fossa) despite excellent dry skin care can be counseled to apply a medium-potency topical corticosteroid, such as triamcinolone 0.1%, to flare-prone areas three times weekly, even in the absence of rash.

Topical calcineurin inhibitors, such as tacrolimus or pimecrolimus 0.1%, can be used for maintenance therapy or for patients experiencing cutaneous adverse events from topical corticosteroid use.

- Topical calcineurin inhibitors can be applied to flare-prone areas three times weekly to decrease flares.
- Topical calcineurin inhibitors should not be applied to actively inflamed skin because they can cause severe stinging and burning.
- This treatment is not recommended by the U.S. Food and Drug Administration (FDA) for infants and children between 2 and 15 years of age; instead, tacrolimus 0.03% should be used.
  - Given their relatively higher cost and lack of conferred benefit over medium-potency

topical corticosteroids, topical calcineurin inhibitors should not be used in lieu of topical corticosteroids as a first-line antiinflammatory.

- Another steroid-sparing alternative, crisaborole (commercially available as Eucrisa), is a phosphodiesterase-4 inhibitor that is an ointment approved for the use of AD in patients older than 2 years of age.
- Using steroid-sparing agents intermittently is advised in those patients with chronic persistent AD to avoid the side effects of topical steroids.

## Trigger Avoidance

Identifying triggers in patients with AD can be very difficult but is necessary to avoid flares. There are now smartphone-based applications (colloquially known as "apps") that can help patients track disease activity and input exposures to help identify possible triggers and predict possible flares.

- Patients should be questioned about their bathing and personal care regimens at every visit to identify behaviors that may be contributing to the worsening of AD.
- All patients who are not responding to appropriate therapy should undergo patch testing to assess for concomitant ACD.

## Itch Management

The most bothersome symptom of AD is intractable pruritus. Control of cutaneous disease correlates with itch control; however, itch-directed therapies are currently frequently ineffective.

- Oral H1 antihistamines (both sedating and nonsedating) are commonly used to treat AD-related itch; however, recent evidence suggests that histamine is not a primary mediator of itch in AD and that H1 blockers are ineffective. Sedating antihistamines are still considered to have a role as adjuncts for sleep.
  - Other agents, including naltrexone and neural modulators (e.g., gabapentin, amitriptyline, mirtazapine), are also occasionally used for itch control.
  - Topical antihistamines (such as Benadryl cream) and other soothing topical antipruritic agents (e.g., doxepin cream, creams with menthol, creams with colloidal oatmeal) might help.

## Other Therapies

- Bleach baths can be used.
  - Twice-weekly dilute bleach baths (one-half cup of household bleach mixed into a 40-gallon bath of water) have long been recommended to prevent pathologic bacterial growth on patients with AD; however, recent evidence suggests that routine use of bleach baths is unnecessary.
  - Bleach baths are indicated for patients with recurrent skin and soft tissue bacterial infections or who are known to be colonized with *Staphylococcus aureus.*
- Wet wraps are used to improve both skin hydration and the efficacy of topical corticosteroids.
  - Wet wraps are very effective for treating severe AD; however, compliance is often poor. Wet wraps should be considered for any patient who has an acute flare that cannot be managed with traditional topical therapies alone.
  - Written instructions on how to properly perform a wet wrap are available from the National Eczema Association at: https://nationaleczema.org/eczema/treatment/wet-wrap-therapy/.
- Phototherapy, pills, and injectables for AD can be prescribed by a specialist.
  - Patients with disease that is refractory to topical management and those who present with disease affecting more than 10% BSA should be referred to a dermatologist who specializes in the use of phototherapy, systemic medications, or biologics for the treatment of AD.

## Warning Signs/Common Pitfalls

The biggest pitfall when managing AD in any location is failure to promote patient adherence to a dry skin care management regimen. Such a regimen is essential for achieving disease control and maintaining disease control in patients with AD; failure to implement a daily dry skin care regimen ensures treatment failure.

- Patients must specifically be counseled that twice-daily use of their prescription topical antiinflammatory is not a substitute for frequent moisturization.
- Avoidance of harsh soaps and irritating cosmetics/perfumes is essential. Patients need specific product recommendations because the cosmetic aisle in drugstores is confusing and the internet is full of misinformation on this subject.

Failure to identify coexisting dermatoses, such as ICD to soaps and ACD (including to topical corticosteroids), can interfere with successful AD management.

Many patients with AD develop superinfections of their AD lesions because their skin barrier is impaired. The most common are impetigo and eczema herpeticum.

- Impetigo, a bacterial superinfection most commonly caused by *S. aureus*, is characterized by the development of yellow crusts superimposed on AD lesions. Impetigo can trigger a full-body AD flare.
  - Impetigo should be treated with oral or topical antibiotics (depending on the severity) that provide *S. aureus* coverage.
  - Patients with recurrent impetigo should consider undergoing *Staph* decolonization with topical mupirocin 2% or initiating bleach baths.
  - Oral antibiotics should not be prescribed to AD patients in the absence of clinical evidence of superinfection.
- Eczema herpeticum, or superinfection of AD lesions by herpes simplex virus (HSV), is a dermatologic emergency characterized by the development of punched-out, herpetic lesions within AD plaques and with or without the presence of fever. Eczema herpeticum should be suspected in any patient who develops acute onset of skin pain superimposed on AD lesions.
  - Eczema herpeticum with fever requires hospitalization for intravenous (IV) antivirals.
  - All patients with possible eczema herpeticum should be started on valacyclovir at the first sign of an outbreak.

Many patients or their parents request referral for food allergy testing because they want an explanation for why they or their child have developed AD. Blind elimination diets or use of immunoglobulin E (IgE) testing without confirmation with a double-blind food challenge is not recommended because it is rarely helpful.

A diagnosis of CTCL should always be considered in patients with disease refractory to topicals, with new onset of disease in adulthood, with atypical-appearing patches/plaques, and/or with atypical distribution of patches/plaques. These patients require biopsies of untreated lesional skin. Specimens must be evaluated by a dermatopathologist given the difficulty of rendering a histologic diagnosis of CTCL.

## Counseling

You have atopic dermatitis, also known as "eczema." Atopic dermatitis is usually an inherited chronic skin condition (meaning there is no cure) that occurs in people who have skin that does not retain enough water and that does not adequately protect itself from outside allergens. Your skin is sensitive, prone to dryness, and susceptible to becoming itchy and developing rashes.

Individuals with atopic dermatitis develop skin inflammation in response to the environment around them. This inflammation makes the skin red and itchy. Importantly, there is no one allergen that causes your skin disease. Additionally, dietary changes have not been reported in the medical literature to cure your disease.

Treating your skin disease requires that you keep your skin healthy by moisturizing it and by avoiding exposing it to things that may irritate it. To keep your skin healthy, it is important that you have a special bathing regimen that promotes your skin health. When you shower, it is important that you use tepid water and that you limit your shower to less than 10 minutes. In the shower, you should use a gentle, unscented bar soap and should only apply soap to the armpits, groin, and areas that are visibly dirty. Do not use a luffa or a washcloth to apply soap because this may further irritate your skin. Pat, rather than rub, yourself dry with a towel. Immediately after drying off, you should apply a moisturizer to lock in the hydration that your skin received while you were showering. It is important that you not only hydrate your skin with a moisturizer after showering, but also that you moisturize at least twice a day. While your skin is still red and irritated, it is important that you do not apply any cosmetics or fragrances because these can inflame or irritate your skin.

Your doctor has prescribed a topical steroid cream that you should use twice daily only for 7 to 10 days, at which time the redness and irritation should be gone. Do not apply this cream to your face, groin, underarms, or under your breasts unless told specifically to use the cream in these locations. Alternative steroid-sparing creams may also be prescribed for more chronic or intermittent use.

These prescription creams are not a substitute for your moisturizer and should be used with your moisturizer, not instead of your moisturizer. Once the redness and irritation has resolved, you can stop the prescription cream, although you may want to restart it when the redness and irritation return. The topical steroid prescribed cream can cause side effects if you use it too frequently or if you use it for too long. These side effects include potential thinning of the skin, dilatation of blood vessels that can become more visible in the area of application, discoloration of the skin, and even an acne like rash. Continue your routine of twice-daily lubrication and shortened tepid bathing as part of your skin regimen.

Atopic dermatitis is cyclical, meaning you will have times when your rash is much better and times when it is much worse. Different people flare for different reasons. You should try your best to identify things that are unique triggers for your atopic dermatitis. You will have to work with your doctor over time to find a skin care regimen that is right for you and that keeps your skin disease under control.

# ALLERGIC CONTACT DERMATITIS—TRUNK

**Christian Gronbeck and Diane Whitaker-Worth**

## Clinical Features

ACD is a delayed-type hypersensitivity reaction to immunogenic agents that come into contact with the skin. Many patients who develop ACD have an impaired skin barrier, allowing small compounds to penetrate the skin and initiate an antigenic response. After initial allergen exposure, affected individuals progress through a sensitization phase, which involves the proliferation of antigen-specific T cells. After reexposure, activation of these T cells leads to an inflammatory response, which prompts more immediate cutaneous symptoms.

Although the skin can be allergic to an innumerable number of compounds, the most common causes of ACD are nickel, fragrance mixtures, preservatives (e.g., formaldehyde), detergents, dyes (often in hair products), sunscreens (especially those containing benzophenones), topical medications (e.g., minoxidil, neomycin, bacitracin), acrylates, and urushiol (a chemical in poison ivy, poison sumac, and poison oak). Although ACD occurs equally among all races, it is more commonly seen in female patients, likely because of the higher prevalence of piercings and the increased number of personal care products used by women.

## Course of Development

### Initial exposure
- After exposure to a new allergen, individuals become sensitized to the particular antigen over the course of 10 to 14 days.

- After 2 weeks, some patients may develop a mild inflammatory dermatitis, consisting of erythematous plaques and papules in the exposed skin region.
- In some cases, continuous low-grade exposure to an allergen can incite sensitization over an extended period of time.

### Subsequent exposures
- Because of the persistence of memory T cells in the dermis, subsequent antigen exposure leads to a more profound and immediate dermatitis, generally within 12 to 48 hours of exposure.
  - Affected individuals will classically develop intense pruritus in exposed areas, along with the development of erythematous, edematous plaques that may develop scale and vesiculation in the following days.

### Chronic allergic contact dermatitis
- Repeated exposures to the allergen can lead to chronic disease, in which the skin becomes thickened, lichenified, hyperpigmented, and hyperkeratotic.
  - Reexposure once every 28 days is frequent enough to maintain ACD.
  - Chronic disease is more likely to occur in individuals who do not receive proper treatment for acute episodes.

## Common Clinical Presentations
- ACD can present with different patterns based on the most likely cause of exposure and the specific body region.
  - ACD on the face may be the result of cleansing products, hair products, cosmetics, or airborne allergens.
    - A rinse-off pattern that affects the sides of the face and upper chest may be the result of shampoos, conditioners, and other cleansing products.
    - A hairline pattern that impacts the superior forehead and nape of the neck may be caused by dyes and perming solutions.
    - Patchy, bilateral plaques on the bilateral cheeks are typically caused by application of a cosmetic product.
    - Involvement of the upper eyelids, nasolabial fold, and submental region generally signifies exposure to airborne allergens (e.g., small particles like powder or gas).
  - ACD on the hands may stem from objects in everyday use or occupational exposures.

- Plaques on the palms may be incited by use of computer mice, cell phones, or stair rails.
- Isolated involvement of the thumb and ring ringer can signify ACD from occupational exposures, such as from using acrylates (dentists) or handling plants (florists).
- ACD on the trunk and extremities may be the result of a nickel allergen or textile products.
  - Involvement of the earlobes, neck, wrists, and skin beneath the umbilicus are likely caused by a nickel allergen.
  - Textile products typically incite reactions along the inferior neck, axillae, and internal surface of the arms and thighs because of more frequent friction from clothing in these regions.
- Regardless of location, the identification of several patterns should clue the clinician in that ACD is the likely culprit:
  - A geometric pattern (e.g., an adhesive reaction that is clearly square shaped).
  - Linear and other so-called "outside job" morphologies (i.e., where the morphology of the rash-like lines can only be explained by exogenous contact with something).
    - This pattern is particularly common in ACD caused by poison ivy, sumac, and oak (Fig. 3.3).
  - Disease isolated to one anatomic unit (e.g., just hands) may be ACD.
- The rash typically develops at the site of primary contact with the allergen (e.g., application of eye shadow leading to periocular dermatitis); however, in some cases, dermatitis occurs at a site distant from where the allergen is applied to the skin (e.g., nail polish causing eyelid dermatitis from touching thin eyelid skin).
- ACD often becomes superimposed atop other background skin diseases (e.g., atopic dermatitis, venous stasis ulcers).
  - In these settings, ACD usually develops to an ingredient in a topical formulation used for treating the background disease (e.g., neomycin, lanolin, topical corticosteroid).

## Differential Diagnosis

The differential for ACD includes AD, ICD, psoriasis, and seborrheic dermatitis.

- The primary morphology of both AD and ACD is an eczematous dermatitis that can vary in appearance

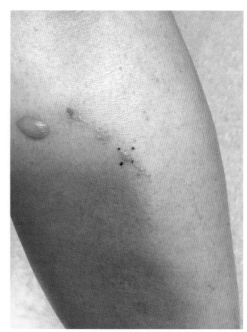

**Fig. 3.3 Allergic Contact Dermatitis.** Poison ivy. (From the UConn Grand Rounds Collection.)

depending on chronicity. ACD can be distinguished from AD by distribution (AD typically affects all flexural areas, whereas ACD is typically more localized), age at onset (AD typically presents in early childhood), and presence/absence of other atopic features (e.g., nasal salute, thinning of lateral third of eyebrow). Many individuals with AD develop ACD to the topical creams used to treat their AD, which is suggested by the development of treatment-refractory disease.

- ICD can also present with the development of erythematous, scaly plaques; however, it can be distinguished from ACD because it is frequently painful and not pruritic and has an irritated rather than inflamed appearance characterized by fissuring. In reality, distinguishing between these two entities is frequently very difficult and patch testing may be required.
- Psoriasis is another mimicker of ACD; however, it should be distinguishable from ACD clinically because psoriasis is well circumscribed, has thick overlying silvery scale, and has a characteristic distribution overlying the extensor surface. Psoriasis is most frequently confused with ACD when it affects the eyelids.

- ACD can be distinguished from seborrheic dermatitis by distribution and morphology.
  - Seborrheic dermatitis affects predominantly seborrheic areas (e.g., scalp, eyebrows, nasolabial folds, beard, chest).
  - Seborrheic dermatitis presents with thin pink plaques with overlying greasy scale.

## Work-Up

A total-body skin examination and patient history is necessary to support the diagnosis of ACD. Patch testing is the gold standard in confirming the diagnosis of ACD and identifying likely allergens:

- A total-body skin examination may reveal classic ACD lesions, including well-circumscribed, pruritic, eczematous plaques and papules in areas that were recently exposed to allergens.
  - Acute reactions may further exhibit vesiculation or weeping, whereas chronic lesions are typically lichenified.
  - A patient history of a chronic, multi-year course that follows contact with specific allergens will further support a diagnosis of ACD.
  - Nevertheless, it is important to recognize that patients' susceptibility to certain allergens may vary over time and that they may develop new-onset sensitization to products they previously tolerated.
- If a single offending agent is strongly suspected, removal can be both therapeutic and diagnostic (if the patient demonstrates resolution of symptoms).
  - If a particular allergen is suspected, it is recommended to provide patients with a list of products containing this allergen so that they can perform targeted removal of the offending agent.
  - Importantly, if a particular allergen or product is not strongly suspected, it is not recommended to blindly remove potential allergens because many products share similar allergens and this does not frequently lead to identification of the allergen.
- Patch testing is typically indicated: (1) when distributions are highly indicative of ACD; (2) when clinical history, as described previously, is consistent with ACD; (3) when the patient is involved in high-risk occupations for ACD, including health care professionals, florists, and cosmetologists; (4) when the cause for the dermatitis cannot be otherwise established; (5) if there is acute worsening of an underlying dermatitis; and/or (6) if the patient proves refractory to initial treatment efforts.

- Patch testing is typically performed through a dermatologist and involves securing several potential allergens to the skin surface for 2 days with subsequent monitoring for signs of an eczematous reaction.
- Note that patch testing is unique from prick testing, which is an alternative allergy test performed by an allergist.
  - Patch testing is the necessary test to identify allergens for ACD (delayed hypersensitivity reaction) as opposed to those causing an immediate (Type 1) hypersensitivity reaction.

## Initial Steps in Management
### General Management Comments

- Definitive management involves avoidance of allergen-containing products, if successfully identified through patch testing (see indications for testing in "Work-Up").
- For existing lesions, antiinflammatory medications are used to prompt symptomatic improvement and resolution of lesions.
- Patients with chronic or persistent ACD or extensive skin involvement may benefit from the use of oral immunosuppressive agents or referral to a dermatologist for further management.

### Allergen Avoidance and Protection

Patients should be counseled to avoid identified or highly suspected allergens.

- Patients should be educated that many products share similar allergens, and they should reference manufacturer websites to identify common household products that may contain their allergen.
- If possible, an informational leaflet can be provided to patients to educate them on common uses of their identified allergen.
- If patients are at risk for workplace exposures, they should be advised to use personal protective equipment (PPE; e.g., laminate gloves).
- Emollients (e.g., Vaseline, Aquaphor) can offer additional skin protection by acting as barriers against external allergens.

### Minimization of Existing Skin Inflammation

- To target skin inflammation of the hands, feet, or nonflexural surfaces, we recommend high-potency topical corticosteroids (clobetasol propionate 0.05% cream) twice daily for 2 to 4 weeks.

- To target the skin inflammation of the flexural surfaces or face, we recommend treating patients with mild- to moderate-potency topical corticosteroids (fluocinolone acetonide 0.01% cream) twice daily for 2 to 4 weeks.
- Patients with ACD of the hairbearing scalp may benefit from high-potency corticosteroids (clobetasol propionate 0.05% solution or fluocinonide 0.05% solution) nightly.
- As an alternative to steroids, topical calcineurin inhibitors (tacrolimus 0.1% cream) can be used twice daily for 2 to 4 weeks

### Management of Chronic Allergic Contact Dermatitis

Patients with chronic ACD may require more extensive management that includes oral immunomodulatory drugs (e.g., methotrexate, mycophenolate) or ultraviolet (UV) light treatment. Nevertheless, these patients are typically best referred to a dermatologist for close management and to ensure their allergens have been adequately identified through patch testing.

### Partial but Inadequate Response

If there is a partial but inadequate response after a 4-week trial of topical corticosteroid monotherapy:

- Confirm patient compliance with the recommended treatment regimen and address any compliance barriers.
- Reconsider the diagnosis of ACD and ensure that the patient has received patch testing.
- For extensive or severe skin involvement that is secondary to an acute exposure (e.g., poison ivy), a 20-day course of oral corticosteroids (e.g., prednisone) is suggested alongside referral to a dermatologist.
  - Dosing should be weight-adjusted at a rate of 1 mg/kg.
  - A typical 20-day taper of oral prednisone for an average-weight patient would include 40 mg daily for 5 days, 30 mg daily for 5 days, 20 mg daily for 5 days, and 10 mg daily for 5 days, with all doses taken in the morning.
  - Shorter, 5- to 7-day doses typically result in rebound flaring after cessation.
  - Systemic comorbidities, such as heart failure, glaucoma, poorly controlled hypertension, and diabetes mellitus should be taken into account when prescribing oral corticosteroids.

## Warning Signs/Common Pitfalls

- Patients with extensive skin involvement or severe plaque formation warrant referral to a dermatologist.
- It is important to monitor patients with ACD for secondary bacterial infection, which may be indicated by warmth, swelling, extensive erythema, or discharge from involved areas.
  - In these cases, oral or topical antibiotics targeting the secondary bacterial infection are warranted.
- Although patch testing can be useful in identifying potential allergens, any identified allergens should fit in the patient history. For example, patients may test positive for certain preservative compounds that they do not readily encounter in their daily life, so these findings are therefore less relevant for future management.
- Prick testing is not equivalent to patch testing and is not suitable to identify the allergens that are causing the ACD.

## Counseling

Allergic contact dermatitis is a skin rash caused by a skin allergy to certain products, chemicals, or medications in your day-to-day environment. Common allergens include shampoos, soaps, nickel (on your watch or pants button), fragrances, cosmetic agents, creams, and some plants, such as poison ivy. Importantly, this type of allergy is not life-threatening.

We generally manage this rash in a few ways. First, we want to identify what you are allergic to. To determine this, we will refer you to a dermatologist for patch testing. Patch testing is a painless procedure in which small pieces of potential allergens will be taped to your back and left in place for 2 days. If we identify what you are allergic to, we recommend that you avoid that allergen to see if your symptoms resolve.

We also have treatments available that can help to resolve your skin rash while we are waiting to determine what you are allergic to. We have prescribed you a topical corticosteroid cream, which you should apply to the rash twice daily. The most common side effect people notice from this cream is that it can cause the skin to thin slightly and the blood vessels to become more noticeable in the surrounding area. Most patients see their rash begin to resolve within a few weeks of consistently using the cream. In addition to using these treatments, you may also find it helpful to hydrate your skin with moisturizers.

# NUMMULAR DERMATITIS

**Christian Gronbeck and Diane Whitaker-Worth**

## Clinical Features

Nummular dermatitis (eczema) is an inflammatory skin condition that derives its name from its characteristic coin-shaped lesions (Fig. 3.4). Nummular dermatitis is likely a clinical variant of atopic eczema and ACD because it shares features of both conditions.

### Geographic Morphology

- The earliest lesions begin as erythematous papules and/or vesicles that enlarge and coalesce to form characteristic, coin-shaped, round, or oval plaques.
- Lesions fall into one of two categories: exudative acute or subacute lesions and dry/lichenified chronic lesions.
- Lesions tend to be well demarcated.
  - Intense pruritus is often present and may worsen during the evening hours.
  - Plaques most commonly occur on the extremities and trunk.
- Subacute lesions may develop a yellowish crust or even frank pustules because of secondary infection with *S. aureus.*
- Chronic plaques typically develop an annular appearance with central clearing, which can eventually flatten to form patches and macules and finally develop a brown pigment felt to be the result of postinflammatory hyperpigmentation (PIH).
- Nummular eczema is a chronic disease, with lesions lasting for weeks or months with a potential for a waxing and waning course or recurrent exacerbations after improvement.

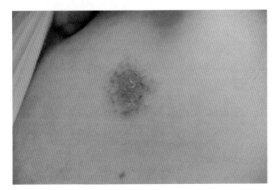

**Fig. 3.4 Nummular dermatitis.** (From the UConn Grand Rounds Collection.)

- Men are generally affected with the condition in later life and often on the legs, whereas women may develop the condition in their second or third decade, commonly on the arms.
- It is more frequently seen throughout the winter months. In some cases, AD, ACD, and stasis dermatitis may play a role in impairing the skin barrier and predisposing the person to nummular dermatitis.

## Differential Diagnosis

The differential diagnosis for nummular dermatitis includes other pruritic skin conditions, such as AD, ACD, psoriasis, tinea corporis, CTCL, and lichen simplex chronicus (LSC). In all cases, geographic morphology (well-circumscribed, coin-shaped lesions) and a patient history of skin irritation/xerosis are helpful in supporting the diagnosis of nummular dermatitis.

- Although AD can present with pruritic and eczematous patches on the upper extremities, these plaques are typically less circumscribed and widespread. Typically, AD presents early in life and is associated with an atopic diathesis (e.g., allergic rhinitis, asthma). In clinical practice, these conditions may occur in an overlap state.
- Plaques from ACD are often less symmetric and monomorphous than those of nummular eczema. Patients with ACD may be able to identify a direct contactant that triggered their skin eruption. Additionally, it would be very unusual for ACD to present with multiple, discrete, coin-shaped lesions.
- Subacute and chronic skin lesions from nummular eczema may mimic psoriasis. In these cases, it is important to question patients regarding the initial appearance of their skin lesions (e.g., vesicular or eczematous). Additionally, pruritus is characteristic of nummular eczema and less typical in psoriatic lesions. Psoriatic lesions also have a strong predilection for extensor surfaces.
- During the early stages, tinea corporis is pruritic, erythematous, and well-circumscribed, sharing a similar geographic morphology to nummular dermatitis. Tinea lesions are typically localized and unilateral, whereas nummular dermatitis is usually bilateral and symmetric. A potassium hydroxide (KOH) preparation can be useful in ruling out tinea when available.
- LSC is characterized by the development of hyperpigmented, thickened, lichenified plaques incited by frequent skin rubbing and scratching. Although LSC most frequently presents with a solitary lesion, it can

present similarly to chronic nummular dermatitis because nummular dermatitis may become lichenified over time because of how itchy it can be.

- CTCL can mimic many eczematous conditions. Generally, CTCL plaques are polymorphic and affect sun-protected areas (e.g., the buttocks). Biopsy can be helpful in distinguishing between the two entities.

## Work-Up

Nummular dermatitis is a clinical diagnosis based on patient history and examination. In general, a skin biopsy is not necessary to make the diagnosis.

- A total-body skin examination is recommended to demonstrate the presence of well-circumscribed, eczematous, coin-shaped plaques located in classic skin regions (upper and lower extremities).
  - Identification of diffuse xerosis may support the diagnosis of nummular eczema.
- A targeted patient history should be obtained to assess for the presence of a relapsing pattern of skin involvement; pruritus that is worse during the evening hours; and recent history of skin irritation, trauma, or bites.
- In patients with excessive exudation or crusting, a skin swab and culture may be used to identify the presence of secondary bacterial infection.
- Although rarely performed on initial presentation, patch testing (through a dermatologist) may be suitable for individuals with persistent skin lesions to better characterize whether ACD is contributing to the patient's rash.

## Initial Steps in Management
### General Management Comments

Nummular dermatitis is managed similarly to atopic dermatitis; nevertheless, it frequently requires higher potency topical steroids than AD and many patients often benefit from the use of systemic immunosuppressive agents.

### General Recommendations for Dry Skin

- Hot water should be avoided during showering and bathing, and patients should use gentle cleansers when possible. The use of cleansers and washcloths should be limited to axillae and groin areas when possible. After bathing, skin should be patted dry and bland emollients should be applied liberally.
  - Given that atopic dermatitis is a potential cause of nummular dermatitis, it is advisable to use fragrance-free, hypoallergenic emollients.

### Recommended Initial Pharmacologic Treatment

- The use of high-potency topical steroids is warranted for severely inflamed lesions once or twice daily for 2 to 4 weeks. Patients should be instructed explicitly that this should not be used as a moisturizer on non-involved skin.
  - Less erythematous areas of inflammation can be treated with a medium-potency topical steroid, such as triamcinolone acetonide 0.1% ointment.
- Secondary bacterial infections should be considered in the presence of excessive crusting or weeping of the skin lesions and should be promptly treated with a course of oral or topical antibiotics.
  - Swab cultures of weepy areas should be performed to select the appropriate antibiotic regimen.

### Partial but Inadequate Result

If there is a partial but inadequate response after a trial of potent topical corticosteroid monotherapy:

- Patients failing to respond to topical therapies should be questioned about compliance barriers or difficulty in obtaining medications.
- In truly refractory cases, it is advisable to consider referral to a dermatologist for initiation of systemic immunosuppressants, phototherapy, or patch testing given the refractory nature of this condition to topicals.
- Patients with refractory disease and few isolated lesions may benefit from intralesional injection of a corticosteroid at the sites of involvement (e.g., triamcinolone acetonide 10 mg/cc).

## Warning Signs/Common Pitfalls

The biggest pitfall when managing nummular dermatitis is prescribing systemic corticosteroids because the patient will flare after they are discontinued.

Other pitfalls include misdiagnosis and failure to use potent enough corticosteroids.

- Misdiagnosis as tinea corporis and subsequent treatment with a topical antifungal medication will delay the improvement of skin lesions. Therefore, when there is diagnostic uncertainty, we recommend testing for the presence of tinea through a KOH preparation.
- Failure to use high-potency corticosteroids (e.g., clobetasol, halobetasol) to affected areas is another potential pitfall.
- Failure to re-enforce the importance of skin barrier protection through the use of emollients may result in further relapses of nummular eczema. Although

patients may be inclined to restrict emollient use to areas with active involvement, they should be counseled on using emollients in all areas of xerosis to prevent the development of skin fissures and entry points for allergens.

## Counseling

You have a skin rash called "nummular eczema." This is an especially itchy type of eczema that occurs more often in people who have dry skin. Although there is no cure for your rash, we can take steps to improve it.

Your doctor is prescribing you a topical corticosteroid ointment. You should apply this ointment to areas of your skin that are affected by the rash two times per day for 2 to 4 weeks. This is a very strong medication and therefore should not be applied to normal-appearing skin.

In addition to the prescription cream, you should also hydrate your skin with a moisturizer. You should moisturize your entire body, including unaffected areas. It is important to use the moisturizer even after your rash improves. We recommend that you shower in warm (not hot) water, pat your skin dry, and apply the emollient liberally on your skin while it is still damp. Additional moisturizing during the day can be helpful.

If your rash fails to improve in the next few weeks, we may consider referring you to a dermatologist for further testing and treatment.

## PSORIASIS

### Clinical Features

Psoriasis is a chronic, immune-mediated disease that presents with a waxing and waning course and is characterized by hyperplasia of the epidermal keratinocytes. It predominantly affects the skin, nails, and joints. It impacts approximately 2% of the U.S. population, and roughly one-third of impacted patients have moderate to severe disease characterized by involvement of more than 10% BSA. Onset typically occurs in two age ranges: 20 to 30 years old and 50 to 60 years old. Evaluation for family history is essential in patients with psoriasis because approximately 30% of individuals with psoriasis have a first-degree relative with the disease. The goal of treatment for psoriasis is to achieve complete or near-complete skin clearance and improve patient quality of life.

Most cases of psoriasis are readily identifiable based on the presence of well-demarcated (i.e., a circle can easily be drawn around the plaque), scaly plaques on extensor surfaces (e.g., elbows, knees, scalp, lower back).

There are several major subtypes of psoriasis that are classified based on skin morphology, with some patients demonstrating overlap between classification types.

- Plaque psoriasis presents with well-demarcated, scaly, and erythematous patches and plaques (Fig. 3.5).
  - The plaques are typically symmetric, bilateral, and are most commonly found on the scalp, extensor elbows, knees, and gluteal cleft.
  - Clinical findings include pinpoint bleeding after removal of scale (Auspitz sign), as well as lesions appearing after trauma (Koebner phenomenon).
- Inverse/flexural psoriasis is characterized by erythematous patches primarily localized to the skin fold regions (axilla, groin) with minimal scaling.
- Guttate psoriasis presents with small, inflammatory plaques (raindrop-sized) with a fine scale that may follow streptococcal pharyngitis.
  - It is more common in children and young adults with no prior history of psoriasis. It may follow Group A Streptococcus infections.
- Pustular psoriasis involves a pustular cutaneous eruption, which may be generalized (von Zumbusch) or localized to the palms and soles (palmoplantar) and often follows infection or withdrawal from corticosteroids.
- Erythrodermic psoriasis is defined by cutaneous erythema and scale covering a large portion of the body

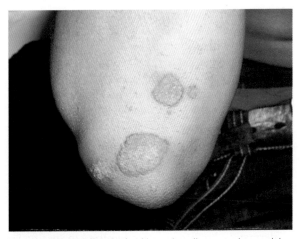

**Fig. 3.5 Plaque Psoriasis.** Note the silvery scale overlying plaque on the extensor surface. (From the UConn Grand Rounds Collection.)

area; it is often associated with systemic manifestations of illness (e.g., fever, chills, malaise).

Patients with psoriasis may also develop manifestations in special sites, including the nails, periocular area, skin folds (intertriginous, inverse psoriasis), and palms/soles (palmoplantar).

- Nail psoriasis can occur in adults or children and is seen in 10% to 55% of patients with psoriasis and 80% to 90% of patients with psoriatic arthritis. It is clinically distinguished by the presence of pitting, onycholysis (separation of the nail from the nail bed), subungual hyperkeratosis, and nail plate crumbling (Chapter 16], "Nail Psoriasis"). In cases where psoriasis is suspected, fingernail examination is incredibly helpful for confirming the diagnosis.
- Patients with psoriasis are at an increased risk for ocular disorders, such as blepharitis, conjunctivitis, xerosis, corneal lesions, and uveitis. Patients may also develop psoriatic lesions on the eyelids with eyelid flaking.
- Patients with intertriginous psoriasis present with well-demarcated, shiny plaques with limited scale and must be distinguished from fungal infections, which also commonly present in similar regions.
- Palmoplantar psoriasis presents with erythematous, hyperkeratotic plaques, along with fissures > It is sometimes considered a form of pustular psoriasis.

## Differential Diagnosis

The differential diagnosis for psoriasis depends on the subtype. For chronic plaque psoriasis (80%–90% of patients), alternative considerations include LSC, seborrheic dermatitis, AD, and cutaneous fungal infections.

- Patients with LSC can also develop plaques with overlying scale, but they are typically less erythematous than those from psoriasis, are incited by chronic scratching, and are therefore more likely to be located in regions that patients can reach (e.g., the scalp, nape of the neck, extensor forearms, thighs).
  - In any event, a patient history of excessive scratch–itch cycles can help distinguish LSC from psoriasis.
- Both plaque psoriasis and seborrheic dermatitis may involve the scalp and intertriginous areas. Seborrheic dermatitis, however, is often localized to specific facial regions (eyebrows, nasolabial folds, postauricular

areas), occasionally involves the trunk and upper chest, and rarely involves the extremities.
  - Additionally, lesions from seborrheic dermatitis are poorly-circumscribed and are characterized by patchy scaling or crusting that has a greasy texture, unlike the well-circumscribed plaques with abundant scale seen in psoriasis.
- AD classically presents with pruritic papules and patches with erythema and scale, but the raised, well-defined borders of plaque psoriasis are not typically seen. Involvement of the flexural surfaces is also common in AD, whereas chronic plaque psoriasis involves the extensor surfaces.
  - Furthermore, patients with AD frequently have a history of involvement from a young age and may have associated atopic conditions, such as asthma and allergic rhinitis.
- Cutaneous fungal infections, such as tinea, can present with erythematous plaques and with nail changes (onychomycosis) similar to those in nail psoriasis. Like psoriasis, tinea can involve the scalp (tinea capitis) or body (tinea corporis), but there are typically a limited number of lesions. Plaques may be further distinguished by their fine scale with a well-defined, reddish margin. Importantly, onycholysis (separation of the nail from the nail bed) is frequently seen in nail psoriasis but less commonly noted in fungal infections of the nail.
  - A KOH preparation can be useful in distinguishing these two etiologies.

## Work-Up

The diagnosis of psoriasis can typically be made through physical examination and supported by patient history, with skin biopsy reserved for challenging cases.

- A total-body skin examination is warranted and should include an assessment of the scalp and nails.
  - Visualization of well-demarcated, inflamed plaques in characteristic skin regions (elbows, areas, scalp, knees) with significant scaling supports the diagnosis of plaque psoriasis.
- Routine biopsy and histologic confirmation is not indicated, except in atypical-appearing cases or in cases that fail to respond to treatment as expected.
  - Importantly, a biopsy should not be obtained from plaques that are actively receiving treatment with topical corticosteroid.

- A patient history indicative of specific risk factors, including family history and obesity, can support a diagnosis of plaque psoriasis.
- Worsening of longstanding psoriasis should prompt a review of medications to identify exacerbating factors.
  - Frequently implicated medications include lithium, beta blockers, antimalarials (e.g., chloroquine, hydroxychloroquine), nonsteroidal antiinflammatory drugs (NSAIDs), and tetracycline.
- A KOH preparation can be employed to rule out a superficial fungal infection if this is suspected, especially in the case of intertriginous lesions, but this examination only has utility if performed by an experienced user.
- It is critical to evaluate for the presence of psoriatic arthritis at the time of initial diagnosis to avoid irreparable joint disease. Even a 6-month delay in treatment of psoriatic arthritis can result in irreversible joint damage.
  - Patients should be questioned regarding the presence of joint pain, joint stiffness, and back pain.
    - Screening tools for psoriatic arthritis exist; however, their sensitivity is limited. Patients who have any joint symptoms whatsoever should be referred to a rheumatologist or dermatologist for evaluation.
- It is not necessary to evaluate for the presence of systemic triggers, such as HIV or streptococcal pharyngitis, in the absence of clinical suspicion (e.g., presence of guttate psoriasis).

## Initial Steps in Management
### General Management Comments

Management of psoriasis has been revolutionized in the 21st century with the emergence of biologic agents. Nearly all patients with psoriasis can now obtain satisfactory disease control with the available treatment armamentarium. This has changed the way management of the disease is conceptualized.

- All patients with psoriatic arthritis must promptly receive systemic therapy that treats psoriatic arthritis. These patients should be referred to a specialist.
- The goal of treatment is patient satisfaction. This typically correlates with a BSA less than 1% and improvement in disease severity of at least 75% from baseline.
- Patients with psoriasis may suffer from psychological disorders, such as depression, and reassurance

regarding the appearance of the skin can be helpful to convey at follow-up appointments.
- Treatment regimens broadly consist of topical and systemic therapies. Choice of a particular treatment regimen is generally based on disease severity (limited/mild to moderate/severe) and disease location.
  - Now that the treatment armamentarium of psoriasis has expanded to include many well-tolerated, highly-effective agents, moderate to severe psoriasis is classified as psoriasis affecting more than 3% body surface area (a patient's palm is around 1%) or special sites (e.g., genitalia, palms) that are not adequately controlled with topical therapy.
    - All patients with moderate to severe psoriasis qualify for systemic therapy.
- Patients with localized plaque psoriasis can generally be adequately managed through their primary care provider.

### Recommended Initial Regimen

- For limited to mild psoriasis on the trunk and extremities, a high-potency topical steroid for a limited time and topical vitamin D can be used.
  - Resolution of the acute flare can be handled with a high-potency topical steroid (clobetasol propionate 0.05% cream, betamethasone propionate 0.05% cream) twice daily for 2 to 4 weeks, tapering afterward.
  - Maintenance therapy involves topical Vitamin D analog five times per week, alternating with a topical steroid on the weekend.
  - Topical tazarotene cream 0.05% to 0.1%, a topical retinoid, can be added twice daily for patients with thickened plaques.
- For limited to mild psoriasis on the face and body folds (intertriginous regions), a low-potency topical steroid or topical calcineurin inhibitors can be used.
  - A low-potency topical steroid (hydrocortisone 1% or 2.5% cream) twice daily for 2 to 4 weeks can be used.
  - Topical calcineurin inhibitors (tacrolimus 0.1% or pimecrolimus 1%) can be alternatively used twice daily to avoid long-term corticosteroid use.
  - Emollients can be applied immediately after showering to keep skin hydrated and minimize friction in affected regions.

- For moderate to severe disease, systemic treatment is recommended, in addition to the previously described topical treatments. It consists of phototherapy, oral medications, and biologic agents.
  - In all cases, systemic treatment should be given after consultation with a dermatologist.
  - Phototherapy consists of in-office treatment in a phototherapy booth indefinitely two to three times per week.
  - Oral medications include methotrexate, cyclosporine, acitretin, apremilast, and tofacitinib.
  - Biologics include tumor necrosis factor (TNF)–alpha inhibitors (e.g., etanercept, adalimumab); interleukin (IL)-17 inhibitors (e.g., secukinumab); IL-12/23 inhibitors (e.g., ustekinumab); and IL-23 inhibitors (e.g., guselkumab, risankizumab).

### Partial but Inadequate Response

If there is a partial but inadequate response after a 4-week trial of potent topical corticosteroid monotherapy:

- In patients who fail to respond to treatment with topical therapies, it is important to review medication compliance and potential compliance barriers.
- If patients express good medication compliance and do not exhibit symptomatic improvement, they should be trialed on the systemic approaches previously described, such as phototherapy, after a dermatology consultation.
- Reconsider the diagnosis. If you are not confident in the diagnosis of psoriasis, it is reasonable to consider a punch biopsy of an affected area at this time. Additionally, we recommend referral to a dermatologist for patients who demonstrate good compliance and fail to respond to initial treatment efforts.

### Other Treatment Options

- Topical coal tar preparations and anthralin have also been reported for the treatment of psoriasis. These treatments, however, are antiquated and not as frequently used now that we have a broad systemic armamentarium for this condition. Additionally, tar preparations are typically messy and can be frustrating for patients to use.

## Warning Signs/Common Pitfalls

- It is highly recommended to screen patients with psoriasis for psoriatic arthritis at regular intervals. If

this is deemed a diagnostic possibility, urgent referral to a rheumatologist is necessary. There are validated screening tools (e.g., the Psoriasis Epidemiology Screening Tool [PEST]) that can easily be implemented in the clinical setting.
- It is important to ask patients about prior experiences with treatment efforts to guide current efforts. Additionally, it is recommended to discuss with patients how they plan to incorporate treatment into their daily routine to gauge medication compliance.
- After initiating treatment, having the patient return for a follow-up visit in 1 to 2 weeks can be useful in increasing rates of compliance.
- Oral corticosteroids should never be used in psoriasis because flare-ups are inevitable after medication tapering. Some patients develop erythroderma or pustular psoriasis from this, which can require hospitalization.
- It is critical to screen patients for the psychosocial aspects of their disease because some patients can develop depression or low self-esteem as a result of the appearance of their skin. Reassurance can be an important tool at follow-up visits, and referral to a psychiatrist or counselor may be useful in some cases.
- In the case of intertriginous psoriasis, we recommend the use of low-potency topical steroids to avoid skin atrophy of the flexural surfaces.

## Counseling

Psoriasis is a skin condition that occurs because your immune system is inappropriately attacking your own skin. Although psoriasis is not curable, meaning it will be present for years, it can be managed with certain medications that can relieve the symptoms and improve the rash. Almost all patients can achieve satisfactory disease control with appropriate therapy. Although psoriasis is not life-threatening, it can increase your risk of several other diseases that are harmful to you.

I have prescribed you a topical corticosteroid. You should apply the corticosteroid twice daily to skin areas that have the rash on them. You should continue using this cream until the rash is no longer red and raised. The inflammation caused by psoriasis may discolor your skin. This discoloration should not be treated with the cream. Once you take a break from using the cream, your psoriasis will come back. You can then continue to use the cream up to twice daily as needed to keep it under control. The major side effect of the corticosteroid is that it can cause the skin to become a bit thinner and therefore cause some of the blood vessels to show more than usual. Taking breaks when the rash has gone away can help to prevent this side effect from happening. It is important to use the medication consistently each day because it is most effective that way. Patients say that they start to see an improvement within a week of using the medication.

## URTICARIA

### Clinical Features

Urticaria (or hives) is characterized by the sudden development of swollen-appearing, variably pink-red papules or plaques on the skin, which are referred to as wheals and/or angioedema (Fig. 3.6).
- Urticarial wheals have three key features:
  - They have a central swelling with or without surrounding erythema.
  - They usually itch, but they can also tingle or burn.
  - They are evanescent, lasting from 30 minutes to 24 hours.

- Urticarial angioedema has three key features as well:
  - It presents with sudden dermal, subcutaneous, and/or mucous membrane swelling.
  - It is typically more painful than itchy.
  - It resolves in less than 72 hours.
- Urticaria is divided into two major subtypes based on the duration of symptoms.
  - Acute urticaria lasts less than 6 weeks.
    - It frequently has an inciting trigger (e.g., illness, medication, food).
  - Chronic urticaria lasts longer than 6 weeks.
    - It can be further subdivided into chronic spontaneous urticaria and chronic inducible urticaria (CIU).
      - Chronic spontaneous urticaria has no known or identifiable specific eliciting trigger.
      - CIU consistently and reproducibly occurs in response to a specific eliciting trigger.
        - Subtypes of CIU include dermographism, delayed pressure urticaria (Fig. 3.7), vibratory angioedema, contact urticaria, aquagenic urticaria, solar urticaria, cholinergic urticaria, cold urticaria, and heat urticaria.

### Differential Diagnosis

The differential for urticaria is broad and includes dermal hypersensitivity reaction, urticarial bullous pemphigoid (BP), urticarial vasculitis, and autoinflammatory disorders (e.g., familial Mediterranean fever [FMF]).
- Dermal hypersensitivity reactions can clinically and histologically overlap with CSU; however, dermal hypersensitivity skin lesions last longer than 24 hours and present with erythema throughout the area of

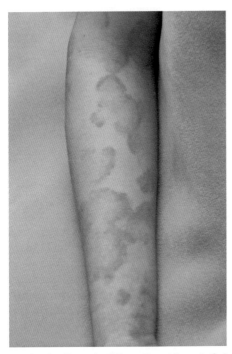

**Fig. 3.6 Urticaria.** (From the UConn Grand Rounds Collection.)

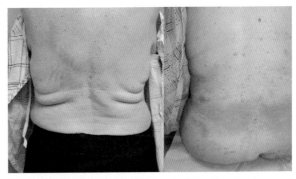

**Fig. 3.7 Delayed Pressure Urticaria.** Note the development of urticarial plaque at the site of the waistband. (From the UConn Grand Rounds Collection.)

dermal swelling rather than at the periphery of the swelling, as is typically seen in urticaria. Furthermore, dermal hypersensitivity reactions are much less responsive to antihistamines than urticaria is.

- Urticarial BP has an urticaria-like appearance, as its name suggests. It can be distinguished from urticaria because its lesions last longer than 24 hours; there can be a history of bullae development; BP is not antihistamine responsive; and a direct immunofluorescence examination of the perilesional skin will reveal a linear deposition of immunoglobulin G (IgG) with or without C3 at the basement membrane zone.
- Urticarial vasculitis is a form of leukocytoclastic vasculitis that presents with urticaria-like lesions. It can be distinguished from urticaria because it burns more than it itches; its lesions persist longer than 24 hours; its lesions are typically dusky/purpuric appearing; and a histopathologic examination shows small-vessel vasculitis.
- Patients presenting with angioedema without concomitant wheals should be evaluated for non-mast cell–related angioedema, of which there are many etiologies (e.g., hereditary angioedema, angiotensin-converting enzyme [ACE] inhibitor–induced angioedema). The presence of both wheals and angioedema differentiates urticaria from other causes of angioedema.
- Many autoinflammatory conditions (e.g., FMF, Muckle-Wells syndrome) present with urticarial lesions. These are unlikely to be misdiagnosed as urticaria because these patients present with fever and other systemic findings and often have a family history of their condition.

## Work-Up

Acute urticaria does not usually require any work-up because frequently, the history elicits the precipitating allergen. Nevertheless, in some cases, referral for allergy testing may be helpful for identifying the culprit and thereby preventing recurrences.

The work-up of patients with suspected chronic urticaria is divided into confirmation of the diagnosis and identification of the triggers/underlying causes.

- A thorough history ascertaining lesional history; concomitant systemic symptoms; inciting/exacerbating factors; personal history of allergies, infections, and autoimmune disease; family history of urticaria; current medications; and prior treatments should be obtained from all patients.

- Extensive laboratory work-up is not recommended in patients with acute urticaria who lack an obvious trigger and who are without systemic symptoms because lab work is unlikely to reveal an underlying cause; those with chronic urticaria should have an age-appropriate cancer work-up, a thorough review of systems, and a physical examination.
  - Patients with chronic fever and/or systemic symptoms in addition to their urticarial lesions should be referred to an allergist for evaluation for an autoinflammatory syndrome.

Patients with angioedema who do not have concomitant wheals should be worked up for non-mast cell–induced angioedema. This work-up is broad and includes but is not limited to a search for external agents such as a drug or food; history of previous treatment with an ACE inhibitor; an underlying autoimmune disease or infection; and C1 inhibitor deficiency. Referral of these patients to a specialist is recommended if the identifying cause is not easily identified.

## Initial Steps in Management

The first-line treatment for chronic urticaria is second-generation antihistamines (e.g., loratadine, cetirizine, fexofenadine, levocetirizine, desloratadine).

- Antihistamines should be initially dosed daily at their usual dose (e.g. cetirizine 10 mg BID).
  - Dosage should be increased up to 4 times the recommended daily dose (20 mg BID) if symptoms are not adequately controlled within 2 weeks of initiating the antihistamine.
    - The same treatment algorithm is used for children; however, lower doses are recommended (e.g., cetirizine 5 mg instead of 10 mg).
    - High-dose antihistamines are effective in around 70% of cases.
  - Mixing different antihistamines is not recommended (e.g., loratadine and cetirizine).
  - Use of a nightly sedating first-generation antihistamine (e.g., hydroxyzine) is not recommended.
  - Previously, H2 blockers (e.g. ranitidine, cimetidine) were added when H1 blockers were inadequate; however, this is no longer recommended.
- Patients who are not successfully controlled with a trial of high-dose H1 blockers should be referred to a dermatologist or an allergist for a trial of high-dose varied and disparate antihistamines and, if that fails, initiation of omalizumab.

## Warning Signs/Common Pitfalls

Most patients with chronic urticaria are antihistamine responsive and respond quickly. Initiation of systemic corticosteroids is almost never indicated because most patients have chronic urticaria for around a year and discontinuation of corticosteroids often results in significant disease flare.

- Similarly, first-generation antihistamines (e.g., diphenhydramine, hydroxyzine) are not generally recommended as first-line therapy because of their side effects.

Many patients with urticaria want an explanation as to why they have urticaria. Extensive laboratory evaluations and allergy testing are expensive and typically add to patient anxiety and therefore should not be performed unless the patient history suggests a specific trigger.

CIU represents only approximately 15% to 25% of all cases of chronic urticaria. Nevertheless, many patients (around two-thirds) with chronic urticaria have a component of CIU. Identification of this component is essential for successfully managing these patients.

Fever and/or systemic symptoms in the setting of chronic urticaria can represent a serious underlying illness. These patients should be referred urgently for additional evaluation.

## Counseling

You have chronic urticaria, which is also known as "hives." Hives are a type of skin reaction that occur from either an allergy, an autoimmune condition, an underlying disease, an infection, a medication, or something in your environment. Although we do not know why you are developing these hives, they often go away on their own within about a year.

You should attempt to identify what brings out your hives or worsens them. For example, some people's hives worsen with they take nonsteroidal antiinflammatory medications, such as ibuprofen; other people have their hives brought out by emotions and sweating.

There are an almost infinite number of causes of hives. We do not perform blood work or allergy testing to try to figure out why you have hives because it is almost never helpful.

Fortunately, most hives dramatically improve with antihistamines. You should take over-the-counter (OTC) cetirizine 10 mg by mouth twice daily. If your symptoms are not satisfactorily improved in 2 weeks,

then you should increase the dose of the cetirizine to 20 mg twice daily.

If you do not improve despite taking antihistamines, we will refer you to a hive specialist for additional treatment options.

# ID REACTION/AUTOECZEMATIZATION

**Christian Gronbeck and Diane Whitaker-Worth**

## Clinical Features

Autoeczematization, or id reaction, is a secondary skin eruption that results from a primary, inflammatory disorder in another part of the body. It is generally thought to be the result of hyperirritability of the skin elicited by immunogenic stimuli.

- In terms of geographic morphology, it presents with symmetric, erythematous, and pruritic papules and plaques with associated scale.
- It may be located at various sites on the body, either close to or distant from the inciting inflammatory disorder.

The type of primary skin infection varies and classically includes ACD, dermatophyte infections, and stasis dermatitis.

- Inciting dermatophyte reactions most classically include tinea pedis but may also be the result of tinea manuum, cruris, corporis, or capitis.
  - Patients with tinea pedis (athlete's foot) commonly present with secondary vesicular eruptions on the hands, head, and neck.
  - Patients with dermatophyte infections may develop id reactions shortly after the initiation of antifungals, which should not be misdiagnosed as a medication allergy. Patients should continue on their antifungal and be treated symptomatically for the id reaction.
- ACD frequently occurs in children and commonly results in development of an id reaction distal to the initial site of irritation.
  - Development of an id reaction is particularly common with nickel dermatitis.
- Stasis dermatitis can give rise to an id reaction 1 to 2 weeks after the initial inflammation and is most frequently located on the forearms, thighs, trunk, and face.

## Differential Diagnosis

The differential diagnosis of an id reaction is broad and includes AD, ACD, drug eruptions, and scabies. In all cases, the diagnosis of an id reaction is made more likely by the identification of a primary rash in a separate body location.

- AD is distinguished from id reactions in that it frequently develops during early childhood, co-develops with other atopic conditions (e.g., allergic rhinitis, asthma), and develops in characteristic geographic regions (antecubital fossae, popliteal fossae, other flexural surfaces).
- ACD is distinguished from an id reaction in that it typically is asymmetrical and eczematous appearing.
- Drug eruptions have variable presentations; however, they are often in the differential for an id reaction because patients are started on new medications for their primary dermatoses, and there is suspicion that these new medications are responsible for a subsequent rash. Drug eruptions are typically generalized, usually develop within 1 month of initiating a new medication, and usually resolve with de-challenge.
- Patients with scabies primarily present with secondary lesions (i.e., excoriations) that develop from the intense pruritus that they experience. These lesions most frequently affect the interdigital web spaces of the hands, the wrists, and the genitals. The face is characteristically spared. Patients with scabies may also demonstrate linear burrow markings in the skin (see following section, "Scabies").

## Work-Up

The diagnosis of an id reaction is a clinical diagnosis based on history and examination.

- In cases where an id reaction is suspected, patients should be questioned about whether they have a different rash elsewhere; however, history is typically not fruitful.
- A total-body skin examination should be performed to identify the primary dermatosis; if a primary rash is identified, management involves treatment of the primary dermatosis.
  - Patients with a primary fungal infection may exhibit erythematous, scaling plaques with central clearing (tinea corporis), erythematous patches affecting the medial thigh and intertriginous areas (tinea cruris), or erythematous erosions and scales between the toes (tinea pedis). If identified, a KOH preparation can be used to diagnose the presence of a primary fungal infection (see following section, "Tinea Corporis").

- Patients with primary stasis dermatitis will typically demonstrate erythematous, scaling, and hyperpigmented lesions on the lower legs, along with a history of venous insufficiency, varicosities, or pitting edema (see Chapter 4).
- A patient with an id reaction secondary to primary ACD will exhibit erythematous, scaling plaques with intense pruritus in regions exposed to allergen exposures (see section, "ACD Overview").
  - Patch testing can be performed if there is suspicion for a contact allergy; however, this is typically deferred until after the acute phase of the id reaction.
- If a work-up is not indicative of a primary etiology, we recommend referral to a dermatologist to pursue further testing, including a skin biopsy.

## Initial Steps in Management
### General Management Comments

- The treatment approach for any id reaction involves targeted therapies toward the primary rash and symptomatic management of the secondary skin eruption.
- Recommended initial treatment of the primary rash is based on the underlying etiology. Specific treatment recommendations can be found in the chapters discussing these primary dermatoses.

### Recommended Initial Treatment of The Id Reaction

- The id reaction may be highly pruritic, and treatment is therefore geared toward both relieving symptoms and resolving the rash.
- High-potency topical corticosteroids (e.g., clobetasol propionate 0.05% cream) can be applied at the sites of the rash twice daily for 2 to 4 weeks.

### Partial but Inadequate Response

If there is a partial but inadequate response after a 4-week trial of potent topical corticosteroid monotherapy:

- In patients who fail to respond to treatment with topical therapies, it is important to review compliance with medications and address any compliance barriers.
- Oral corticosteroids are typically reserved for severe or refractory cases and not recommended as first-line efforts. Treatment with oral corticosteroids does not supplant the need to treat the primary dermatosis.
  - In these cases, we suggest a 3-week oral prednisone taper (50 mg for 4 days, 40 mg for 4 days, 30 mg for 4 days, 20 mg for 4 days, and 10 mg for 4 days).

- Dosing should be weight-based; therefore, heavier individuals may initially require prednisone 60 mg.
- Patients with refractory skin involvement may benefit from wet dressings at sites with extensive weeping or oozing; however, this approach is rarely considered as a first-line option because of the burden wet dressings place on the patient.
  - Patients should first soak their skin in a warm bath, followed by application of a topical corticosteroid and emollient cream (e.g., Aquaphor).
  - Bandages should be soaked in warm water and then applied to the areas of skin involved. Tubular-shaped bandages can be useful because they are typically easier for patients to apply.
  - Dry bandages are applied on top of the wet bandages to keep clothing from becoming damp.
  - Wraps are typically left on throughout the night.

### Warning Signs/Common Pitfalls

The biggest pitfall when managing an id reaction is failure to identify the primary dermatosis and to manage it appropriately. Resolution of an id reaction can lag behind improvement of the primary dermatosis and therefore aggressive symptomatic management can be employed.

### Counseling

You have an id reaction. This is a type of skin rash that occurs because your skin is developing inflammation in response to another skin condition present elsewhere on your body. This occurs because your body's immune system is reacting to the first rash. Both the rash that your body is reacting to (the primary rash) and the rash that has developed in response to the first rash (the id reaction) have to be treated separately.

For your id reaction, your doctor has prescribed you a topical corticosteroid cream called "clobetasol," which you should apply to the affected area twice daily. Most people see a full resolution of both rashes within 2 to 4 weeks; however, if you fail to treat the rash that caused this second allergic rash, the rash will come back.

In addition to using these treatments, you may find it helpful to apply wet wraps or dressings to your rash if it starts to ooze or weep fluid. To do so, you should first soak your skin in a warm bath for several minutes. Afterward, you should apply the clobetasol steroid cream that you have been prescribed to the affected areas,

followed by a layer of emollient cream, such as Aquaphor. You should then wrap a layer of wet cotton bandages, followed by a layer of dry bandages, to the affected areas. We recommend using cotton clothing, such as socks or t-shirts for bandages, but you can also find custom-made wraps at your local pharmacy. Dressings should be left on throughout the night.

## XEROSIS CUTIS

### Clinical Features

Xerosis cutis (also called "dry skin," "winter itch," "asteatotic eczema," "erythema craquele," or "eczema for excessively dry skin") involves skin that is dry, scaly, and cracked and that may be inflamed. It results from dysfunction of the skin barrier, which allows for increased epidermal water loss or changes to the skin, most often associated with an environment of low humidity.

- Xerosis presents with variable degrees of dryness (appreciated by accentuation of natural skin lines), scaling and flaking, cracking and fissuring, and actual inflammation of the skin.
  - Patients with more pronounced skin findings can present with curvilinear patterning to their scaling and fissuring.
- Xerosis results in pruritis that is out of proportion to examination findings and can significantly impair patients' quality of life.
  - Patients with cracking and fissures may experience skin pain.
- Xerosis can occur in all age groups but is most common in young children and the elderly, who do not have prominent sebaceous gland secretions.
- Xerosis can affect any area of the body but most commonly affects, in decreasing order of frequency, the hands, the feet, the extremities, and the trunk.
- Although some individuals are more predisposed to developing xerosis than others (e.g., people with AD, those with diabetes, older adults), modifiable external factors play a major role in the development of xerosis.
  - Bathing habits, skin moisturization, chemical exposures, cold weather, and a dry environment are the most common contributors to xerosis.
  - Internal factors, such as medications (e.g., diuretics, statins) and medical conditions (e.g., hypothyroidism, HIV, nutritional deficiencies), can further predispose a patient to xerosis.

## Differential Diagnosis

The differential for xerosis includes AD, ichthyosis vulgaris, ICD, stasis dermatitis, nummular eczema, and tinea pedis.

- Most patients with AD have background xerosis, but not all patients with xerosis have AD. AD can be differentiated from xerosis because it presents with true inflamed, eczematous plaques, predominantly located in the flexural areas (e.g., antecubital fossae, popliteal fossae, flexural neck); on the other hand, xerosis is frequently poorly localized and affects the extremities in patients without known atopy.
  - Although AD can develop in adulthood, the most common cause of eczema in the elderly is xerosis.
- Ichthyosis vulgaris is an autosomal dominant genetic condition characterized by the development of fish like scaling (hence the name), which arises in adolescence and is most appreciable on the lower extremities but can affect the skin on any part of the body. Regular and diffuse patterning of the scales and presence of scaling from adolescence often suggests ichthyosis rather than xerosis.
- ICD overlaps with xerosis because both occur when exogenous factors result in epidermal barrier dysfunction. ICD is distinguished from xerosis because it typically occurs more focally at the site of a known exposure (e.g., hand washing), whereas xerosis is a more generalized process that (while contributed to by external factors) cannot be explained by a single exposure.
- Stasis dermatitis frequently overlaps with xerosis in the elderly because many elderly patients with xerosis complain of itchy legs and have background venous stasis. On the legs, the processes should be assumed to coexist in cases where true eczematous plaques are forming on the legs. Look for varicosities or pitting edema and, if present, address both the stasis issues and the xerosis.
- Nummular eczema presents with many coin-shaped eczematous plaques that predominantly affect the extremities and are intensely pruritic. This is opposed to the curvilinear fissures frequently seen in inflamed xerotic skin.
- Tinea pedis frequently presents with scaling and inflammation of the plantar foot and interdigital web spaces with or without onychomycosis. It can be very difficult to distinguish from xerosis; however, scaling with or without maceration within the interdigital web spaces suggests a diagnosis of tinea pedis, as does the presence of nail involvement.

## Work-Up

Xerosis cutis should be expected in any patient presenting with dry skin in the absence of a primary pathology or who has a bothersome itch and minimal examination findings.

- The work-up for xerosis involves identifying modifiable environmental factors that may be contributing to a patient's xerosis and identifying internal processes that may either be contributing to the patient's xerosis or better explain the patient's symptoms.
  - A work-up for internal causes of xerosis is usually not performed until after a patient fails to improve with dry skin management.

## Initial Steps in Management

Management of xerosis predominantly involves teaching patients a comprehensive dry skin care routine; however, topical antiinflammatory medications can also be helpful for symptomatic and inflamed areas.

### Dry Skin Care Management

Obtain a list of all personal care products and gain an understanding of an individual's bathing techniques (e.g., use of a luffa).

Patients should be counseled that it is okay/encouraged to bathe daily as long as they use appropriate bathing techniques followed by lubrication.

- Patients should be counseled to use a mild, unscented bar soap such as Dove White Unscented Bar Soap, CeraVe Hydrating Cleanser Bar, or Cetaphil Gentle Cleansing Bar.
- Soap should only be routinely applied to the axilla, groin, and overtly dirty areas. A luffa should not be used to apply soap because it may harbor bacteria and is abrasive.
- Hot water should be avoided and showers should be limited to less than 10 minutes in length.
- Patients should pat dry with a towel rather than rub the towel against their skin.
- Immediately after bathing, individuals should moisturize.
- Barrier care should be performed by moisturizing at least twice daily (including immediately after showering). Thick moisturizing creams (e.g., Vanicream, CeraVe Moisturizing Cream, Eucerin Advanced Barrier Repair, etc.) or ointments (e.g., Vaseline, Aquaphor, Vaniply, Healing Ointment) should be applied to the entire body. Some patients prefer using oils or products

containing natural ingredients. Patients should be provided with a list of acceptable moisturizers so they can identify the products that they are willing to use.

- Patients with significant fissuring and/or scaling should be encouraged to use a product containing 10% urea, such as Eucerin Dry Skin Intensive or Aquacare.
- Creams containing ceramides (e.g., CeraVe, Eucerin Advanced Repair Cream) are recommended to help replace ceramides in the stratum corneum, a frequent finding in xerosis and AD.
- Very dry and scaling or hyperkeratotic skin may be more responsive to creams with lactic acid, like amlactin cream, or creams containing alpha hydroxy acids. These creams may result in transient burning or tingling after application if the patient has dry, fissured skin.

### Topical Antiinflammatory Agents

For inflamed skin, first-line treatment should include a medium-potency topical corticosteroid, such as triamcinolone 0.1% cream, applied twice daily for several weeks (with avoidance of application to facial skin or intertriginous areas to avoid skin thinning).

- Patients who have difficulty complying with twice-daily corticosteroid applications can be offered a slightly more potent topical corticosteroid for once-daily application (e.g., mometasone 0.1% cream).
- Patients should be prescribed 1 gram of cream per day for each percentage of BSA affected.

### Itch Management

Pruritis is typically the most bothersome symptom of xerosis cutis.

- Restoration of the skin barrier in patients with xerosis with dry skin care typically leads to itch resolution.
- Topical anti-itch agents can be used in extremely symptomatic patients.
  - Storing pramoxine-containing lotions and creams (e.g., Sarna Anti-Itch, CeraVe Itch Relief) in the refrigerator can improve their efficacy at curbing itch.
- Xerosis-induced itch is not predominantly mediated by histamine; therefore oral antihistamines typically do not have a role in therapy.

### Fatty Acid Replacement

The loss of lipids that make up the natural moisturizing factor in the skin contributes to the development of xerosis. As a result, some providers recommend oral supplementation.

- Oral supplementation with Omega-3 fatty acids (1 gram/day) has been shown to have some benefit in select patients and can be considered.

## Warning Signs/Common Pitfalls

The biggest pitfall when managing xerosis cutis is underestimating the impact that dry skin can have on a patient's life. Failure to emphasize that the patient's symptoms are resulting from dry skin and that dry skin care can improve their symptoms is a common cause of noncompliance with dry skin lifestyle changes.

Itch management with antihistamines is ineffective and therefore should not be recommended. Sedating antihistamines can be dangerous in the elderly and promote falls.

Pruritis can be the heralding sign of significant internal disease (e.g., liver failure, HIV). Patients with pruritus that is refractory to dry skin care lifestyle modifications should be referred to a dermatologist for additional work-up.

## Counseling

You have xerosis cutis, which is a severe form of dry skin. This means that your skin is not hydrated well enough, which is causing it to breakdown and became itchy and/or painful. Xerosis cutis is very common and is often made worse by things your skin is coming into contact with. Xerosis cutis is frequently cyclical, meaning that it gets better at times and worsens at other times. Its cyclicality is frequently associated with changes in the seasons, with the winter being the hardest time of the year for many people.

Treating your skin disease requires that you keep your skin healthy by moisturizing it and by avoiding exposing it to things that irritate it. To keep your skin healthy, it is important that you have a special bathing regimen that promotes your skin health. When you shower, it is important that you use tepid water and that you limit your shower to less than 10 minutes in length. In the shower, you should use a gentle, unscented bar soap and should only apply soap to the armpits, groin, and areas that are visibly dirty. Do not use a luffa or a washcloth to apply soap because this may further irritate your skin. Pat, rather than rub, yourself dry with a towel. Immediately after drying off, you should apply a moisturizer to lock in the hydration that your skin received while you were showering.

It is important that you not only hydrate your skin with a moisturizer after showering but that you also moisturize at least twice a day. While your skin is still irritated, it is important that you do not apply any cosmetics or fragrances because these can inflame or irritate your skin.

Many people who have xerosis cutis are very itchy. We recommend that you use an anti-itch cream (such as Sarna Anti-Itch or CeraVe Itch Relief) in addition to your moisturizing creams. You should store this anti-itch cream in the refrigerator and apply it anytime that you are itchy to soothe the itch and keep you from scratching.

You may notice some areas of your skin that become red and inflamed from your skin condition. To treat these areas, your doctor has prescribed a topical steroid cream that you should use twice daily only for 7 to 10 days, at which point the redness and irritation should be gone. Do not apply this cream to your face, groin, underarms, or under your breasts unless told specifically to use it in these locations.

This prescription cream is not a substitute for your moisturizer and should be used with your moisturizer, not instead of your moisturizer. Once the redness and irritation has resolved, you can stop the prescription cream, although you may need to restart it when the redness and irritation return. The topical steroid prescribed cream can cause side effects if you use it too frequently or if you use it for too long. These side effects include potential thinning of the skin, dilatation of blood vessels that can become more visible in the area of application, discoloration of the skin, and even an acne like rash. Continue your routine of twice-daily lubrication and shortened tepid bathing as part of your skin regimen.

# SCABIES

Christian Gronbeck and Diane Whitaker-Worth

## Clinical Features

Scabies results from skin infestation by the *Sarcoptes scabiei* mite. It is extremely common worldwide, affecting all ages and socioeconomic levels, and is classified as a Neglected Tropical Disease by the World Health Organization (WHO).
- Scabies is most often seen in individuals living in crowded conditions, in those who are institutionalized (e.g., in nursing homes, prisons), and in those living in endemic areas.
  - Hygiene does not play a significant role, despite the perception that people with scabies are dirty.

The scabies mite is very small and therefore cannot be seen without magnification.
- The mite is an obligate parasite and cannot live without a viable host for more than 24 to 36 hours at normal room temperature.
  - Therefore, direct transmission from prolonged skin-to-skin contact is the primary mode of transmission and indirect transmission is uncommon.
- Once a mite finds a new host, the female mite quickly burrows into the epidermis, laying 2 to 3 eggs per day, which subsequently hatch 2 to 3 days later in the epidermis.
- Larvae leave the burrow and mature on the skin surface for several weeks before repeating the cycle.
- Infestation causes pruritus and rash through development of a delayed-type hypersensitivity to the mite and its feces.
- The extent of the rash is not indicative of the number of mites inhabiting the skin.
- Symptoms of itch usually do not appear until at least 3 to 4 weeks after initial exposure, although subsequent infestations can present within a few days because of host sensitization.
- Many individuals with infestations are asymptomatic, which contributes to the spread of scabies, especially in institutionalized settings.

Clinical presentation is often divided into classic, crusted, and nodular and can vary based on the adequacy of the patient's immune response.
- Classic scabies is characterized by diffuse, exquisitely pruritic pink papules with overlying linear excoriations.
- Scabies is typically diagnosed based on characteristic distribution and burrow identification.
  - An itchy rash involving the finger webs, wrists, and/or genitals (especially in men) should raise heavy concern for a diagnosis of scabies.
    - Scabies almost always spares the head in immunocompetent adults. Scalp and facial pruritus suggest an alternate diagnosis.
  - Identification of burrows is diagnostic of scabies; however, it can be difficult for less experienced providers to identify them.
    - Look for linear tunnels on the palms, web spaces, and wrists. They look like very small, gray-white, serpiginous, scaly plaques.
    - It may even be possible to visualize a dark speck with the naked eye at the tip of the burrow, which represents the adult female mite.

- Dermoscopy can also be helpful in visualizing the mite. When applied to the distal portion of the burrow, a dark triangular structure may be visualized and represents the adult mite.
  - Identification of burrows is important because these are the areas that are scraped during a scabies preparation.
  - Burrows can be difficult to identify because, despite the diffuse nature of the rash, there are generally only about 10 to 15 mites present on the host.
- Nodular scabies is much less common than classic scabies.
  - It is characterized by the same intractable itch; however, it presents with reddish-brown nodules, often on the genitals, breast, axillae, or buttocks.
    - Nodular scabies is slow to resolve, even with appropriate treatment.
- Crusted scabies is the most dramatic of the clinical presentations of scabies (Fig. 3.8).
  - It occurs in immunocompromised hosts and in patients who are severely debilitated and therefore cannot scratch themselves.

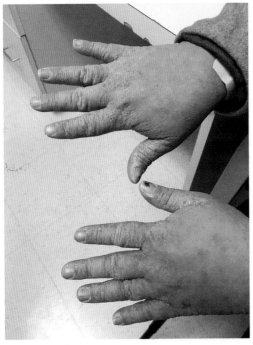

**Fig. 3.8 Crusted Scabies.** Note the crusted plaques on the wrist and interdigital web space. (Courtesy Jonas Adalsteinsson, MD.)

- Lesions are characterized by thick, scaly, white-gray plaques with minimal pruritus on the scalp, face, back, buttocks, and feet.
- Generalized lymphadenopathy may be present.
- Open fissures can increase the risk for bacteria entry, creating a higher risk for secondary infection.
- Because of impaired immune function, these patients can harbor thousands to millions of mites at a single time and may shed large numbers of mites into the environment, making this form highly contagious.
- Infants and children more commonly have lesions on the scalp and neck than adults. These areas are often uncommonly involved in adult patients, and treatment in children may require special attention to applying topicals in these areas.
- Secondary infection is a possible complication of all types of scabies. Bacterial infection is common and may present as impetigo, furunculosis, or even cellulitis.

## Differential Diagnosis

The differential for scabies includes AD, ACD, dermal hypersensitivity reaction, arthropod assault, BP, dermatitis herpetiformis (DH), and delusions of parasitosis (DOP).

There should always be a high suspicion for scabies in all patients with new-onset pruritus and diffuse rash, especially when the rash affects the finger web spaces and genitals.

A history of contacts with a similar rash or itch can be helpful but is not essential to making the diagnosis, given the lag time between infection and symptoms.

In general, if the examination is suggestive but not diagnostic of scabies, it is still recommended to treat patients for scabies, given the frequency with which this diagnosis is missed and the benignity of treatment.

- Scabies is often mistaken for AD and ACD. Unlike these conditions, scabies does not present with eczematous skin lesions. It is also uncommon for AD and ACD to subacutely present with near-diffuse rash, except in scenarios where patients have baseline eczema that has flared because of recent exposure (e.g., oral corticosteroid withdrawal). Involvement of genitalia and finger web spaces strongly suggests a diagnosis of scabies.
- A dermal hypersensitivity reaction either to a drug or another exposure is the most difficult diagnosis

to distinguish from scabies because the rash in scabies infestation is a form of a dermal hypersensitivity reaction. New drug exposures; failure to respond to antiscabetic agents; absence of burrows; and lack of involvement of finger webs, wrists, and genitalia are suggestive of a dermal hypersensitivity reaction.

- Scabies may also be confused with arthropod assault (e.g., bed bugs), although the latter generally will show monomorphous edematous papules, often with a central punctum, and tend to be asymmetrically distributed. Bug bites tend to crop together in a localized distribution.
- Scabies and BP are both commonly seen in the elderly and can be pruritic, of sudden onset, and widespread. In the early phase of BP, it presents without blisters, making the distinction between these two conditions difficult; however, the presence of tense bullae on examination is suggestive of BP. In general, the plaques of BP seem to be more discrete than those of scabies. BP can be distinguished from scabies by direct immunofluorescence examination of perilesional skin and by enzyme-linked immunosorbent assay (ELISA) testing for BP180 and BP230 antibodies.
- DH may be misdiagnosed as scabies because of the degree of pruritus patients with DH experience; however, DH presents with localized, symmetric, excoriated papulovesicles on extensor surfaces and the buttocks. Histologic examination of lesional skin also easily differentiates between these two conditions.
- DOP is a delusional disorder where patients falsely and unwaveringly believe that they are infested by bugs, parasites, or mites. These patients frequently endorse seeing the infestation and will often bring in samples they have collected (the so-called "matchbox sign"). These patients have excoriations in the absence of any primary dermatosis on examination. This is distinguished from scabies by the lack of a primary dermatosis, the failure to respond to antiscabetics, and the clear odd behavior during examination. A positive matchbox sign is near-diagnostic for DOP.

## Work-Up

In all cases, the gold standard for diagnosis is direct visualization of mites, eggs, or burrows. This can be done via dermoscopy or by skin scraping. Skin scraping is often unavailable in primary care settings because of the lack of access to a microscope.

- To perform a skin scraping:
  - Identify a burrow (if burrows are not seen, scrapings can be performed in areas such as the wrist, fingers, and axillae).
  - Apply mineral oil or Surgilube to the burrow.
  - Scrape the burrow with a #15 blade until pinpoint bleeding is observed.
  - Mount scrapings on a slide and examine with a microscope on low power to visualize mites, feces, and eggs (Fig. 3.9).

When definitive visualization of the mite is not possible, the presumptive diagnosis of scabies is clinical and relies on a total-body skin examination and thorough patient history.

If there is uncertainty regarding the diagnosis, a punch biopsy of lesional skin can be performed. Biopsy frequently demonstrates a dermal hypersensitivity pattern with eosinophils, which is nondiagnostic. Rarely, scabies mites are identified on biopsy.

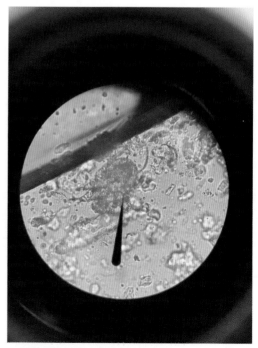

**Fig. 3.9** Mineral Oil Preparation Showing Scabies Mite. (Courtesy Jonas Adalsteinsson, MD.)

## Initial Steps in Management
### General Management Comments

- It is recommended to treat scabies if there is a high suspicion of the disease, regardless of diagnostic confirmation through visualization of mites and eggs.
- All close contacts, even if asymptomatic, should be treated alongside the patient.
  - If a patient who is institutionalized (e.g., in a nursing home or prison) has a confirmed diagnosis of scabies, mass treatment with ivermectin should be considered.
- All patients should be advised to dry all clothing and linens used within the last week at 60° C for 10 minutes to destroy remaining mites and eggs. Because the mite cannot live for prolonged periods in the environment without a host, any clothes, furniture, and the like that are not used for 2 to 3 days should be free of mites after that time. Vacuuming of floors can also be helpful, but extermination using chemicals is generally not necessary.
- Initial management differs in children weighing less than 20 kg, pregnant women, and immunocompromised hosts.

### First-Line Treatment for Classical Scabies

- There are two first-line treatment options for scabies. Both treatments need to be repeated 1 week after the initial treatment.
  - Permethrin 5% cream is applied to skin areas caudal to the neck and left on overnight.
    - In children, the elderly, and immunocompromised patients, treatment should include the face and scalp.
    - Special attention must be paid to applying permethrin under the fingernails because this is a common reservoir for recurrence.
    - Permethrin should be used preferentially in pregnant women and children weighing less than 20 kg.
    - The most common side effects of permethrin treatment include localized erythema and burning.
    - Patients may return to work, daycare, or school the day after the first treatment.
  - Ivermectin 200 mcg/kg by mouth is the authors' preferred first-line treatment.
    - Compliance is much better than it is for permethrin and recent high-quality evidence suggests it is superior for mass treatment protocols.

### Treatment for Pregnant Women

- Topical permethrin is believed to be safe for pregnant and breastfeeding women.
- Ivermectin is classified as pregnancy category C.

### Treatment for Children

- Topical permethrin is recommended for children, with ivermectin less suitable for children weighing less than 20 kg.

### Management of Crusted Scabies

Crusted scabies is best addressed with combination topical permethrin and oral ivermectin treatment.

- We recommend 5% topical permethrin cream (once daily for 7 days), followed by twice weekly until cure alongside oral ivermectin (200 mcg/kg on days 1, 2, 8, 9, and 15).
- These patients are especially prone to secondary infections and may require antistaphylococcal oral antibiotics if signs of cutaneous infection are present.
- Importantly, patients with moderate or severe crusted scabies have very high mite burdens and are likely to spread the infestation.

### Management of Institutionalized Patients

- Oral ivermectin should be provided to all other institutionalized individuals. This has been done on an islandwide scale in the Solomon Islands, which demonstrated both the safety and efficacy of such an approach.

### Inadequate Treatment Response

The biggest cause of treatment failure in the first 6 weeks after treatment is postscabetic pruritus. As previously mentioned, the itch in scabies is caused by a hypersensitivity reaction to infestation. The itch from this reaction persists for up to 6 weeks after successful treatment and is not a sign of continued infestation or reinfestation.

- Patients with persistent itch can be managed with mid-potency topical corticosteroids (e.g., triamcinolone 0.1% cream) to affected areas twice daily.

Itch persisting beyond 6 weeks can occur for several reasons.

- Non-compliance is especially common with permethrin and should be assessed for. Improper application of permethrin is a common form of noncompliance.

- Reinfestation is especially common in institutionalized settings or when close contacts are not treated.
- Treatment failure occurs rarely when patients are truly refractory to treatment.
  - These patients should be treated with combination ivermectin and permethrin.
- Misdiagnosis can also happen and the patient may, in fact, not have scabies

## Warning Signs/Common Pitfalls

The biggest pitfall when managing scabies is failing to treat close contacts or to mass eradicate it in an institutionalized setting.

Scabies should always be considered in patients with new-onset severe itch. Examination of the genitalia and finger web spaces is crucial in these patients.

Monitoring for superinfection of skin lesions is important because these infections can result in bacteremia.

Patients who continue to request antiscabetics may have DOP. These patients need antipsychotic medications, although they frequently refuse them.

## Counseling

Your rash is caused by a small insect that is spread from person to person. This is called "scabies." Although the mite is unlikely to cause a serious disease, it lives in the upper layers of your skin and can cause irritation and itching, which can be very uncomfortable. It typically likes to live in skin areas that are located in creases, such as between the bases of your fingers, your armpits, or your genital area. You did not do anything in particular to acquire this infestation; however, it was likely transmitted from someone else who was in close contact with you. Scabies is not a result of poor hygiene. Washing vigorously will not eradicate the mite.

We have several treatments available that can help remove the mites. Some treatments are in pill form and others are in cream form. Your doctor will have chosen the best treatment for your situation. If a topical cream is prescribed, you will apply it to the skin below your neckline before going to bed. Sometimes, your doctor may tell you to apply this cream to the scalp and face as well. You should leave this cream on overnight while you sleep (approximately 8 hours) and remove it in the shower the next morning with normal cleansing. Take care to ensure that all skin surfaces are covered, including the wrists, fingers, and even nails. If nails are long, trimming them before applying the cream can be

helpful. We may recommend that you repeat this once more in 1 week. Although this treatment is typically effective in removing the mites, your itching may persist for another few weeks after your second treatment. This is generally normal and is because of your body's lingering reaction to the mites. It does not mean that you are contagious or that the treatment did not work.

We may also recommend that you follow up with us after your second treatment so that we can reevaluate the rash. Also, because the mite can continue to live in your home for a few days, we recommend that you dry all of your clothes and linens that you have used within the last week at 60° C for 10 minutes to kill any remaining mites. Using a dryer on high heat is usually adequate. It is not necessary to isolate yourself from other individuals, and you should be able to return to work/school the morning after your first treatment. Please let us know if any of your skin rash develops signs of infection, such as warmth, tenderness, swelling, or unusual discharge.

# BULLOUS PEMPHIGOID

**Savannah Alvarado and Jun Lu**

## Clinical Features

BP is an autoimmune condition that manifests as tense, subepidermal blistering of the skin and/or mucous membranes; it is the most common autoimmune blistering disorder in adult patients. This condition most often appears in elderly patients with neurologic disease, particularly stroke, dementia and Parkinson disease, with onset generally at or above age 60. There is no difference in prevalence based on ethnicity or sex.

- Lesions commonly appear on the trunk and proximal extremities, including flexor surfaces, axillae, and inguinal areas.
- Lesions often present as pruritic, large, tense, serous, or sanguineous blisters (bullae) or as crusted superficial ulcers or erosions (Fig. 3.10).
- Twenty percent of patients with BP do not develop blisters; in these patients, the common features are urticarial plaques and/or papules. Many patients with blistering BP will also present with concomitant urticarial plaques and/or papules
- A small subset of patients with BP will develop mucosal lesions. Mucosal involvement is much less common and milder than is seen in patients with pemphigus vulgaris (PV).

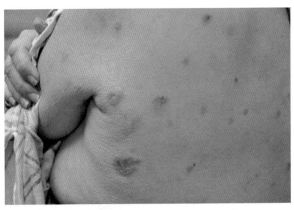

**Fig. 3.10 Bullous Pemphigoid.** Note presence of many tense bullae. (From the UConn Grand Rounds Collection.)

- The prognosis of BP is generally good with a relapsing and remitting course over the span of months to years.
- Several factors are associated with a higher likelihood of relapse in patients not being treated:
  - Advanced age
  - Comorbid health problems (especially neurologic disease)
  - Extensive disease involvement
- Lesions generally heal without scarring, although patients may experience temporary PIH.

BP can be fatal in some patients without adequate treatment. One-year mortality rates vary geographically and range from 6% to 40%.

## Differential Diagnosis

The differential diagnosis should include other autoimmune blistering disorders (subtypes of pemphigus, including PV and pemphigus foliaceus) and drug-induced or infectious blistering disorders. Laboratory analysis, as well as the physical examination, can help to distinguish BP from other blistering disorders. It can be clinically distinguished from the autoimmune intraepidermal disease PV because the blisters in PV are flaccid rather than tense and painful rather than pruritic.

## Work-Up

The two main components of the work-up for patients with suspected BP are histology and immunofluorescence/ELISA. The work-up requires one biopsy from an active lesion (used for histology) and either an additional biopsy from a perilesional site (used for direct immunofluorescence [DIF]) or a sample of the patient's serum (used for indirect immunofluorescence [IIF] or ELISA).

- Histology from an active lesion will demonstrate separation of keratinocytes from the basement membrane, forming a subepidermal blister with eosinophils.
- DIF of a perilesional biopsy will demonstrate the presence of IgG and/or C3 in a linear deposition along the basement membrane.
- IIF or ELISA will detect autoantibodies to BP180 and BP230 in the patient's serum.
  - This provides a quantitative measure of autoantibody levels.
  - Levels correlate with the severity of the clinical course and can indicate the likelihood of relapse.

As always, histology and immunofluorescence should be used in combination with clinical presentation to make the most accurate and clinically significant diagnosis.

The association of a malignant neoplasm with BP is controversial and has never been definitively established. The patient population is usually elderly and therefore age-appropriate screenings and work-up of suspicious symptoms are recommended.

## Initial Steps in Management

Treatment for patients with BP depends on the extent and clinical severity of the disease, as well as the patient's comorbidities. In general, the mainstay management is with corticosteroids or alternative immune suppressants.

- Mild to moderate focal disease is treated with high-potency topical steroids.
- Oral lesions can be treated with 0.05% clobetasol propionate ointment or gel or with a dexamethasone (0.1 mg/mL) swish and spit preparation.
- Severe disease requires treatment with systemic corticosteroids.
  - Therapy is initiated with 0.75 to 1 mg/kg QID and patients are monitored for a response within 2 to 3 weeks.
    - Patients requiring long-term steroids may also require osteoporosis prevention and pneumocystis prophylaxis.
- Discontinuation or tapering of therapy should be considered in patients who demonstrate an adequate

response to medication. An adequate response is defined as complete remission for 2 consecutive months.

- Before discontinuation, patients should be slowly tapered to a minimal systemic corticosteroid therapy (<0.1 mg/kg/day of prednisone) or minimal topical corticosteroid therapy (<20 g/week of clobetasol propionate).
- Several glucocorticoid-sparing agents are used to preserve remission while glucocorticoids are being tapered. These agents are also available for patients who do not respond to or cannot tolerate corticosteroid therapy.
  - The most commonly used alternative therapies are mycophenolate mofetil, azathioprine, and methotrexate.
  - Other options for alternative therapy include tetracycline with nicotinamide or dapsone.
  - Therapies used only in refractory cases include rituximab, intravenous immunoglobulin (IVIG), dupilumab, omalizumab, and plasmapheresis.

Patients receiving therapy need to be closely monitored for adverse effects of medication.

- Common side effects of chronic systemic corticosteroid therapy include cardiovascular, hematologic, orthopedic, metabolic, and neurologic side effects.
- Severe infection and sepsis can also occur.
- Thrush may present in patients receiving oral steroid preparations either topically or systemically.

Providers should use a conservative approach to treatment because the complications associated with BP are commonly caused by side effects of the medications in conjunction with the primary disease processes. Even in patients receiving only topical therapy, high-dose steroids can be absorbed and have a systemic effect, especially in highly susceptible patients and patients with comorbidities.

## Warning Signs/Common Pitfalls

It is important to consider the entire clinical picture when working up a patient with possible BP.

- Twenty percent will not develop the cutaneous manifestations classic of BP.
- Five percent of the general population will demonstrate positive BP180 autoantibodies without any clinical signs of disease.
- Several conditions are classically associated with pemphigoid, especially neurologic and psychiatric disease/mood disorders.

There are several possible triggers of BP; at the time of diagnosis, patients should be evaluated for exposure to:
- UV light
- Radiation therapy
- Medical conditions that have been reported to trigger BP, such as psoriasis, lichen planus, diabetes, rheumatoid arthritis, ulcerative colitis dementia, Parkinson disease, stroke, epilepsy, multiple sclerosis, and psychiatric diseases (especially schizophrenia)
- Certain medications
  - There is a long list of pharmaceuticals that have a known association with BP. A full review of medications must be obtained and assessed to identify possible disease triggers.

BP can also mimic other conditions, including:
- Drug eruptions such as erythema multiforme, Stevens-Johnson syndrome, and toxic epidermal necrolysis (see Chapter 18)
- Infectious causes of blistering such as bullous impetigo and *Staphylococcal*-scalded skin syndrome (see Chapter Y)
- Pemphigus and several variants of pemphigus, including paraneoplastic pemphigus associated with internal malignancies

Providers must use both clinical presentation and laboratory analysis (histology, immunofluorescence, and ELISA) to correctly distinguish between these conditions. Referral to a dermatologist for this work-up and management is recommended.

## Counseling

Your blistering is caused by an autoimmune disorder, which means that your immune system is attacking cells in your own skin as if these cells were dangerous to the body.

If you develop a blister, you should gently clean the area well with soap and water and puncture the blister with a clean needle that has been boiled. You should leave the skin on top of the blister intact because it will act as protection for the sensitive skin under the blister. Afterwards, apply clean petroleum jelly to the area to keep the skin moist. You can apply a small amount of topical steroid directly to the affected area twice daily.

If you have blisters in your mouth, you should avoid eating hot (temperature) or spicy foods, as well as foods with sharp edges (like chips). It is important that you maintain good oral hygiene to prevent infections in your mouth. Brush your teeth using a bland toothpaste twice daily and floss between your teeth at least once daily. If you frequently get blisters in your mouth, you can use a topical steroid (gel or mouth rinse) two to three times daily to aid in healing and preventing new blisters from forming. If the blisters in your mouth are very painful, you can use a gel or solution to help numb the area.

It is important that you protect yourself from sunlight because UV radiation from the sun can worsen your blistering. Make sure you wear sunscreen and protective clothing on a daily basis. Remember that you are regularly exposed to the sun, even if you are not sitting in direct sunlight.

The medications that you take for your blisters can cause dangerous side effects. If you experience any of the potential side effects, you should contact your doctor immediately.

# SEBORRHEIC DERMATITIS—TRUNK

## Clinical Features

Seborrheic dermatitis (seb derm) of the trunk occurs in both infants and postadolescent patients.

- Seb derm most frequently affects areas rich in sebaceous glands (e.g., the presternal area, axilla, groin, anogenital area, inframammary area, and umbilicus).
- Truncal seb derm is characterized by the presence of thin, red-pink plaques with overlying large greasy scales.
  - Presentation can range from pruritus and barely perceptible patches to deep red plaques encroaching past the classic seborrheic distribution.
  - Scale is less perceptible when seb derm occurs in intertriginous areas. In these locations, shiny pink plaques are more common.
  - Infants typically present with scalp cradle cap with or without axilla and diaper involvement.
- Seb derm is frequently pruritic; however, scaling (dandruff) is often the most bothersome symptom for patients.
  - Scale can be so prominent that white scale is visible on the patients' clothing. If asked, many patients report that they avoid wearing dark clothing because their scale can be seen on it.
- Isolated truncal seb derm is relatively rare. An examination of other seborrheic areas, such as the face, retroauricular area, and scalp, often helps clarify the diagnosis.
- Severe, subacute-onset seb derm can be a sign of an underlying disease such as Parkinson disease or HIV infection.

## Differential Diagnosis

The differential for truncal seb derm includes xerosis, ACD, intertrigo, Darier disease, and Grover disease. In infants, napkin psoriasis, ICD from urine and feces, and Langerhans cell histiocytosis (LCH) must also be considered.

- Identifying that a rash presents with a seborrheic distribution is essential for diagnosing seb derm, especially in subtler cases characterized by barely perceptible pink patches or thin plaques, pruritus, and mild flaking.
  - Looking for flaking on the patient's clothing can help confirm a diagnosis of seb derm in adults.
- In general, response to a trial of treatment with a topical azole antifungal is suggestive of a diagnosis of seb derm.
- Truncal xerosis can be misdiagnosed as seb derm because xerotic skin can appear scaly and may also affect the presternal area; however, unlike seb derm, xerosis is much more diffuse, affects nonseborrheic areas, and should not present with any true inflammatory plaques.
- ACD can affect the central chest and neck; however, unlike seb derm, it is rarely localized to a seborrheic distribution and lacks the greasy scaling that is characteristic of seb derm.
- Intertrigo can be almost clinically indistinguishable from seb derm; however, presence of seborrhea elsewhere is suggestive of seb derm; in infants, pink plaques in intertriginous are almost always seb derm; and intertrigo almost exclusively occurs in overweight patients where skin-on-skin maceration is clearly playing a contributory role.
- Darier disease can look almost indistinguishable from seborrhea; however, presence of verrucous lesions, disease severity, nail changes, family history of Darier, treatment refractoriness, and presence of disease in nonseborrheic areas should all suggest a diagnosis of Darier disease.
- Grover disease also presents as thin, pink, often pruritic lesions on the trunk; however, these lesions typically affect the abdomen and lower back, are usually scattered, fixed papules or papulovesicles rather than coalescent, dynamic plaques as seen in seborrhea, and lack significant scaling.
- Napkin psoriasis (diaper area psoriasis) can be distinguished from seb derm by its beefy red appearance, sharp circumscription, drier scale, and by the

presence of characteristic seborrhea or psoriatic lesions outside of the diaper area.

- Diaper ICD predominantly affects the convex areas of the diaper areas and typically spares the intertriginous fold where seborrhea is almost always identified.
- In infants, LCH, a potentially fatal malignancy of Langerhans histiocytes, is a feared mimicker of seborrheic dermatitis. LCH typically has a more severe presentation, may be associated with failure to thrive, is treatment refractory, and may present with eroded papules and/or petechiae/purpura. Importantly, the presence of cradle cap does not rule out a diagnosis of LCH because of how ubiquitous cradle cap is in children. Because of the significant implications of a diagnosis of LCH, children with refractory seb derm or seb derm plus failure to thrive should be urgently evaluated by a pediatric dermatologist.

## Work-Up

- Total-body skin examination should be performed to look for characteristic skin lesions elsewhere.
- Adults who present with subacute onset severe seb derm affecting the face and chest should be screened for HIV unless another obvious trigger for development of seborrheic dermatitis is identified (e.g., organ transplant immunosuppression, Parkinson disease)
- Seb derm is generally a clinical diagnosis and rarely is a biopsy required to make the diagnosis. Nevertheless, biopsy should be performed in children in whom there is a concern for LCH.

## Initial Steps in Management

There is no cure for seb derm. The course is chronic with waxing and waning. Failure to emphasize the importance of using a maintenance therapy virtually guarantees disease recurrence and patient dissatisfaction.

Treatments for seb derm are primarily divided into topical antiinflammatory agents and topical antifungals.

## Antifungals

- Seb derm is not considered contagious. A normal body yeast, *Malassezia*, is associated with this eruption, probably secondary to the fact that this yeast in affected patients precipitates an abnormal inflammatory immune response to these yeasts.
  - For truncal seborrhea, topical antifungals formulated either as shampoos or a cream can be used.

In cases where a shampoo is used, the shampoo must be left in contact with the skin for at least 5 minutes. Application of shampoo to the trunk can be drying and therefore regular moisturizer use is recommended.

- Shampoos are preferable in hairy patients and in patients with concomitant scalp and face involvement.
- Azole creams (e.g., ketoconazole 2%, clotrimazole 1%) can be applied twice daily to affected areas; shampoos (e.g. ketoconazole 2%), on the other hand, are used two to three times per week during acute management and once weekly for management and suppression. More frequent application of azole shampoos does not confer additional benefit because the medication binds to hair shafts and is present for around 72 hours after application. OTC azole shampoos (e.g., miconazole) are less effective than prescription ketoconazole shampoo.
  - Azole creams (ketoconazole 2% cream) are typically used preferentially over shampoos in children because creams allow for more focal application and decrease the risk for systemic absorption of the topically applied drug.
  - Oral azoles (e.g., fluconazole 200 mg weekly over 4 weeks) can be considered in patients with severe disease; however, these patients frequently are taking many systemic medications that have cytochrome P45 (CYP) interactions with systemic azoles, making this approach less desirable.
- Ciclopirox is a reasonable second-line antifungal. It is formulated as both a cream and a shampoo. Even though it is equally as effective as topical azoles, it is more likely to cause irritation and is typically more expensive. In patients who are bathed infrequently, ciclopirox shampoo is preferential to ketoconazole as less frequent applications (1 to 2 times/week have been demonstrated to be effective).
- Selenium sulfide (active ingredient in Selsun Blue).
- Zinc pyrithione (active ingredient in Head and Shoulders).

## Antiinflammatories

- Topical corticosteroids are equally as effective and possibly more effective than antifungals, although they are more likely to cause cutaneous adverse effects and more likely to cause early disease rebound after discontinuation.

- Medium-potency topical corticosteroids (e.g., triamcinolone 0.1% cream twice daily) are recommended but only intermittently and for a short course for the chest and back; only low-potency topical corticosteroids (e.g., hydrocortisone 1% or 2.5% cream twice daily) should be used in intertriginous areas.
  - Hairy patients frequently prefer liquid, lotion, or foam formulations of topical steroids, such as fluocinolone 0.01% body oil, because it is easier to apply.
  - Once-daily application of slightly more potent topical corticosteroids, such as mometasone 0.1%, may be helpful for patients who struggle to comply with twice-daily applications.
  - All topical steroids should only be used intermittently and for short courses to avoid side effects.
- Topical calcineurin inhibitors are equally as efficacious as topical corticosteroids; however, they are more expensive and typically require failure of topical corticosteroids before insurance approval.
  - Topical pimecrolimus 0.1% cream is the only calcineurin inhibitor formulated as a cream, which makes it more desirable for application to hairbearing areas; however, it may be too weak for initial treatment of seborrhea in severe cases.
    - Topical tacrolimus 0.1% is equally as potent as triamcinolone 0.1% cream; however, it is only formulated as an ointment, which may be too messy to apply to hairbearing areas.
- Other agents are rarely necessary and lack substantial evidence supporting their use.
  - Crisaborole is only available as an ointment and has not been demonstrated to be particularly efficacious for seb derm.
  - There is not one single active ingredient in Promiseb. It is a combination of nonsteroidal antiinflammatory agents. It is often very expensive but can be considered in refractory cases.

## Warning Signs/Common Pitfalls

There is no cure for seb derm; therefore all patients require maintenance treatment and should be warned that the disease is chronic with waxing and waning.

For seb derm affecting hairbearing areas, cream or liquid or foam (i.e., shampoos, oils, solutions) formulations are preferable to ointments because they are typically easier to spread and more cosmetically acceptable.

Patients with acute-onset of severe and recalcitrant seborrheic dermatitis should undergo HIV testing unless they have been recently diagnosed with Parkinson disease.

Children with refractory seb derm or who have petechiae, purpura, or erosive lesions on examination should be referred urgently to a pediatric dermatologist for evaluation for LCH.

Diapers occlude topical corticosteroids and therefore only low-potency and intermittent topical corticosteroids (e.g., hydrocortisone 2.5% or 1%) should be used in the diaper area.

Checking the patient's medication list for significant CYP interactions is essential before starting an oral azole antifungal.

Patients using antifungal shampoos should alternate each day between shampoos to decrease the likelihood of secondary treatment failure (tachyphylaxis).

## Counseling

You have a rash called "seborrheic dermatitis." It is a form of dandruff that can involve areas of the skin with oil glands, such as the face, ears, scalp, chest, axillary areas, and groin. It is a chronic, recurrent, waxing and waning type of rash, which means that there is no cure. Most importantly, it is a self-limited type of rash, meaning that it will not cause you internal harm. This rash is caused by inflammation caused by your immune system. The exact reason that you have developed this rash is unknown. Some experts think that it develops because your immune system overreacts to fats made by a yeast called "*Malassezia*" that lives on your skin; however, other experts do not think this is the case. Because this is a normal skin yeast, this is not a form of infection and is not contagious.

I have prescribed you an antifungal (yeast) shampoo. You should use this shampoo from the belt line up 3 times per week for 4 weeks. It is important that you let the shampoo remain on your skin for at least 5 minutes before rinsing it out. In 4 weeks, you can decrease the frequency with which you use this shampoo to once per week. It is important that you continue to use this shampoo every week because if you do not, it is likely that the rash will come back. On the days that you do not use the antifungal shampoo, I recommend that you use an OTC shampoo containing either selenium sulfide or zinc pyrithione because these products also have antifungal properties. Examples of brands that contain these ingredients include Selsun Blue and Head & Shoulders. If one of these shampoos that you have been using chronically loses effectiveness, switch to another type of shampoo; always use at least two different types of shampoos, alternating which one you use, during the week to reduce this possibility.

## Polymorphous Light Eruption

### Victoria Stoj and Jun Lu

- Polymorphous light eruption (PMLE) is an idiopathic photodermatosis characterized by acute recurrent polymorphic eruptions (Fig. 3.11).
- Most commonly affected are fair-skinned females in their third decade, but all skin types can be affected. Prevalence is highest between 10 to 21 years of age with an average age of onset of 23 years.
- It is the most common photodermatosis.
  - It is thought to be because of an inflammatory, delayed-type hypersensitivity reaction to a photo-induced endogenous antigen. The photoantigen responsible has yet to be identified.
  - There appears to be a genetic component highlighted by twin studies.
  - UVA radiation, which can penetrate window glass, is most commonly implicated in the pathogenesis of PMLE, but UVB radiation and visible light may also induce PMLE.

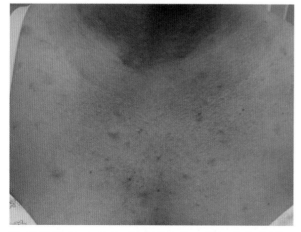

**Fig. 3.11 Polymorphous Light Eruption.** Note photodistribution on the chest. (From the UConn Grand Rounds Collection.)

## Clinical Features

- PMLE most commonly appears in the spring or early summer with typical onset within hours after sunlight exposure.
- It persists for days to weeks before it resolves with good sun protection. If the sun cannot be avoided, PMLE will improve as the summer progresses and the patient becomes tan (a result known as "hardening"). It tends to resolve in the autumn or winter. The lesions do not scar.
- Erythematous papules and papulovesicles are the most common morphologies; however, as its name suggests, PMLE can present with several different morphologies, including erythematous macules, patches, papules, plaques, vesicles, targetoid lesions, and lichenoid plaques.
- The eruption is usually pruritic, which can be painful when scratched. Itch can occur without primary cutaneous lesions. Systemic symptoms are rare.
- The eruption is confined to sun-exposed sites, although it often spares habitually sun-exposed areas like the face and dorsal aspects of the hands because chronic sun exposure in these areas results in tanning and tolerance to light. The most common distribution is on the arms, forearms, legs, chest, and neck.
- Although PMLE is typically recurrent and chronic, continued sun exposure throughout the summer can lead to a hardening of the skin in which increased exposure leads to built-up tolerance and moderation or even resolution of the eruption.

## Differential Diagnosis

- The differential for PMLE includes other photodermatoses such as actinic prurigo, chronic actinic dermatitis, solar urticaria, porphyria cutanea tarda, photo allergy, and variants of lupus erythematosus.
  - Unlike PMLE, actinic prurigo tends to occur in children, characteristically involves the lips, and may last into the winter months.
  - Chronic actinic dermatitis has a male predominance and although it may worsen in the summer, it often persists year-round for years. It is hallmarked by its sharp cutoff at typically clothed sites, such as the shirt line on the nape of the neck.
  - Solar urticaria typically occurs in young adults with a female predominance similar to PMLE; however, the characteristic lesions are urticarial plaques that are evanescent and resolve within 24 hours. Solar

urticaria is distinguished from other photoderma-toses because it characteristically occurs within minutes of sun exposure and is consistently induc-ible with visible light exposure.

- Porphyria cutanea tarda (PCT) often presents with skin fragility, crusts, and scarring. It is identi-fied clinically based on the presence of tense and flaccid bullae on sun-exposed areas (predomi-nantly dorsal hands and forearms) and scarring sequelae, including milia and hypertrichosis. Lab tests will show elevated porphyrins in the urine and stool.
- Photoallergic reactions can occur at any age and typically present as pruritic, eczematous lesions 1 to 2 days after exposure to sunlight in association with an inciting (usually topical) agent. The most common photoallergen is sunscreen. It often re-solves after discontinuing the inciting agent.
- Cutaneous lupus erythematosus (CLE):
  - Early subacute cutaneous lupus erythematosus (SCLE) lesions may appear similar to those of PMLE; however, they are more likely to be an-nular with scale and not as pruritic as those in PMLE. Additionally, although SCLE is photoex-acerbated, it may occur in protected areas (e.g., the trunk). Serologic tests and other associated symptoms will help make the diagnosis.
  - Lupus tumidus is an uncommon variant of lupus erythematosus (LE), rarely associated with systemic symptoms or positive serologic tests. It presents with erythematous, nonscar-ring plaques in sun-exposed areas, but the course is typically longer than PMLE. It affects men and women equally, and biopsy is neces-sary to confirm the diagnosis.

## Work-Up

- Diagnosis is usually made clinically based on patient history and physical examination findings.
- Sometimes a skin biopsy is necessary to exclude other photodermatoses in the differential, particu-larly if CLE cannot be ruled out clinically.
- Provocative phototesting performed by exposing the patient's forearms or neck to suberythemal doses of UVA for 3 to 5 days can elicit a PMLE to confirm the diagnosis. In clinical practice, this is rarely per-formed because it is only available in a small number of centers.

## Initial Steps in Management

### Prevention

- Sun protection is first line.
  - Sun avoidance: Seek shade and avoid peak hours between 10 AM and 2 PM. Avoidance of sunlight even through windows is usually required.
  - Sun block: Broad-spectrum sunblock of at least SPF 30 should be recommended to all patients to help prevent recurring PMLE.
  - Sun-protective clothing: Wearing long sleeves, long plants, and wide-brim hats is recommended.
- For systemic photoprotection, prophylactic regimens before sun exposure are recommended.
  - Beta-carotene, 60 mg three times per day for 2 weeks before sun exposure.
  - Polypodium leucotomos 480 mg daily, split into two doses of 240 mg, continuously.
  - Systemic corticosteroids:
    - Prednisone 20mg per day 2 days before and 2 days during sun exposure.
    - Intramuscular triamcinolone acetonide 0.5 mg/kg several days before sun exposure.
      - Systemic corticosteroids should only be used in select patients who do not have comorbid-ity-related contraindications to their use.
- Hardening can also be induced.
  - Tolerance can be induced by photochemotherapy with PUVA and narrow-band UVB, often given in the early spring two to three times per week for 4 to 6 weeks.

### Treatment

- PMLE typically will resolve on its own over the course of approximately 10 days.
- Oral antihistamines can be helpful to patients with pruritus.
- For mild to moderate PMLE, topical corticosteroids creams can be used.
  - Groups 1 to 3 topical corticosteroid, such as clo-betasol propionate cream .05%, can be applied twice daily for 5 to 7 days.
    - If PMLE affects the face, use group 6 or 7 topi-cal corticosteroids, such as OTC hydrocorti-sone cream.
- For severe cases, a short course of oral corticosteroids may be required for acute episodes of PMLE.
  - Usually, 30 mg prednisone for 4 to 5 days is ade-quate for most severe episodes of PMLE.

- Given the side effect profile of chronic systemic corticosteroid use, frequent courses are contraindicated and discouraged.

## Warning Signs/Common Pitfalls

- Rarely, patients with PMLE have positive antinuclear antibody (ANA) titers, and this subset of patients may be at increased risk for connective tissue disease.
- A positive ANA and photosensitivity rash may make it difficult to distinguish PMLE from lupus.
  - PMLE may precede the development of lupus in some cases, but this relationship has not been adequately studied in long-term follow-up studies.
- Studies have shown positive ANA titers in 3% to 19% of PMLE patients.
- Patients with PMLE and positive ANA titers may be at an increased risk for developing autoimmune disorders; therefore clinical and, when appropriate, laboratory follow-up are recommended.

## Counseling

- PMLE is a hypersensitivity reaction to the sun that should clear on its own over the next couple of weeks. It will not leave permanent scars.
- It is usually chronic, which means it can recur every spring and summer for years.
- Sun protection is the most important preventative treatment, which includes wearing a wide-brimmed hat, protective clothing, and broad-spectrum sunscreens with an SPF of at least 30. Because sunlight through glass can also cause this rash, be careful in the car and indoors near windows.
- Your doctor may prescribe topical corticosteroid cream and oral antihistamines to help with symptoms. In severe cases, you may need to take a short course of oral corticosteroids.
- The condition tends to go away on its own after several years.

# NOTALGIA PARESTHETICA

Katalin Ferenczi

## Clinical Features

Notalgia paresthetica (NP) is a sensory neuropathy that presents as unilateral pruritus involving the upper or mid-back. There is a strong association between NP and significant degenerative or traumatic spinal or musculoskeletal disease and many patients relate a prior history of motor vehicle accident, degenerative disc disease, neck trauma, vertebral fracture, or herniated disc. Degenerative or traumatic changes in the spine or spasms in the paraspinal musculature result in nerve entrapment. Impingement of the spinal nerve roots in the T2 to T6 distribution can lead to alteration of the cutaneous sensory nerves of the upper back and pruritus, which is characteristic of NP.

NP is most common in adults aged between 40 and 80 and is more often seen in women. NP can be associated with multiple endocrine neoplasia type 2a (MEN2a). In this case, it occurs in younger patients and is not associated with underlying spinal or muscular disease.

In some patients, NP can be associated with brachioradial pruritus, another sensory neuropathy. In brachial radial pruritus, patients complain of itching involving the forearms, which is often exacerbated by sun exposure.

NP can persist for many years with periods of remission and flares.

- Patients present with unilateral pruritus affecting the midback or upper back in the distribution of T2 to T6 dermatomes.
- Burning sensation, dysesthesia (hypoesthesia or hyperesthesia), or pain may be associated.
- A hyperpigmented patch is often seen involving the scapular area, representing postinflammatory pigmentary change secondary to chronic rubbing and scratching.
- Lichenification and/or macular amyloidosis (MA) can also develop as a result of chronic rubbing or friction.

## Differential Diagnosis

The differential diagnosis for NP includes tinea versicolor (TV), LSC, MA, and PIH.

- TV, also known as "pityriasis versicolor," is a common skin condition characterized by hypopigmented or hyperpigmented macules and/or patches involving the chest and back. It is caused by *Malassezia*, a type of yeast found on the surface of the skin. Microscopic examination of skin scraping for KOH can help with the diagnosis. TV responds well to topical or oral antifungal treatment.
- LSC, or neurodermatitis, is a skin condition characterized by thickened plaques and pronounced skin lines occurring as a result of chronic itching and scratching. LSC is typically worsened by scratching. Treatment consists of avoiding constantly rubbing the affected areas, moisturizing, and applying topical steroids.

- MA is another skin condition that is the result of chronic scratching because of itching. It can occur in association with NP. In fact, some consider that MA involving the back is part of the spectrum of NP. It presents as a hyperpigmented patch demonstrating a rippled pattern on the upper back and sometimes the arms. The amyloid deposits are thought to be keratinocyte derived, likely in this scenario because of trauma such as rubbing and scratching. Biopsy of MA shows the presence of amyloid deposition in the dermis. Treatment can be challenging because macular amyloidosis is very resistant to topical therapy. UVB light therapy can provide some relief.
- PIH is a common condition that occurs after an inflammatory skin disorder, skin irritation, or injury. It is more common in patients with darker skin types. It presents as a hyperpigmented patch that can affect any area of the body. Depending on the etiology, management could include observation, hydroquinone, azelaic acid, or topical steroids. If the precipitating rash or injury has resolved, PIH is asymptomatic.

## Work-Up

Diagnosis of NP is typically made through history and physical examination.

- A thorough history is critical and should include history of motor vehicle accident, cervical disc disease, neck trauma, vertebral fracture, degenerative disc disease, or musculoskeletal conditions. Physical examination should include an examination of the skin in the scapular area and assessment for the presence or absence of cervical muscle spasm/tenderness.
- Spinal imaging is not necessary, unless the patient has other neurologic or musculoskeletal symptoms. Cervical or thoracic radiographs or magnetic resonance imaging (MRI) should be a consideration in patients with a history of spinal trauma or injury and spine symptoms.
- Biopsy is usually not needed in cases with classic presentation, but it can be done if other conditions are considered in the differential diagnosis. Biopsy in NP is nonspecific and may show dermal melanophages, a finding that is consistent with PIH. In some cases, amyloid deposition in the dermis may be seen.
- In pediatric patients with NP, their calcitonin level may be obtained to rule out the possibility of underlying MEN2a.

## Initial Steps in Management

NP is difficult to treat because typical pruritus treatments, such as antihistamines or topical steroids, are not effective. Some topical therapies can help temporarily alleviate cutaneous symptoms; however, they often fail once the treatment is stopped and systemic medications become necessary. If there is evidence of cervicothoracic or musculoskeletal disease, treatment should be aimed at managing the underlying condition because this approach results in significant improvement or resolution of the symptoms.

### Topical and Oral Treatments

- Topical capsaicin 0.025% cream (a derivative of chili peppers) can be applied 4 to 5 times a day for 1 week, then 4 to 5 times a day for 3 to 6 weeks. Alternatively, an 8% capsaicin patch could also temporarily help with the itch sensation. Symptoms, however, return after cessation of the treatment. Alert patients to a burning sensation that might be felt when first applying the capsaicin. Also educate patients to wash their hands after applying. Other topical options could include a eutectic mixture of lidocaine 2.5% and prilocaine 2.5% (EMLA) cream used twice daily, pramoxine cream, or a camphor/menthol combination lotion.
- Botulinum toxin type A injections in a single subcutaneous administration and narrow-band UVB light therapy three times a week have been shown to result in improvement of the symptoms.
- Systemic medications that may help alleviate symptoms are gabapentin, pregabalin, oxcarbazepine, and amitriptyline. Gabapentin is given at a dose between 300 mg and 600 mg per day. Pregabalin is a new oral medication, related to gabapentin. The dose is 50 to 75 mg, and it can be increased up to 300 mg a day.

### Treatment of the Underlying Spinal and Musculoskeletal Disease

- Nerve block, such as a paravertebral local anesthetic block with bupivacaine and corticosteroids, can be used to treat the underlying spinal and musculoskeletal disease.
- Another option is surgical decompression of the paraspinal nerve.
- Osteopathic manipulative treatment, acupuncture, physiotherapy, and transcutaneous electrical nerve stimulation (TENS) can also be used.

- Electrical muscle stimulation (EMS) of the neck and exercises aimed to strengthen cervical and back muscles and extend the spine can also be useful.

## Warning Signs/Common Pitfalls

- The intense pruritus and discomfort associated with NP may negatively impact the patient's quality of life. The lack of definitive treatments and unpredictable, chronic course can lead to ongoing frustration.
- In a subset of patients, certain activities, such as forward bending of the head or forward movement of the arms (such as typing), can worsen muscle spasm and NP symptoms.
- Intense scratching can sometimes lead to the development of erosions and secondary infections.

## Counseling

You have a condition called "notalgia paresthetica," which is a chronic but benign disease that can be challenging to treat. It is important to try to avoid constant scratching and rubbing of the affected area because this will result in the itch-scratch cycle that is very difficult to break.

The course can be unpredictable and it may last for years, with periods of remission and flares of itching and discomfort. There are currently no specific targeted therapies available, but certain topical or oral medications can help reduce your symptoms. If you have any evidence of spinal or musculoskeletal disease, in that case, management should be aimed at treating the underlying condition because it can lead to significant improvement.

The itching you experience may become severe. Let your physician know if it begins to negatively impact your quality of life so that your treatment plan can be adjusted accordingly.

## TINEA CORPORIS

**Campbell Stewart**

### Clinical Features

Tinea is caused by dermatophytes, which are fungi attracted to the skin. The disease is typically broken down by body site: corporis for the body, manuum for the hands, pedis for the feet, and cruris for the groin folds. The clinical appearance of tinea can vary based on these body sites. Tinea is commonly referred to as ringworm, athlete's foot, or jock itch by patients. The three most common causes of tinea include the genera *Trichophyton*, *Microsporum*, and *Epidermophyton*.

- The classic clinical features of tinea corporis include an annular red or pink plaque with an elevated border and central clearing. The plaques should be scaly, particularly around the border.
- In tinea manuum, the hands may take on a more diffuse scaling appearance with a background of sharply demarcated erythema. Often, only the dominant hand is affected, and this is likely from scratching of affected feet (tinea pedis). This process creates the clinical picture of two-foot, one-hand tinea. Annular plaques may also occur and extend up the wrists and arms.
- Tinea cruris presents as bright red annular plaques that affect the medial and lateral groin folds, classically sparing the scrotum, penis, and female genitalia. These plaques can extend onto the buttocks as well. The fungus may present as scattered red papules or plaques with only an almost imperceptible scale or no scale at all. Other forms show maceration, vesicles, or pustules.
- In tinea pedis, the lesions appear as diffuse scaling that lines the plantar surface and typically spares the dorsal foot, causing a moccasin distribution. Annular aspects are common on the medial and lateral aspects of the feet. Occasionally, petechiae may be seen. Interdigital scale is white and macerated. It is most seen between the fourth and fifth digits on the toes. Tinea can coinfect with yeast and bacteria, particularly in the web spaces. Tinea pedis is often associated with onychomycosis/tinea unguium (see Chapter 16, Onychomycosis).
- Bullous tinea is an uncommon presentation. It can present with bullae, vesicles, or pustules, often within a background of a more classic scaling patch or plaque. It is more common in immunosuppressed patients.
- Majocchi granuloma is a fungal folliculitis caused by dermatophytes. It is normally caused by the application of medium- to high-potency steroids applied to a rash, but disruption of the follicles from shaving (legs, beard) can induce it as well. It is characterized by studded pustules that often arise in a broader pruritic patch or plaque.

## Differential Diagnosis

The clinical differential diagnosis depends on the body location. For tinea corporis, the differential includes granuloma annulare, TV, psoriasis, and eczema.

- Granuloma annulare is an idiopathic inflammatory reaction pattern in the skin that presents with annular plaques without scale. A KOH prep can help distinguish these, as can skin biopsy.
- TV normally presents as a disseminated hyperpigmented or hypopigmented macular eruption with minimal scale on the trunk, which may involve the intertriginous sites as well. A KOH test will show scattered yeast and pseudohyphae (the so-called "spaghetti and meatballs" pattern). A biopsy with a periodic acid–Schiff (PAS) stain will also distinguish TV from tinea corporis.
- Psoriasis presents with sharply demarcated bright red plaques with adherent silvery scale. Normally, it affects extensor surfaces, such as the elbows and knees; however, it can impact multiple body sites. A KOH prep will distinguish these two entities, as can a skin biopsy with a PAS stain.
- Eczema has a highly variable clinical presentation. Classically it presents as patches and plaques with fine scale, lichenification, erosions, and crust if it is traumatized or secondarily infected. These lesions are often distributed in adults along the neck, antecubital fossae, and popliteal fossae but can be widespread. Patients who use topical steroids chronically for eczema treatment can easily develop a secondary fungal infection such as tinea. KOH is negative in the setting of eczema.

For tinea manuum, the differential includes hand dermatitis secondary to eczema, contact dermatitis, and palmar psoriasis.

- In hand dermatitis caused by eczema, there is diffuse erythema and scale that lacks the annular aspect of tinea manuum. Hand eczema shows fissuring and hyperkeratosis, and although it can be very itchy in the acute stages, it is often painful (because of fissuring) and interferes with daily activities. Dyshidrotic eczema causes tender deep papulovesicles on the palmar aspects of the hands and fingers. A KOH prep is negative in the setting of hand eczema.
- Contact dermatitis can cause a primary hand dermatitis; however, it often presents as an exacerbation of underlying AD on the hands. It is caused by personal care products, excessive hand washing, and lack of emollient use. Patch testing can be performed to identify triggers. A KOH prep is negative in the setting of contact dermatitis.
- Palmar psoriasis is challenging to differentiate from tinea manuum if there are no other body sites affected by psoriasis. It presents as painful, red, hyperkeratotic plaques with fissures and pustules. KOH prep and skin biopsy with a PAS stain can differentiate these entities.

Similarly, the differential diagnosis for tinea pedis is contact dermatitis, psoriasis (particularly if there are nail changes), and plantar eczema. These entities can be distinguished as previously described.

The differential diagnosis for tinea cruris includes erythrasma, candidiasis, ACD/ICD, inverse psoriasis, and intertrigo.

- Erythrasma typically presents as well-demarcated, hyperpigmented or erythematous, reddish-brown patches. There can be accentuation of skin lines and some fine scale. A Wood lamp examination should reveal a coral red/pink color. A KOH prep is negative in erythrasma. Erythrasma can coinfect with tinea; therefore a positive diagnostic test for one entity does not exclude the other.
- Candidiasis normally presents with a deeper red plaque with satellite lesions and pustules. A KOH can be performed to detect yeast forms as opposed to the hyphae seen in tinea. Fungal culture can also be performed to differentiate from tinea.
- Contact dermatitis can be either allergic or irritant in nature and is not uncommon in the groin or perineum. Common causes include fragrances, household cleansers, elastic products, and clothing dyes. It presents as geometric, well demarcated, and classically symmetric patches and plaques with scale. In acute forms, vesicles may be present. A KOH is negative in ACD/ICD. A skin biopsy with a PAS stain can also help distinguish it from tinea.
- Inverse psoriasis presents with well-demarcated red plaques with wet, macerated scale in intertriginous sites. Fissuring can occur. It typically lacks the annular appearance of tinea cruris. A KOH examination and skin biopsy can be used to distinguish these two entities.

## Work-Up

A thorough physical examination to look for other sites of involvement is essential. For example, if a patient presents with only a single hand involved with an itching rash, it is important to examine their feet and groin/buttocks because the patient may not connect the separate sites himself or herself.

A KOH prep can be performed in the office to confirm the diagnosis. This test is best performed by lightly swiping the advancing border of the lesion with an alcohol swab and then immediately using a 15-blade off the handle to lightly lift the scale and spread it onto a slide. KOH should be dropped on (do not flood the slide) and the slide coverslipped and allowed to sit for at least 10 minutes. Examination should reveal branching septate hyphae. If not present, the KOH prep should be allowed to sit for another 10 minutes. Gently heating the specimen can accelerate the reaction; however, direct heat can ruin the prep by crystallizing the solution.

A culture for fungus can be sent to a microbiology lab. For this test, scraping the advancing border of a lesion (without the alcohol prep) and placing loose scale into a sterile urine cup is sufficient. Culture takes several weeks to give a definitive result. This test carries the advantage of providing a species of fungus, and if necessary, sensitivities to antifungal medications.

A skin biopsy can be performed to confirm the diagnosis. A punch is preferred in light of the inflammatory disorders in the clinical differential. The sample may not reveal significant changes; however, a PAS stain can easily highlight hyphae if present. Be sure to notify your pathologist that you are considering tinea as a diagnosis to ensure the PAS stain is performed.

## Initial Steps in Management
### General Management Comments

A KOH test is a simple way to provide an immediate diagnosis. Do not skip this step in favor of trials of treatment because this can lead to a delay in diagnosis and worsening of the patient's eruption.

### Recommended Initial Regimen

A 4-week course of topical ketoconazole (applied twice daily) to the affected lesions is normally curative. It is important to treat around the lesion to manage the subclinical aspect of the disease. Other topical options include clotrimazole, miconazole, oxiconazole, sulconazole, sertaconazole, luliconazole, terbinafine, and ciclopirox.

### Partial but Inadequate Response

What to do if there is a partial, but inadequate response after a 4-week trial of topical antifungal monotherapy:
- Make sure the diagnosis is correct. A KOH may be limited after a 4-week trial of topical antifungals, especially if the disease involves the hair follicles. A culture should be performed.
- Two weeks of oral terbinafine daily (250 mg for adults) is normally curative unless the patient has widespread disease, is immunosuppressed, or has Majocchi granuloma.
- Oral itraconazole is a suitable alternative, as long as it does not interact with the patient's other medications. It is taken as 100 mg daily for 2 weeks or 200 mg daily for 1 week.

### Continued Inadequate Response

What to do if the response continues to be inadequate:
- A biopsy to confirm diagnosis is recommended. If the biopsy shows hyphae after the above treatments, consider longer courses or long courses of pulsed oral agents, such as terbinafine or itraconazole, coupled with the regular use of topicals. The patient should also be questioned about the possibility of an untreated vector in the home (i.e., a pet, child, or partner), as well as exposures outside of the home, such as the gym.
- If the rash is responsive, but persistent itch is a concern, low-potency topical steroid (hydrocortisone 1%–2.5% cream) may be used in addition to antifungal treatment, but no medium- or high-potency steroid is recommended.

### Other Treatment Options

Oral fluconazole may also be used at 50 to 100 mg daily for up to 4 weeks.

Oral griseofulvin may be used but should be dosed at least at 20 mg/kg per day in partially responsive disease. Normally, 6 to 12 weeks is needed for stubborn lesions.

## Warning Signs/Common Pitfalls
- A warning sign for tinea is an annular, pruritic rash, with scale and central clearing.
- Skipping a KOH test, or a culture if KOH materials are unavailable, is a common pitfall.
- Another pitfall is treating tinea with a combination cream such as clotrimazole-betamethasone. These

combinations provide enough local steroid-induced immunosuppression to allow the fungi to persist and spread, without an effective counter from the antifungal. They can also give the appearance of improvement without clearing the infection. There is no clinical role for the combination agents if tinea is suspected or diagnosed. The steroid is potent enough to induce Majocchi granuloma (tinea invading the hair follicle), which generally needs treatment with oral agents.

## Counseling

You have a superficial infection of the skin called "tinea." Tinea is caused by a fungus. It is very rare that this fungus is dangerous or life-threatening; however, the infections are often persistent and recurrent. If you are immunosuppressed, then it can become more serious. Similarly, if you have diabetes, it is important that we treat you quickly to avoid any possible secondary infection from bacteria.

The fungus is very contagious and easily spreads between humans in close contact and those who share common bathing areas. Certain forms of the fungi can cross between you and your pets so if you are a pet owner, it is important to get them checked by a veterinarian.

Tinea can usually be treated with OTC topical products, such as clotrimazole or terbinafine creams. If these agents are not effective, we can prescribe antifungal creams as well, such as ketoconazole. It is essential to apply these creams twice a day for 4 full weeks to see results, and all areas that are affected must be treated at the same time. If a family member also has tinea, you both should be treated at the same time to prevent reinfection (pets included).

If topical creams do not work, then oral medication can be used. Oral terbinafine can be taken once daily for 14 days to clear most infections. Oral itraconazole may also be used. These pills are normally well tolerated; however, they can interact with other medications you may take. Blood work may be needed for extended courses of treatment to make sure your blood counts, liver, and kidney are tolerating the medication.

If your rash is not responsive to these treatments, further testing may be needed, including a culture or biopsy of your affected skin.

# PEMPHIGUS

## Clinical Features

Pemphigus is an autoimmune condition that manifests as blistering of the skin (intraepidermal) and/or mucous membranes.

- This condition most often appears in mid- to late adult life, with onset ranging from 40 to 70 years of age.
- There is a slightly increased prevalence in female patients (sex ratio 1.33 to 2.25).

Severity of this condition ranges from nearly asymptomatic to pruritic to excruciatingly painful and potentially life-threatening; generalized involvement can lead to protein and fluid loss, serious infection, sepsis, and death.

There are several subtypes of pemphigus; the two most common subtypes are pemphigus vulgaris (PV) and pemphigus foliaceus (PF).

### Pemphigus Vulgaris

#### Savannah Alvarado and Jun Lu

PV can involve both cutaneous (Fig. 3.12) and mucosal surfaces (Fig. 3.13). Mucosal lesions are often the presenting sign and can persist for months as the only sign of disease.

- Lesions can be large, flaccid blisters or painful or pruritic erosions of various sizes.
- The oropharynx is the most commonly involved mucosal site. Patients with oropharyngeal lesions may be unable to tolerate food and liquids, leading to

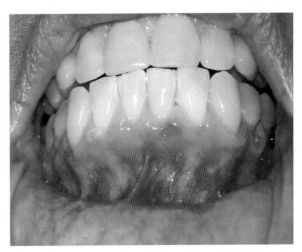

**Fig. 3.12 Pemphigus Vulgaris Presenting as Desquamative Gingivitis.** (From the UConn Grand Rounds Collection.)

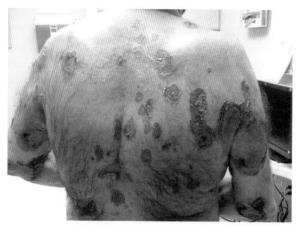

**Fig. 3.13** Pemphigus Vulgaris Presented With Flaccid Bullae And Denuded Epidermis. (From the UConn Grand Rounds Collection.)

significant complications requiring hospitalization for resuscitation.

- Other common mucosal sites include the nasal and laryngeal mucosa.
- Less common mucosal sites include the vulvovaginal, ocular, and gastrointestinal mucosa.

There are several other findings seen in patients with PV. Patients often demonstrate the ability to cause a blister at a distant site (Nikolsky sign) or easily extend a blister (Asboe-Hansen) by applying pressure or friction to the skin. Roughly 5% of patients with PV will experience hair loss, which is generally temporary.

The prognosis of PV varies based on the extent of cutaneous and mucosal involvement.

- In some patients, PV is potentially fatal without treatment. Patients with comorbidities are at a significantly higher risk for developing serious complications.
- With treatment, mortality rate is 0.023 deaths per 100,000 cases.
- Patients may achieve long-term remission with few or no flares.
- Some patients require long-term therapy

## Pemphigus Foliaceus

PF is a milder variant of pemphigus that affects only cutaneous surfaces and does not involve mucosal surfaces. Patients with PF tend to have focal, rather than generalized, disease.

- Lesions can be small, coalescing blisters or painful, crusted, or scaly erosions (Fig. 3.14).

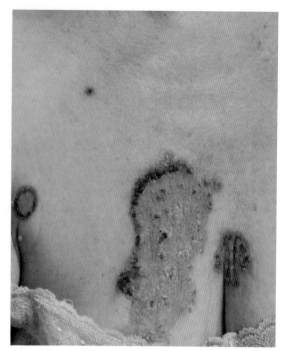

**Fig. 3.14** Pemphigus Foliaceous. Notice the cornflake like scale. (From the UConn Grand Rounds Collection.)

- Lesions generally develop over erythematous skin.
- Lesions commonly appear on the face, scalp, and upper trunk.
- The prognosis is better than in PV.

## Differential Diagnosis

The differential diagnosis should include other variants of pemphigus (endemic pemphigus, immunoglobulin A [IgA] pemphigus, paraneoplastic pemphigus, neonatal pemphigus, drug-induced pemphigus, and diet-related pemphigus) and drug-induced or infectious blistering disorders. Laboratory analysis, as well as the physical examination, can help to distinguish pemphigus from other blistering disorders. It can usually be clinically distinguished from the autoimmune subepidermal disease BP because the blisters in pemphigoid are tense rather than flaccid, pruritic rather than painful, and more commonly diagnosed in a more elderly population.

## Work-Up

The two main components of work-up for patients with suspected pemphigus are histology and IF/ELISA. Work-up requires one biopsy from an active lesion (used for histology) and either an additional biopsy from a perilesional site (used for DIF) or a sample of the patient's serum (used for IIF or ELISA).

- Histology from an active lesion will demonstrate separation of keratinocytes within the epidermis (acantholysis), forming an intraepidermal blister.
- DIF on a perilesional biopsy will demonstrate the presence of antibodies targeting the surface of keratinocytes.
  - DIF on a biopsy from an active lesion can produce a false negative result.
- IIF or ELISA will detect autoantibodies to desmoglein 1 and desmoglein 3 in the patient's serum.
  - This provides a quantitative measure of autoantibody levels (desmoglein 1 and desmoglein 3). Although high antibody levels do not provide reliable information regarding prognosis, very low or absent antibodies indicate a favorable prognosis for remission.
  - ELISA has a higher sensitivity; therefore it might be a better test when no or few active lesions are present.
  - ELISA can be used to distinguish PV (desmoglein 1 and 3) from PF (desmoglein 1 only) because it provides specific information regarding the nature of autoantibodies.

As always, histology and IF should be used in combination with clinical presentation to make the most accurate and clinically significant diagnosis.

## Initial Steps in Management

There is currently no consensus on optimal initial management of pemphigus. In general, patients with focal disease can be treated with topical steroids, whereas patients with widespread disease require systemic treatment and should be immediately referred to a dermatologist. Patients with PV generally require systemic therapy at presentation because of the severity of oropharyngeal involvement and the high likelihood of generalized involvement.

Corticosteroid therapy is very effective in treating pemphigus and is the mainstay of medical management, although there is an increasing trend to start all PV patients on rituximab at the time of diagnosis because of its efficacy, superior safety profile when compared with long-term systemic corticosteroids, and possible disease-modifying properties.

- Prednisone dosing is initiated with 0.5 to 1.0 mg/kg per day and patients are monitored for response within 2 to 3 weeks.

- Administration can be split into BID or TID dosing in patients who fail to respond to QD dosing.

In severe cases (including severe mucous membrane involvement) and in cases where steroids cannot be easily weaned, rituximab is the first-line steroid-sparing agent.

- Rituximab is a monoclonal antibody that targets CD20 on B cells.
  - Rituximab is well tolerated but requires IV administration, which is not available to all patients.
    - Our recommended dosing of rituximab is 375 mg/m$^2$ per week for 4 weeks.
  - Rituximab's effects take around 2 months to work and last for around 6 months.
    - Redosing rituximab every 6 months is recommended by some authorities.

Local therapy can be used in addition to systemic treatment.

- Potent topical corticosteroids can be applied to highly involved sites.
- Intralesional triamcinolone injection can be used for particularly severe or persistent lesions.
- Swish and spit preparations can be made for patients with oropharyngeal involvement.

If patients are unable to adequately control their condition on minimal systemic corticosteroid therapy (5–10 mg/day) or if they are poor candidates for corticosteroid therapy, alternative treatments can be added on or used as a substitute.

- As previously mentioned, rituximab is the first-line steroid-sparing agent for PV.
- Mycophenolate mofetil, azathioprine, or methotrexate are alternatives to rituximab that are available to be taken by mouth.
- IVIG or plasmapheresis can be considered in very severe cases and/or in patients who cannot undergo immune suppression.

In patients who demonstrate an adequate response to medication, the dose can be tapered by 0.25 mg/kg per day. Adequate response to therapy is defined as:

- 7 or more days without new onset lesions
- A negative result for the Nikolsky sign
- The healing of active lesions

When attempting to taper a patient on corticosteroids, maintain the full dose of the adjunctive medication. Consider tapering adjunctive therapy only if the patient's disease continues to respond well on minimal or no corticosteroids.

Patients on these medications need to be closely monitored for adverse effects of medication.

- Common side effects of chronic systemic corticosteroid therapy include cardiovascular, hematologic, orthopedic, metabolic, and neurologic effects.
- Severe infection and sepsis may also occur.
- Patients taking oral steroid preparations may contract thrush.

It is also important to discuss birth control with patients because many of these medications are highly teratogenic. These patients require frequent lab monitoring according to medication regimen and comorbid conditions.

## Warning Signs/Common Pitfalls

Several classic associations with pemphigus include:
- Myasthenia gravis and/or thymoma
- Personal history of autoimmune disease (thyroid, rheumatoid arthritis, diabetes mellitus 1)
- History of autoimmune disease in a first-degree relative Management of associated conditions is not associated with improvement in pemphigus.

Pemphigus can also mimic other conditions.
- It can resemble drug eruptions, such as Stevens-Johnson syndrome and toxic epidermal necrolysis (see Chapter 18).
- It can mimic infectious causes of blistering, such as bullous impetigo and Staphylococcal scalded skin syndrome.
- It can look like BP and other variants of pemphigus, such as paraneoplastic pemphigus associated with internal malignancies.

Providers must use both clinical presentation and laboratory analysis (histology, IF, and ELISA) to correctly distinguish between these conditions. Referral to a dermatologist for this work-up and management is recommended.

## Counseling

Your blistering is caused by an autoimmune disorder, which means that your immune system is attacking cells in your own skin as if these cells were dangerous to the body.

If you develop a blister, you should gently clean the area well with soap and water and puncture the blister with a clean needle that has been boiled. You should leave the skin on top of the blister intact because it will act as protection for the sensitive skin under the blister.

Afterwards, apply clean petroleum jelly to the area to keep the skin moist. You can apply a small amount of topical steroid directly to the affected area twice daily.

If you have blisters in your mouth, you should avoid eating hot (temperature) or spicy foods, as well as foods with sharp edges (like chips). It is important that you maintain great oral hygiene to prevent infections in your mouth. Brush your teeth using a bland toothpaste twice daily and floss between your teeth at least once daily. If you frequently get blisters in your mouth, you can use a topical steroid (gel or mouth rinse) two to three times daily to aid in healing and preventing new blisters from forming. If the blisters in your mouth are very painful, you can use a gel or solution to help numb the area.

It is important that you protect yourself from sunlight because UV radiation from the sun can worsen your blistering. Make sure you wear sunscreen and protective clothing on a daily basis; you are regularly exposed to the sun, even if you are not sitting in direct sunlight.

The medications that you take for your blisters can cause dangerous side effects. If you experience any of the following, you should contact your doctor immediately:
- Fever
- Rapid worsening of your blistering or sloughing of skin
- Changes in your vision
- Pregnancy

## PITYRIASIS ROSEA

**Sonal Muzumdar and Jun Lu**

### Clinical Features

- Pityriasis rosea is a common papulosquamous skin disease, with an estimated incidence between 0.5% and 2.0%. It most frequently affects young adults between 15 to 30 years of age but may be seen in any age group.
- Although pityriasis rosea can occur at any time of year, it is most commonly seen in the winter months.
- Prodromal symptoms may precede pityriasis rosea in more than two-thirds of cases. Common prodromal symptoms include fever, malaise, sore throat, and lymphadenopathy.
- The etiology remains unknown but the seasonal presentation suggests the possibility of an infectious etiology.

- In classic cases, pityriasis rosea initially presents with a 2 to 10 cm round, erythematous (salmon to pink in color), scaly patch on the trunk or proximal extremities, which is called the "herald patch" (Fig. 3.15).
  - One to two weeks after the appearance of the herald patch, patients develop an eruption of macules and papules over the trunk, neck, and proximal extremities. This eruption is distributed symmetrically along Langer lines of cleavage and classically resembles a Christmas tree in distribution.
  - Lesions demonstrate light scaling. Scale is classically adherent at the periphery of the lesion and lifted up towards the center in a collarette pattern.
  - In approximately 25% of patients, lesions are pruritic.
  - The eruption typically lasts less than 8 weeks before resolving.
  - Most patients only get pityriasis rosea once in their lives.

## Differential Diagnosis

The differential diagnosis for pityriasis rosea includes psoriasis, eczema (particularly nummular eczema), pityriasis lichenoides, and secondary syphilis.

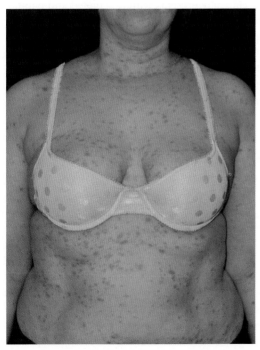

**Fig. 3.15** Pityriasis Rosea. (Courtesy Justin Finch, MD.)

- Pityriasis rosea can be differentiated from psoriasis by lesion location, lesion morphology, and associated findings.
  - In psoriasis, the extensor surfaces and scalp are classically involved. In contrast, pityriasis rosea typically presents on the trunk.
  - Although the lesions in pityriasis rosea are associated with a light, often peripheral scale, those in psoriasis typically have thicker, silvery, adherent scale.
  - Psoriasis may be associated with arthritis, as well as nail findings such as pitting, nail bed hemorrhages, and oil drop spots.
- Pityriasis rosea can be differentiated from nummular eczema by lesion location and morphology.
  - Lesions of nummular eczema are more commonly found on the arms and legs compared with the primarily truncal involvement of pityriasis rosea.
  - Lesions in nummular eczema are typically pruritic and may ooze liquid or have crusting.
- Pityriasis rosea can be differentiated from pityriasis lichenoides by lesion morphology.
  - Pityriasis lichenoides classically presents with a sudden-onset eruption of bright red papules, which then may ulcerate and develop scale. Lesions may coalesce into a widespread rash. Multiple stages of lesions are often present at a given time.
- Pityriasis rosea can be differentiated from secondary syphilis by lesion location, lesion morphology, and associated symptoms.
  - In secondary syphilis, the palms and soles are commonly affected. In contrast, the eruption of pityriasis rosea typically spares the acral surfaces and is classically distributed on the trunk and proximal upper extremities.
  - The lesions of pityriasis rosea are papulosquamous, whereas those of secondary syphilis are polymorphous.
  - Secondary syphilis may have a number of manifestations, including mucocutaneous lesions, alopecia, and condyloma lata. These are not present in pityriasis rosea.

## Work-Up

- Pityriasis rosea is usually diagnosed based on clinical presentation. Patients typically present with the features previously described.

- Dermoscopy may also aid in diagnosis. Under dermoscopy, lesions present with a yellow background, loosely arranged pinpoint vessels, and peripheral scale.
- Rarely, a biopsy is undertaken if the presentation is atypical. Histologically, it demonstrates a spongiotic dermatitis with mounds of parakeratosis and extravasated red blood cells.

## Initial Steps in Management

- Pityriasis rosea is a self-limiting condition which typically resolves within eight weeks even without treatment.
- Antihistamines and topical or oral corticosteroids may be used for symptomatic treatment in patients complaining of pruritus.
- Pregnant patients with pityriasis rosea should be counseled on the risks of the disease and monitored closely throughout their pregnancies.

## Warning Signs/Common Pitfalls

- Pityriasis rosea may present atypically in as many as 20% of cases. Common atypical forms to consider include pediatric pityriasis rosea, forms with atypical lesion location, forms with atypical lesion morphology, and forms with atypical disease course.
  - Papular lesions are more common in pediatric pityriasis rosea. Lesions erupt approximately 4 days after the appearance of the herald patch and resolve in approximately 2 weeks.
  - Forms with atypical lesion location may be unilateral, flexural, or acral.
  - Forms with atypical lesion morphology may be erythema multiforme-like, papular or vesicular, and/or purpuric or hemorrhagic.
  - Forms with an atypical disease course may be relapsing, recurrent, or persistent.
- In pregnancy, pityriasis rosea may lead to premature delivery or fetal demise. Pregnant women with pityriasis rosea should be monitored closely by their obstetrician and counseled about the risks of pityriasis rosea.

## Counseling

You have a condition called "pityriasis rosea." This is a benign condition that usually resolves on its own. Most patients get better within 8 weeks without any treatment. Nevertheless, if you are uncomfortable or itchy, we can treat you with steroids or antihistamines to make you more comfortable until the rash resolves. Although the etiology of pityriasis rosea remains a mystery, it is not contagious and therefore you cannot pass it on to those around you. Most people only get this condition once in their lives. If your rash persists beyond 8 weeks, you should contact your physician for further evaluation.

# CONFLUENT AND RETICULATED PAPILLOMATOSIS

## Clinical Features

Confluent and reticulated papillomatosis (CARP) is a disorder of keratinization that presents with asymptomatic, reticulated (configured in a net like pattern), warty papules coalescing into plaques that affect, in descending order of frequency, the trunk, axilla, and neck.

- It affects both men and women and presents as early as adolescence.
- Characteristic lesions typically have overlying epidermal changes (i.e., scaling, flaking).
- It is typically responsive to antibiotics; however, it runs a chronic course and frequently recurs on treatment discontinuation.

The presence of the following criteria is suggestive of a diagnosis of CARP:

- It clinically presents with reticulated and papillomatous, scaly, brown macules/papules and patches/plaques.
- Characteristic lesions involve the trunk (typically above the umbilicus), neck, and/or flexural areas.
- Lesions are either negative for fungi on KOH examination or do not respond to an appropriate course of antifungals.
- Lesions are responsive to antibiotics.

## Differential Diagnosis

The differential for CARP is TV, acanthosis nigricans (AN), Darier disease, and other more rare disorders of keratinization, which will be grouped for the purposes of this chapter.

- TV is distinguished from CARP because: 1) lesions are frequently hypopigmented and most visible during summertime but look more fawn-colored in the winter; 2) lesions are collections of scaly macules and patches that are not warty in appearance; 3) KOH staining of a skin scraping from TV lesions demonstrate *Malassezia sp.*; and 4) lesions are responsive to topical and systemic azole antifungals.

- AN is more common than CARP and therefore CARP is often initially misdiagnosed as AN.
  - CARP is distinguished from AN because it affects the trunk and potentially the axilla and/or neck, whereas AN typically spares the trunk and tends to involve body folds, and CARP is responsive to antibiotics. Histologic examination does not reliably distinguish between the two.
- Darier disease is a genetic condition characterized by the development of greasy, warty lesions in a seborrheic distribution. It can be distinguished from CARP based on family history (autosomal dominant inheritance); widespread distribution; lesional appearance (not reticulated in pattern/distribution, has overlying greasy scale); and steroid responsiveness.
- There are other rare disorders of keratinization (Dowling-Degos disease, Galli-Galli) that can clinically mimic CARP and are typically considered in patients with a family history of these conditions or in patients diagnosed with CARP who fail to respond to multiple rounds of antibiotics and systemic retinoids.

## Work-Up

CARP is diagnosed clinically. No specific work-up is required to make a diagnosis of CARP. Similarly, because CARP is a skin-limited condition, no additional work-up is required once a diagnosis of CARP is made.

## Initial Steps in Management

Oral antibiotics are the treatment of choice for CARP. Their presumed mechanism of action is that they kill *Dietzia sp.*, the gram-positive bacteria pathogen implicated in CARP development.

- Minocycline 50 mg by mouth BID for 6 weeks is the initial treatment of choice. Many patients will respond in this timeframe; however, they relapse after discontinuation is common.
  - Patients should be counseled about minocycline-associated risks, including drug hypersensitivity, drug-induced lupus, vestibular dysfunction, and dyspigmentation.
- Patients who fail minocycline or who are intolerant/allergic to the tetracycline class can be started on azithromycin 500 mg TIW for 3 weeks.
- Patients who are antibiotic nonresponders or relapse quickly can be managed with systemic retinoids. Because isotretinoin is a federally regulated medication,

patients who may benefit from it must be referred to a prescriber that is registered with iPledge, the program that regulates isotretinoin use.

## Warning Signs/Common Pitfalls

The biggest pitfall when managing CARP is failing to reconsider the diagnosis after patients have failed multiple rounds of antibiotics and/or systemic retinoids. Both AN and genetic disorders of keratinization clinically mimic CARP and should be considered when patients are nonresponders to conventional therapy.

Older literature suggests that CARP is fungal mediated and recommends treatment with antifungals. This is no longer recommended and will result in treatment failure.

## Counseling

You have confluent and reticulated papillomatosis. This condition is caused by a bacterium that lives on the skin called "*Dietzia*." This condition only affects your skin and is not an infection, meaning it is unlikely to be spread from person to person. Additionally, it is a chronic condition, which means that it frequently comes back despite being treated.

Your doctor has prescribed you an oral antibiotic called "minocycline." You should take this medication twice daily for the time period that your doctor has recommended. It may take weeks for you to notice that your skin is improving. Please let your doctor know if your skin has not improved after 2 months because this may suggest that you need a different treatment for your condition.

## HERPES ZOSTER

### Clinical Features

Herpes zoster (HZ), or shingles, is caused by reactivation of the varicella zoster virus (VZV), the causative agent of chickenpox. VZV remains dormant in the dorsal root ganglia until reactivation occurs. Not all patients with HZ recall having chickenpox as children.

There are three truncal variants of HZ.

- Dermatomal is the most common presentation of HZ and is the acute development of painful and/or itchy papulovesicles that progress to eroded and crusted papules in a dermatomal distribution (Fig. 3.16).

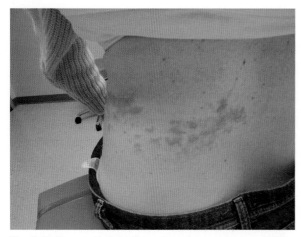

**Fig. 3.16 Herpes Zoster.** Note sharp demarcation at midline. (From the UConn Grand Rounds Collection.)

- HZ is frequently preceded by a prodromal period, which is characterized by paresthesia and/or itch in the subsequently affected area with or without malaise.
- HZ mostly impacts adults over the age of 50; however, young adults and, rarely, even children can develop HZ.
  - HZ is more common and more severe in immunosuppressed individuals, such as those on chemotherapy and those with uncontrolled HIV and advanced lymphoproliferative or hematologic malignancies.
- On the trunk, HZ typically affects the midthoracic trunk from around the spine to around the midline.
- HZ can present in multiple contiguous dermatomes; however, it does not frequently skip dermatomes.
  - HZ does not have to perfectly respect the midline because dermatomes do not perfectly respect the midline; however, a symmetrical bilateral rash is unlikely to be HZ (although bilateral HZ can occur).
- Acute episodes of HZ frequently last around 2 to 4 weeks.
  - Longer episodes can occur in chronically immunosuppressed individuals.
- Individuals who received the VZV vaccine as children have an almost negligible risk of developing HZ.
- Herpes sine zoster may develop in some individuals and is characterized by acute pain, paresthesia, and/or itch in a dermatomal distribution in the absence of cutaneous findings.
- Rarely, almost exclusively immunocompromised individuals will develop disseminated HZ, which is characterized by the development of classic papulovesicles diffusely with systemic symptoms (e.g., meningoencephalitis, pneumonitis). This variant can be fatal and is almost invariably associated with significant morbidity.
- Postherpetic neuralgia is neuropathic pain at the site of previous herpetic lesions lasting longer than 30 days after resolution of the rash. It is the most common complication of acute HZ.
  - It occurs most commonly in the elderly, in immunosuppressed individuals, and in individuals with prolonged episodes of acute HZ.

## Differential Diagnosis

The differential for truncal HZ includes herpes gladiatorum, varicella (chickenpox), lichen striatus, blaschkitis, postzoster dermatoses, and zosteriform cutaneous metastases.

Acute HZ has such a unique presentation that classic cases are only infrequently misdiagnosed; however, other entities that mimic acute HZ may be misdiagnosed as HZ.

- Herpes gladiatorum is a herpes simplex infection that develops on the trunk from human-to-human contact. It is named thus because it most frequently develops in wrestlers and other athletes who come in close contact with bare skin; however, anyone can develop it.
  - It is distinguished from HZ because it recurs more frequently, it is more common in younger adults, it is less dermatomal, and its papulovesicles are uniform in size.
    - The desire to distinguish HZ from herpes gladiatorum primarily occurs in situations in which a person develops recurrent episodes and there is a question as to whether valacyclovir prophylaxis is indicated. In these cases, a biopsy evaluated with HSV and VZV immunohistochemistry can distinguish between the two conditions.
- Chickenpox is becoming increasingly uncommon as vaccination against VZV becomes more prevalent; however, some parents do not vaccinate their children against VZV and some adults, particularly those

born outside of the United States, may not have been vaccinated against VZV as children.

- Chickenpox (varicella) presents with a febrile prodromal period followed by the development of disseminated vesicopapules all in the same stage of development.
  - In adults, chickenpox is typically more severe and can result in hospitalization.
  - Chickenpox can be distinguished from HZ because it is almost always disseminated and occurs in individuals without a known history of chickenpox or VZV vaccination.
- Lichen striatus and blaschkitis can be grouped together for the purpose of differential diagnosis. These conditions are misdiagnosed as HZ because they present in a dermatomal (so-called "zosteriform") distribution.
  - These entities can be distinguished from HZ based on morphology, chronicity, symptoms, and location.
    - HZ presents with vesiculopapules, whereas lichen striatus and blaschkitis are typically warty in initial appearance.
      - Verrucous HZ occurs after classic HZ and in chronically immunosuppressed individuals.
    - HZ resolves within weeks, whereas these entities resolve over months.
    - HZ almost always is associated with pain, itch, and/or paresthesia; in contradistinction, these entities are almost always asymptomatic.
    - HZ most commonly affects the thoracic trunk, whereas these entities typically develop on an arm or leg and may extend onto hands/feet.
- There are many inflammatory cutaneous complications of HZ that arise after resolution of an acute episode of HZ and that can be misdiagnosed as persistent HZ. These conditions are a reactive phenomenon to the acute infection and can be variable in appearance. They should be considered in cases where new rash develops at the site of healed HZ lesions.
- Zosteriform cutaneous metastases are rare but, given their grave significance, they must be considered in cases of atypical or chronic zoster. As their name suggests, they are a form of cutaneous metastases that present as firm dermal nodules in a zosteriform distribution.
  - Breast cancer is the most common primary cancer that causes zosteriform metastases.

- Zosteriform cutaneous metastases can be distinguished from HZ because they are typically asymptomatic and are not preceded by the classic vesicopapules of HZ.

## Work-Up

In typical cases, diagnosis can be made on clinical grounds alone.

- In cases where the diagnosis is uncertain and HZ is favored, a swab for viral culture or PCR (more sensitive but more expensive) can be performed to confirm the diagnosis.
- In cases where the diagnosis is uncertain and HZ is not favored, a punch biopsy can be helpful. Routine H&E cannot reliably distinguish HZ from HSV. To do so, immunohistochemistry is required.

Patients with severe disease and/or frequent recurrences in the absence of a clear trigger should be evaluated for HIV if clinical suspicion for HIV exists.

### Initial Steps in Management

Management of acute HZ can be divided into antiviral therapy, pain control, and topical anesthetics.

### Antiviral Therapy

Antivirals shorten the duration of symptoms and decrease the likelihood of postherpetic neuralgia

- Valacyclovir 1 gram by mouth TID for 7 days is the recommended initial therapy in immunocompetent individuals and works best if given within the first 48 hours of symptoms or rash.
  - Immunosuppressed patients may require an extended duration of valacyclovir therapy
  - Valacyclovir-resistant HZ is very rare and almost exclusively occurs in immunosuppressed individuals. It may be considered if HZ is persistent despite multiple weeks of adequate doses of valacyclovir therapy. If antiviral resistance is expected, a referral to infectious disease is indicated.

### Pain Control

Pain management for HZ can be divided into oral and topical therapy. For the purposes of this chapter, we will focus on a discussion of pain management during acute episodes of HZ.

- Oral therapy:
  - For the vast majority of patients, adequate analgesia can be achieved with use of scheduled alternating

acetaminophen (1 gram Q8H) and ibuprofen (800 mg Q6H).

- Some patients may require a brief course of opioid analgesics for severe pain. In these cases, opioid prescriptions should be limited to less than 7 days.
- Systemic steroids, once recommended in the elderly to reduce acute pain and potentially the incidence of postherpetic neuralgia, is now controversial and no longer recommended.
- Topical therapy:
  - Some experts recommend using super-high–potency topical corticosteroids as a symptomatic adjuvant therapy.
    - Topical clobetasol propionate 0.05% cream/gel/or ointment can be used twice daily for up to 7 days.

### Topical Anesthetics

- Topical lidocaine jelly is frequently prescribed given its safety; however, its efficacy as an analgesic in this setting is debated.
- Two vaccines are FDA-approved for prevention of HZ. The two-dose recombinant zoster vaccine, Shingrix, is the preferred vaccine by the CDC.
  - The vaccine is recommended for primary and secondary prevention of HZ in immunocompetent adults over the age of 50 (detailed recommendations can be found on the CDC website).
  - Although the vaccine is recommended for adults on low-dose immunosuppressants, it is not yet recommended for immunocompromised individuals.

### Warning Signs/Common Pitfalls

Occasionally, patients will present during the prodromal period. If clinical suspicion for impending HZ is strong, initiation of valacyclovir should not be delayed because early initiation can decrease the severity of the condition and decrease the likelihood of subsequent postherpetic neuralgia.

Profoundly immunosuppressed patients frequently require prolonged courses of valacyclovir. Failure to improve with 7 days of therapy should be considered to be a treatment failure or a sign of antiviral resistance.

During an acute episode of HZ, contact with children who have not yet received the VZV vaccine should be avoided.

- HZ is infectious for varicella and can be transmitted either by direct contact in immunocompetent hosts or potentially by respiratory secretions in immunocompromised hosts.

Rarely, patients develop neurologic involvement from HZ before the development of disseminated cutaneous lesions. Patients with HZ and acute neurologic symptoms should be hospitalized and urgently undergo lumbar puncture with CSF PCR for VZV.

- All patients in whom disseminated HZ is suspected should be hospitalized. Shingles occasionally develops in children and pregnant women. The safety of valacyclovir in these populations is less well established.
- In immunocompetent children, antiviral therapy is typically avoided because the episodes are typically mild and self-limited.
- In immunocompromised children, treatment should be directed by the child's infectious disease physician.
- In pregnant women, the decision to treat with antivirals is based on disease severity and is at the discretion of the patient's obstetrician.

### Counseling

You have herpes zoster, also known as "shingles." Shingles is caused by reactivation of the virus that causes chickenpox. There is no one reason why people develop shingles, although it occasionally develops during periods of stress or illness. Shingles is contagious and can be transmitted to individuals who have never had chickenpox and that were not vaccinated against chickenpox as children. To decrease the likelihood of spreading the virus, you should cover the affected area with clothing and avoid known contact with those individuals.

Shingles is typically self-limited, meaning that it will go away on its own; however, you have been prescribed valacyclovir to help make the shingles go away faster and to decrease the likelihood that you develop pain at the area of your shingles called "postherpetic neuralgia."

Shingles is typically very painful and therefore your doctor has recommended that you take acetaminophen and ibuprofen to help make the pain manageable. You should alternate between these two medications and take them at set times rather than as needed to help manage your pain. You should take 1 gram of acetaminophen every 8 hours alternating with 800 mg of ibuprofen every 6 hours.

You have also been prescribed a strong prescription steroid cream. You should apply this twice daily for 1 week.

Do not apply it to your face or other uninvolved areas because it can thin the skin.

Finally, even though you have shingles, you are still at risk for developing shingles again. To prevent this, you should schedule yourself to receive the shingles vaccine after this acute episode is over. If you previously received the Zostavax, you should still receive the new Shingrix vaccine because these are different vaccines and the Shingrix vaccine is more effective.

# NECROBIOSIS LIPOIDICA

Campbell Stewart

## Clinical Features

Necrobiosis lipoidica (NL) is an idiopathic inflammatory disorder of the skin.

- The classic clinical presentation of NL is sharply demarcated, irregularly shaped, red to brown plaques on the anterior lower legs. In established lesions, there can be an annular indurated border, with central yellow atrophy and prominent telangiectasias. The lesions start small and show expansile growth.
- NL can occur at any age and is significantly more common in female patients.
- NL is typically asymptomatic; however, pain and itch have been reported. Areas of atrophy can have diminished sensation. If lesions ulcerate, they can be painful.
- The disorder was formerly attributed to diabetes mellitus and called "necrobiosis lipoidica diabetacorum."
  - Only a minority of patients with NL either have preexisting diabetes or develop diabetes at the onset of NL or after. The percentage of all people with diabetes who have NL is less than 1%.
- There is a potential relationship between NL and GA. The two conditions can coexist and overlap both clinically and histopathologically.

## Differential Diagnosis
### Granuloma Annulare

- GA and NL can be challenging to differentiate, particularly in early lesions of NL that do not have significant central atrophy. A biopsy will reveal granulomatous dermatitis but may not be able to distinguish GA from NL. In such a scenario, the diagnostic determination should be based on clinical features. The patient may need to be monitored over time for the granulomatous disorder to declare itself. NL tends to leave evidence of scarring, whereas GA does not scar.

### Sarcoidosis

- Sarcoidosis generally lacks the same yellow color and telangiectasias seen in NL but can clinically mimic almost any disease of the skin. The classic histopathology of naked granuloma formation in sarcoidosis is distinct from NL; however, there can be some overlap in skin biopsy results. The patient should be examined carefully for lesions in areas other than the lower extremities (which is rare in NL). A review of systems can help elucidate any extracutaneous sarcoid.

### Necrobiotic Xanthogranuloma

- Necrobiotic xanthogranuloma is an extremely rare condition with similar clinical and histopathologic features to NL. It involves the head and neck, particularly the periorbital face, as opposed to NL, which tends to occur on the anterior lower extremities. Ulceration is not uncommon. This disease is associated with paraproteinemias. If there are multiple sites on the body involved with ulcerative features, screening for hematologic disorders is recommended.

## Work-Up

A full-body skin examination should be done to assess for the presence of other lesions. If multiple lesions are identified away from the anterior lower legs, the diagnosis should be questioned.

Inquire about a family history of diabetes and assess if there are any other concerning symptoms/signs of glucose intolerance. Screen for diabetes based on clinical judgment.

A punch biopsy is usually needed to confirm the diagnosis. Similar to GA, the sample should be taken from the edge of a lesion. Histopathology shows layers of granulomatous inflammation arranged like a layer cake. Multinucleated cells are abundant and involvement of the dermis and subcutaneous fat is seen.

## Initial Steps in Management
### General Management Comments

- Treatment is often ineffective, and there is no preferred agent. The lesions can be highly concerning to patients from an aesthetic perspective. Patients may become understandably frustrated by a lack of improvement and the progressive nature of NL.
- Avoidance of trauma to prevent ulceration is key. Early intervention can slow the progression of disease.

## Recommended Initial Regimen

- Topical steroids applied twice daily for 2 to 3 weeks, followed by a 1-week break, can be effective. This cycle can be repeated until any atrophy secondary to steroid use occurs. Atrophy outside of the central zone of a lesion is rare and is usually related to steroid abuse.
- Intralesional triamcinolone (10 mg/mL) can be injected into the outer edge of active lesions and should be used in a 1 to 2 cm radius around the active site to target subclinical involvement. Injection of atrophic sites should be done with caution because the intralesional steroids can exacerbate the atrophy, making it more prone to breakdown, ulceration, and infection.

## Partial but Inadequate Response

What to do if there is a partial but inadequate response after a trial of topical corticosteroid and/or intralesional therapy:

- Topical tacrolimus ointment can be used long term without concern for steroid atrophy. Twice-daily application for several months may be needed to appreciate any benefit. Topical tacrolimus may also be used as an alternative during the breaks from steroid treatment (see above).
- Topical retinoids can be used to improve atrophy as well.

## Continued Inadequate Response

What to do if the response continues to be inadequate:

- Oral methotrexate, even at low doses, can be effective. Oral mycophenolate and oral cyclosporine have also been used with success.
- Antiplatelet agents, including pentoxifylline, as well as combination aspirin and dipyridamole, have been used with some benefit.

If the disease acutely progresses, particularly in the setting of steroids or other immunosuppressive agents, evaluation for an occult infection of the skin should be pursued. Work-up should include a tissue culture.

## Other Treatment Options

- A low-risk option is oral nicotinamide (500 mg three times daily) taken for 3 to 6 months. Nicotinamide can be used alone or in combination with other oral agents.

## Other Agents

- Biologic agents, such as etanercept, adalimumab, and infliximab, can be used.

- Other agents to try include photodynamic therapy, UVA-1, combination hydroxychloroquine/chloroquine, and thalidomide.

## Warning Signs/Common Pitfalls

Confusion with GA is a common pitfall. GA may show depressed central areas but does not show atrophy and telangiectasia. GA does not heal with scarring and only rarely ulcerates (normally in the setting of perforating GA).

Ulceration in NL is common, and atrophy leads to easily eroded or ulcerated skin in the setting of trauma. Lesions can become secondarily infected. A culture should be performed in the setting of acutely worsening disease, particularly if there is ulceration with crust or drainage.

When injecting triamcinolone, treating the surrounding clinically normal skin can slow the risk for disease progression. Atrophic sites should not be injected directly.

## Counseling

You have an inflammatory disorder in your skin called "necrobiosis lipoidica." The cause is not known, but there is a possible link to diabetes. If you have a personal or history of glucose intolerance, you should be screened for diabetes using a blood test.

Necrobiosis lipoidica tends to only affect the front of the lower legs. The lesions can expand in size, and the central areas can become tissue-paper thin, making them sensitive to trauma. If your skin breaks down, it can become infected and we may need to use topical and/or oral antibiotics.

Treatment for this condition is frustrating and often disappointing. Lesions rarely resolve without treatment and normally leave superficial scars with discoloration that can be long-standing or permanent.

We will start with topical and injected steroids to see if that improves your necrobiosis lipoidica. The goal is to halt the spread of your condition.

If these treatment options do not work, there are numerous oral therapies. You may need a referral to a dermatologist to discuss next steps in treatment if you do not respond to the initial treatments.

# LEUKOCYTOCLASTIC VASCULITIS

**Neelesh Jain, Jonas Adalsteinsson, and Jun Lu**

## Clinical Features

Leukocytoclastic vasculitis (LCV), also known as "cutaneous small-vessel vasculitis," is commonly idiopathic but may present 7 to 10 days after exposure to an offending agent or inciting event.

- In true LCV, there is skin-limited involvement by definition; however, systemic vasculitis must be ruled out with a careful physical examination and diagnostic testing because it can clinically mimic LCV.
- It appears symmetrically on the lower extremities as pink, red, or violaceous macules and papules, progressing to deeper red or purple nonblanching palpable purpura, sometimes followed by hemorrhagic bullae and ulcers.
  - It is most commonly located on the shins and dorsal feet.
  - It is less commonly found on the thighs and buttock; these locations are more typical in bed-bound patients.
  - It least commonly appears on the abdomen, upper extremities, or in localized areas on the upper body.
  - Edema may be present.
  - Skin lesions may cause pruritus, burning, or pain but are most often asymptomatic.
- Systemic involvement may present with symptoms of fever, myalgias, arthralgias, abdominal pain, hematuria, hematochezia, or malaise.

## Differential Diagnosis

Clinically, diseases that present with petechiae or purpura mainly on the extremities mimic LCV. The following differentials are important to keep in mind for LCV.

### Other Types of Vasculitis

- Any size vessel vasculitis should be on the differential; when medium or larger vessels are involved, the skin lesions can be more dramatic with nodules or ischemic-induced ulcers.
- Medium-size vessel vasculitis (such as polyarteritis nodosa and Kawasaki disease) can present with leg purpura, but here you will have signs of organ failure elsewhere, such as in the pulmonary, renal, and gastrointestinal systems.
- IgA vasculitis (Henoch-Schönlein purpura) usually only affects children under 10 years old after an upper respiratory infection and will be accompanied by symptoms of fever, arthralgias, abdominal pain, and hematuria.
- Granulomatosis with polyangiitis (formerly called "Wegener granulomatosis") presents with symptoms related to upper and lower respiratory involvement, as well as renal involvement.

- Microscopic polyangiitis is almost always associated with signs of renal involvement and other systemic symptoms.

### Infection

- In sepsis with DIC, purpura will be more retiform and the patient may exhibit areas of necrosis or frank bleeding. Signs of tachycardia, hypotension, and widespread organ failure will be present.
- In Rocky Mountain spotted fever (RMSF), the petechial rash starts on both the distal upper and lower extremities before spreading centripetally and progressing to purpura on the bilateral extremities, with associated fever, myalgias, and headache. Initiate immediate antibiotic treatment if suspected.
- With a meningococcal infection, the purpuric rash almost always includes the trunk and patients will have signs of meningeal irritation, as well as other systemic symptoms.

### Miscellaneous

- Arthropod bites are often limited in distribution and appear more urticarial with a central punctum. Lesions can often be aligned linearly (the so-called "breakfast, lunch, and dinner sign").
- Capillaritis (pigmented purpuric dermatosis) can be distinguished by the presence of petechial lesions that are classically described as like cayenne pepper in appearance.
- In immune thrombocytopenic purpura, nonpalpable petechiae and ecchymoses are common in a more diffuse pattern.
- Erythema multiforme classically presents with target lesions that begin at acral sites before spreading centripetally.
- Vasculitis can be seen in association with many diverse diseases, including collagen vascular diseases, infections, or an underlying malignancy. A thorough history and physical examination are required to detect one of these underlying diseases.

### Work-Up

Patients in whom LCV is suspected should be referred to a dermatologist for a skin biopsy and further work-up to confirm the diagnosis and etiology. Before consulting a dermatologist, it is of the utmost importance that other diagnoses on the differential with LCV be excluded with a careful history, review of systems, physical examination, and other diagnostic testing.

Around 50% of cases are idiopathic. When a trigger is identified, it is most often attributed to an underlying condition or inciting event.

- Fifteen to twenty percent are because of bacterial and viral infections, including *Streptococcus*, *Staphylococcus*, hepatitis, HIV, and Epstein-Barr virus (EBV).
- Fifteen to twenty percent are secondary to autoimmune connective tissue diseases, including SLE, Sjögren syndrome, and rheumatoid arthritis.
- Ten to fifteen percent are the result of drugs, such as antibiotics, NSAIDs, and diuretics.
- Five percent are because of neoplasms.
- A very rare form of LCV is caused by exercise, particularly in warm weather.

Further testing can be helpful in identifying systemic involvement and elucidating prognostic information. Clinicians should order a CBC, ESR, and C-reactive protein as a baseline. Additional studies should only be ordered appropriately when they are clinically indicated and may be helpful to manage systemic involvement and differentiate possible underlying causes.

- For gastrointestinal involvement, fetal occult blood testing is often positive in HSP.
- In terms of autoimmune diseases, it may be helpful to test ANA and complement levels. Hypocomplementemia is associated with extracutaneous disease.
- For rheumatoid arthritis, it may be helpful to order a rheumatoid factor test.
- When hepatitis is suspected, it may be useful to test cryoglobulins and the hepatitis B and C serologies.
- For a bacterial infection, blood cultures, echocardiogram, and ASO/anti-DNase B tests may be indicated.
- When checking for HIV, an HIV serology may be indicated.
- For Sjögren syndrome, it may be helpful to conduct anti-Ro and anti-La tests.
- When looking at renal involvement, a urinalysis, urine sediment test, or basic metabolic panel may be indicated.
- For pulmonary involvement, a chest X-ray may be needed.
- When looking for malignancy, a serum protein electrophoresis (SPEP)/urine protein electrophoresis (UPEP) or cancer screening may be conducted.
- An antineutrophil cytoplasmic antibody (ANCA) test may also be indicated.

In some cases, one may be able to identify inciting drug agents, infections, neoplasms, history of autoimmune connective tissue disease, or exercise in warm weather. Patients presenting with suspected LCV should be questioned about exposure to the following:

- NSAIDs
- Anticoagulants
- Allopurinol
- Antigout medications
- Antibiotics
- Diuretics
- Infliximab
- Tyrosine kinase inhibitors
- Anticonvulsants

Two punch biopsies should be performed to be sent for an H&E stain and DIF. Both should be performed on lesional skin, preferably on the upper extremities on a lesion less than 24 hours old. For the sample being sent for H&E, the lesion may be up to 72 hours old. The DIF sample is essential to distinguish IgA vasculitis, such as Henoch-Schönlein purpura, from IgG vasculitis.

## Initial Steps in Management

The initial management of LCV should include a detailed history, review of systems, physical examination, and select diagnostic studies. If an underlying trigger can be identified, it should be managed, such as in the case of infection, autoimmune connective tissue disease, offending drug, or neoplasm.

Many patients may be treated only symptomatically and will see resolution over a few weeks to months. For skin-limited disease, consider the following treatments:

- Oral antihistamines can be taken by mouth every 12 to 24 hours for pruritus.
- Compression stockings and leg elevation can be used if edema is present,
- NSAIDs can be taken for pain.
  - NSAIDs should be used with caution because they may be an inciting agent for LCV and are contraindicated in the elderly and if there is renal involvement.

Cases in which there is systemic involvement may require oral steroids or steroid-sparing agents. Closer follow-up and referral to a dermatologist is also recommended. For LCV with systemic involvement, consider the following treatments:

- NSAIDs can be taken for pain, myalgias, fever and arthralgias.

- Prednisone 1 mg/kg by mouth every 24 hours may be prescribed.
  - Consider adding vitamin D and calcium supplements if the patient requires long-term dosing.
  - Certain comorbid conditions may warrant extra caution before prescribing systemic steroids, including diabetes mellitus, poorly controlled hypertension, glaucoma, heart failure, and recent stroke.
- Steroid-sparing agents may also be used.
  - Options include colchicine, methotrexate, mycophenolate mofetil, azathioprine, and cyclophosphamide.

## Warning Signs/Common Pitfalls

LCV is always a diagnosis of exclusion, and if suspected, always warrants a biopsy.

Clinicians should be aware of the purpura differential previously mentioned and should be able to differentiate LCV from these conditions.

Clinicians should be keenly aware of the worsened prognosis in the case of systemic involvement in LCV. If systemic involvement is suspected, further diagnostic testing is required to evaluate for end-organ damage. Swift treatment and close follow-up to avoid long-term sequelae are recommended.

Many cases do not have an identifiable trigger.

Cutaneous involvement alone may not require systemic steroids and will often spontaneously resolve within a few months.

Although LCV usually presents on the lower extremities, it should still be considered when evaluating purpura elsewhere on the body.

## Counseling

The rash on your body may have been caused by an immune reaction to an infection or a medication you have taken or may be the result of an underlying disease. This immune reaction targeted the vessels in your body, producing this rash. In many cases, however, it is not possible to identify a specific trigger. This type of rash is called "leukocytoclastic vasculitis." It can appear anywhere on your body but most commonly presents on the lower body, especially the legs. It is important to discuss what medications you are currently taking with your doctor because certain medications may be an inciting factor in the development of this rash. If your doctor identifies a medication you are taking as a known drug that causes this rash, then they may recommend discontinuing that medication and/or switching to another medication. It is also important to discuss any recent illnesses or history of autoimmune diseases that you may have. If your doctor can identify an underlying condition that might have caused the rash, then they may be able to treat it and resolve both the underlying condition and the rash.

Some people with your type of rash benefit from one or, more likely, two small skin biopsies. These may be performed in a dermatologist's office. The procedure involves taking a small sample of your skin where the rash is. Ideally, the sample should be from a spot that has recently developed in the past 1 to 2 days. There will be a needle used for local anesthetic, but other than the initial pinch from that injection, there should be no pain. The sample of skin will be sent to the laboratory for further testing to definitively diagnose your rash as leukocytoclastic vasculitis.

This rash can also affect your internal organs so it is important to mention any other aches or pains you have developed since noticing the rash. It is also prudent to discuss any changes in your urination or bowel movements because this rash may affect the kidneys and gastrointestinal system. Based on the severity of your rash and other symptoms, the doctor may recommend systemic medications. When deciding which treatment plan is best for you, make sure to discuss with your doctor how a new medication may impact any other health problems you may have.

# 4

# Hand and Foot Dermatitis

## HAND DERMATITIS—WITH A SPECIFIC FOCUS ON IRRITANT CONTACT DERMATITIS, ALLERGIC CONTACT DERMATITIS, AND DYSHIDROTIC ECZEMA

### Clinical Features

Hand dermatitis is extremely common because the hands are exposed to many environmental chemicals and irritants.

- The severity of hand dermatitis ranges dramatically from mild scaling in the absence of erythema to the presence of deep fissures (Fig. 4.1).
- The vast majority (around 90%) of hand dermatitis cases are irritant contact dermatitis (ICD), with a minority of patients presenting with allergic contact dermatitis (ACD).
  - ACD frequently occurs in patients with underlying ICD.
    - Patients with chronic hand dermatitis that becomes unresponsive to treatment over time frequently have developed superimposed ACD.

- There is no clinical finding that definitively distinguishes hand ACD from hand ICD.
- The most common irritants implicated in hand dermatitis are water (from hand washing or wet work) and hand soap.
  - The groups at the highest risk for developing hand dermatitis include hairdressers, mechanics, house or office cleaners, mothers of young children, healthcare workers, and those with atopic dermatitis (AD).
  - Most hand dermatitis results from repetitive low-grade irritant insults (e.g., hand washing).
- Hand dermatitis typically is more bothersome to patients than dermatitis elsewhere because it can significantly affect activities of daily living.
- Hand dermatitis is more common in individuals with underlying AD.
  - Patients with AD who develop hand dermatitis may have concomitant components of ICD and ACD.
  - Isolated hand dermatitis is not a common manifestation of AD.

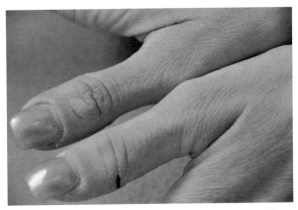

**Fig. 4.1 Fissured Irritant Contact Dermatitis.** (From the UConn Dermatology Grand Rounds Collection.)

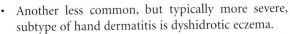

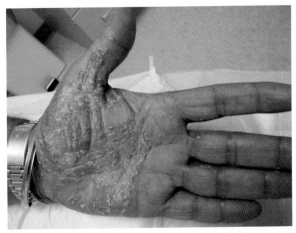

**Fig. 4.2 Palmar Pustulosis, a Variant of Palmoplantar Psoriasis.** (From the UConn Dermatology Grand Rounds Collection.)

- Another less common, but typically more severe, subtype of hand dermatitis is dyshidrotic eczema.
  - Dyshidrotic eczema is an extremely pruritic hand (and sometimes foot) dermatitis variant characterized by the development of small blisters predominantly on the lateral aspects of the fingers.
    - Despite its name, it is not definitively linked to sweating.
    - Patients with dyshidrotic eczema frequently describe pruritus out of proportion to examination findings.

## Differential Diagnosis

The differential diagnosis for hand dermatitis can be divided into true dermatitis (ICD, ACD, AD, dyshidrotic eczema, or nummular dermatitis) and other nondermatitic infection and inflammatory conditions, such as palmoplantar psoriasis, tinea manuum, and contact urticaria. As was previously mentioned, clinical examination alone is often insufficient for distinguishing the different types of true hand dermatitis from each other, with the exception of nummular dermatitis and dyshidrotic eczema, which have skin features that differentiate them from the other diagnoses.

- Nummular hand dermatitis typically presents as circular, erythematous plaques on the dorsal hands that are stable in size and exquisitely pruritic. Examination of the extremities will often reveal lesions of a similar morphology.
- Palmoplantar psoriasis (Fig. 4.2) typically affects both palms and soles with hyperkeratotic plaque, which may or may not have overlying silver-white scale with minimal itch. The presence of large, sterile pustules is characteristic of some forms of palmoplantar psoriasis. Psoriasis may also be present on other extensor surfaces, the scalp, and the lower back. Nail psoriasis is almost always identifiable in cases of palmoplantar psoriasis.
- Tinea manuum is a dermatophyte (fungal) infection that generally only affects the palmar surfaces. It presents predominantly with diffuse scaling, with or without background erythema; however, occasionally it can look like classic ringworm and involve the dorsum of the hand. Onychomycosis of the involved hand and bilateral feet is also often observed. Additionally, examination of the feet is useful because most patients have concomitant bilateral tinea pedis (a two-feet, one-hand presentation).
- Contact urticaria is an acute allergic reaction that involves the abrupt onset of wheals, burning, stinging, and swelling over areas that come into contact with an environmental allergen. When their use was commonplace, latex gloves were a frequent cause of contact urticaria. Food handling is now a more common cause.
- Id reactions are secondary papulovesicular eruptions that occur as the result of a primary skin condition on another area of the body and should be suspected if an initial skin lesion (e.g., tinea, ACD, or stasis dermatitis) is identified at a separate site. Id reactions rarely localize exclusively to the hands and more

commonly involve the dorsal hands and extensor forearms simultaneously.

## Work-Up

Hand dermatitis is typically a clinical diagnosis. All patients with hand dermatitis should have their nails and feet examined. A total-body skin examination for identification of rash elsewhere is also helpful.

History taking should be directed at assessing personal and occupational habits to identify potential irritants or allergens.

- Patients should be questioned regarding exposure to potential irritants or allergens, keeping in mind that occupational and nonoccupational allergens may differ slightly.
  - The most common workplace allergens causing hand ACD include first aid medications, metallic salts, organic dyes, plants, and rubber additives.
  - The most common nonoccupational allergens causing hand ACD are nickel, fragrances, cosmetic agents, and preservatives.
  - Common irritants implicated in hand ACD include detergents, chemicals in household cleaning agents, mild soaps (with repetitive use), metal tools, fiberglass, wood shavings, and dust.
  - Professionals at high risk for exposure to irritants and allergens include hairdressers, cement workers, food processors, florists, chefs, builders, medical workers, and painters.
  - Frequent hand exposure to wet environments (more than 2–3 hours per day), skin trauma, vibration, or pressure can compromise protective barriers in the skin and increase the likelihood of developing either ICD or ACD.

Because ICD cannot be reliably differentiated from ACD based on examination alone, patch testing to assess for contact allergies is recommended in all patients refractory to conservative measures.

- Prick testing is not a replacement for patch testing because it does not assess for Type IV hypersensitivity reactions.

Because patch testing cannot be used to identify irritant exposures, consulting workplace materials safety data sheets may prove helpful in these cases.

In all cases of hand dermatitis, a skin biopsy is rarely necessary and typically is not helpful in differentiating between various types of hand dermatitis.

In cases where tinea manuum is in the differential diagnosis, obtaining a scraping for fungal culture can be fruitful.

## Initial Steps in Management
### General Management Comments

Regardless of the particular etiology, treatment of hand eczema requires a multifaceted approach, involving 1) skin barrier restoration/maintenance; 2) behavioral changes to protect against insults to the skin barrier; and 3) the use of antiinflammatory prescription medications (e.g., topical corticosteroids, topical calcineurin inhibitors, systemic immunosuppressants).

### Irritant/Allergen Avoidance

All patients with chronic hand dermatitis should be offered patch testing to identify allergens because ACD cannot be ruled out on clinical grounds alone.

- Randomly eliminating potential, unconfirmed allergens is rarely indicated unless the patient can clearly associate an exposure with a disease flare.
- Frequent hand washing is an exacerbating factor for hand dermatitis in almost all cases. Patients should be counseled to decrease the frequency of hand washing and to apply emollients after drying.
  - Advising patients to keep a moisturizer near the sinks that they most frequently use improves compliance with skin barrier restoration.
- Vinyl or nitrile gloves can be used if patients are routinely exposed to potential irritants/allergens in their occupational field. If used for extended periods, a thin cotton glove can be worn underneath to absorb excess moisture because moisture under a glove can exacerbate the dermatitis.
- Water-repellent barrier creams can be applied twice daily to block the entry of potential allergens, particularly if patients have already developed fissures or breaks in their skin.

### Recommended Antiinflammatory Treatment

The choice of topical corticosteroid is dictated by the severity of the hand dermatitis.

- Patients with mild to moderate hand dermatitis can use a mid-potency topical corticosteroid.
  - Begin with the mid-potency topical corticosteroid (triamcinolone acetate 0.1% ointment) once or twice daily for 1 month or until the skin lesions resolve.

- Ointment vehicles tend to be more effective, but some patients may not be able to tolerate the greasiness for certain tasks.
- Even for mild-moderate hand dermatitis, steroid-sparing topicals (e.g., tacrolimus, crisaborole) are rarely efficacious.
- After achieving remission, we advise the continued use of a mid-potency corticosteroid cream ointment at a reduced frequency (two or three times per week) to prevent new exacerbations.
- If response to mid-potency topical corticosteroids is inadequate after a 2- to 4-week trial, increase the potency to a Class I steroid (e.g., clobetasol propionate 0.05%).
- Patients with severe hand dermatitis or with dyshidrotic eczema benefit from a stronger topical corticosteroid.
  - Start a super-potent topical corticosteroid (clobetasol propionate 0.05% ointment) once or twice daily for 1 month or until skin lesions resolve.
    - Steroid-induced atrophy is fairly uncommon on acral skin.
    - Patients can be titrated down to a mid-potency topical corticosteroid once their disease is under better control.
  - If there is evidence of secondary infection, topical or oral antistaph antibiotics can be a helpful addition to the therapeutic regimen.

### Partial but Inadequate Response

If there is a partial but inadequate response after a 4-week trial of high-potency topical corticosteroid monotherapy, it may mean that other treatments should be tried.

- Severe hand dermatitis frequently is refractory to topical therapy. Patients may benefit from soak psoralen plus ultraviolet A (PUVA; i.e., phototherapy) treatment, oral immunosuppressants, or dupilumab. These patients should be referred to a dermatologist.

### Warning Signs/Common Pitfalls

If patients do not respond within 2 to 4 weeks of using super-potent topical corticosteroids and skin barrier care, then patch testing should be performed.

It is imperative to counsel patients to continue skin barrier care once their hand dermatitis has improved or it will inevitably recur.

Using gloves inappropriately can worsen hand dermatitis. Gloves should only be worn during periods when patients come into contact with local allergens (e.g., during work) because sweating underneath the gloves can further damage the skin barrier and worsen dermatitis.

- This can be mitigated by wearing a thin cotton liner glove.

Secondary impetiginization and herpetic infections of hand dermatitis are not uncommon. The presence of yellow crusting, blisters, or punched-out ulcerations is suggestive of a secondary infection and requires management with appropriate antimicrobials.

### Counseling

You have been diagnosed with hand dermatitis. There are a number of different reasons why you may have developed this rash; however, typically it is because your hands are coming into contact with something that is either injuring them or that they are allergic to. The most common cause of hand dermatitis is frequent hand washing. The reason for this is that over time, washing your hands removes the protective barrier that your skin produces, thus dehydrating your hands.

The most important thing that you can do to improve your rash is to rehydrate and protect your skin. To do this, you should keep a bland moisturizer near the sinks that you use most frequently and moisturize your hands after you wash your hands. You should also use unscented bar soaps for hand washing because they are less irritating to the skin than most liquid soaps.

If you are unable to avoid prolonged exposure to water or other irritants, you can consider wearing vinyl or nitrile gloves when you are going to come into contact with these irritants. If you are going to wear gloves for a prolonged period of time, then you should wear a pair of white cotton gloves underneath the vinyl gloves so that your sweat does not further irritate the rash.

To decrease the inflammation in your skin, we are prescribing you a topical steroid cream. You should apply this to your skin once or twice daily to affected areas until your rash is no longer visible. Once the rash has gone away, we recommend continuing to apply the cream two to three times per week to keep it away.

If your rash does not improve within the next 2 to 4 weeks, please notify us.

# PALMOPLANTAR PSORIASIS (SEE CHAPTER 3, PSORIASIS)

# TINEA PEDIS

**Douglas Albreski**

## Clinical Features

- Tinea pedis is a dermatophyte infection of the foot that usually involves direct barefoot exposure to an organism. Common organisms include *Trichophyton* and *Epidermophyton*. The infection can involve the dorsal surfaces, the plantar surfaces, and the interdigital spaces.
- Presentation occurs in one of three ways.
  - Interdigital tinea pedis presents with erythema and/or scaling associated with web space maceration. Symptoms include pruritus and possible burning; patients with an adductovarus (rotated and curved hammertoes) deformity have a higher incidence of this condition affecting three to four web spaces.
  - Chronic, or moccasin-type, tinea pedis (Fig. 4.3) presents with a dry scaling plantar surface and, occasionally, erythema is present. One of the main symptoms is pruritus. This type is usually associated with onychomycosis because the nail infection serves as the source of the infection and causes the repetitive skin infection. This condition is mostly seen in the older population.

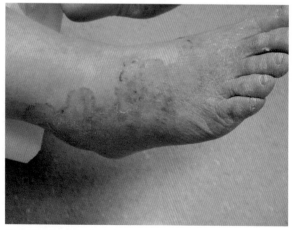

**Fig. 4.3 Tinea Pedis, Inflammatory.** (From the UConn Dermatology Grand Rounds Collection.)

- Acute, or vesiculobullous, tinea pedis presents with bullous eruptions along the medial plantar arch or plantar sulcus. Symptoms include pruritus and pain at the site of bullous lesions. This condition is generally seen in a younger population.
- An uncommon variant of tinea pedis is ulcerative, which can become secondarily infected by bacteria, resulting in a severe infection that can be limb threatening. Interdigital tinea pedis is the most common ulcerative form of tinea pedis and is associated with a secondary bacterial infection.

## Differential Diagnosis

- For interdigital tinea pedis:
  - Erythrasma is a bacterial infection caused by *Corynebacterium* that produces similar symptoms; it can be quickly diagnosed with a Wood lamp, revealing a coral-red appearance.
  - Candida is the most common yeast infection and presents with erythema and scaling.
  - Hyperkeratotic scaling comes from interdigital pressure and skin irritation, causing fibrous callous formation.
- Chronic, or moccasin-type, tinea pedis:
  - Inflammatory dermatitis, including AD or dyshidrotic eczema, presents with erythema and scaling with pruritus. The condition may not include the total plantar surface.
  - Palmoplantar psoriasis usually presents with a well-circumscribed plaque with scaling in a plantar distribution, commonly seen at the site of irritation and friction.
  - Chronic ACD or ICD presents with similar erythema and scaling at the site that has been in direct contact with the allergen or irritant.
  - Pitted keratolysis is a bacterial infection usually involving the ball/sulcus and heel of the plantar foot; this condition can be associated with increased odor and clinically is appreciably pitted in appearance.
  - Juvenile plantar dermatosis, also known as "sweaty sock dermatitis" or "atopic winter feet," is defined as a juvenile condition and is not usually seen in the older population. The skin usually has a shiny, scaling, and waxy appearance with fissures. Associated pain is the result of ambulation on tender fissures. Etiologic causes include occlusive foot wear, hyperhidrosis or sweaty feet, and friction.

- Keratolysis exfoliation is an episodic condition and involves skin peeling; it is usually asymptomatic with an unknown etiology.
- Keratoderma congenita is a hereditary condition causing increased hyperkeratotic buildup on the plantar surface of the foot.
- Acute, or vesiculobullous, tinea pedis:
  - Dyshidrotic eczema, or pustular psoriasis, presents with multiple vesicles or sterile pustules involving the medial arches and medial/lateral heels.
  - Acute contact dermatitis presents with bullous lesion formation at the contact sites with pruritus.
  - Scabies involving the plantar skin presents with the burrowing mites causing slightly raised pink and vesicular lesions.

## Work-Up

- A physical examination of the lower extremity, which includes examining the skin, toenails, and web spaces, is required. In addition, comparing the upper extremity can assist in ruling out dermatitis conditions that may commonly present as palmoplantar.
- A potassium hydroxide (KOH) examination is the most common test to confirm the presence of dermatophyte hyphae in a tissue scraping and confirm the diagnosis.
- Further diagnostic tests include the Dermatophyte Test Medium (DTM) or dermatophyte tissue cultures.
- For interdigital tinea pedis, because of potential maceration, tissue scraping microscopic KOH examination remains the best diagnostic method; swabbing a web space for culture may yield a mixed or contaminated flora and make diagnosis misleading.
- For acute, or vesiculobullous, lesions, tissue examination should include deroofing a lesion and scraping the base for the highest fungal yield. Bullous fluid or abscess drainage could yield sterile fluid and be nondiagnostic.
- In cases of failed therapy or worsening symptoms, a tissue biopsy can help confirm the diagnosis and rule out a secondary diagnosis.

## Initial Steps in Management

- Over-the-counter (OTC) topical antifungal agents have been shown to be very effective in the treatment of tinea pedis when used as directed. These agents include azoles, allylamines, butenafine, ciclopirox, and tolnaftate. They are used once or twice daily and require up to 4 weeks of treatment.
- In severe cases, or for patients requiring an oral antifungal approach, there may be concerns associated with past or existing medical conditions and possible drug interaction risks. Skin involvement requires a shorter therapeutic course. Adult dosing is as follows:
  - Terbinafine 250 mg daily for 2 weeks
  - Itraconazole 200 mg twice daily for 1 week
  - Fluconazole 150 mg daily for 2 to 6 weeks
- Pediatric dosing is available and the length of therapy is similar but requires weight-based dosing. In addition, griseofulvin is available for the pediatric population, but the clinical course is longer and can take up to 8 weeks. In the absence of nail fungal involvement or oral medication indication, topical agents have high success rates.
- Adjunct treatment approaches:
  - The addition of topical keratolytic agents, such as urea or salicylic acid, can reduce dry scales and improve the effectiveness of the topical antifungal agent.
  - Drying agents, such as antifungal gel-based agents, gentian violet, or Castellani paint applied interdigitally, can reduce maceration.
- Inflammatory tinea pedis with residual erythema may require the addition of a topical mid- or high-potency steroid in conjunction with the antifungal agent for complete resolution.

## Warning Signs/Common Pitfalls

The primary pitfall is missed diagnosis and/or secondary fungal infection with an underlying other inflammatory process. The additional use of a different antifungal class or prolonged use of an agent without improvement requires further work-up or proper referral for reassessment of the initial diagnosis. A biopsy should be considered in cases of nonresolving tinea pedis.

## Counseling

Tinea pedis, often referred to as "athlete's foot," is a common skin infection caused by a fungus that affects the young and old. Prevention is the best tool to avoid the symptoms and course of this disease. Symptoms can include skin peeling, itchy feet, and redness.

Prevention begins with reducing exposure to fungus by wearing protective shoes, such as water socks, socks, or sandals when walking in areas of high exposure. Areas of concern include locker rooms, public showers, pools, hotels, or areas where multiple people are walking barefoot. Using topical antifungal powders or sprays can help reduce the chance of infection if your skin is exposed to fungus.

If signs of athlete's foot are present, OTC antifungal agents are effective and can usually resolve the symptoms. Like any OTC medications, if they are used as directed and symptoms still persist, consult your doctor.

# Groin and Inframammary Dermatitis

# INTERTRIGO

**Shivani Sinha, Gloria Lin, and Katalin Ferenczi**

## Clinical Features

Intertrigo is an inflammatory condition commonly found in the intertriginous skin folds and flexures. It can be caused by multiple different conditions within the inflammatory and infectious categories. Many healthcare providers use the word "intertrigo" synonymously with candida intertrigo (CI), so for simplicity, this chapter will mainly focus on intertrigo secondary to infection.

The intertriginous areas are susceptible to friction and excess moisture, leading to subsequent maceration and weakening of the epidermis, which increases the risk for secondary fungal and bacterial infections. This condition is often seen in the geriatric and disabled population or anyone who is bedridden with limited mobility. Other risk factors include obesity; hyperhidrosis; poor hygiene; incontinence; immunocompromised states (e.g., diabetes, HIV); excess irritation in the area (e.g., recurrent allergic contact dermatitis [ACD]); and hot, humid climates.

- Intertrigo has an insidious onset that often starts with pruritus, burning, and/or tingling within the skin folds. Patients often complain of excess sweating and an inability to keep those areas dry.
- Lesions initially present as moist, erythematous patches in areas of opposing skin, such as the inframammary folds, axillae, abdominal folds, and groin. Over time, erosions, maceration, and fissures may develop, and it is common to find more than one anatomic location affected by this condition.
- Secondarily infected areas may present with further signs of inflammation, such as pain, abscesses, vesicles, and crusting. Superimposed candidiasis can lead to foul-smelling lesions and is characterized by the presence of erythematous satellite papules and pustules.

- CI of the interdigital spaces is known as "erosio interdigitalis blastomycetica" (EIB) and often affects the web space between the third and fourth fingers or toes. Although associated with the same aforementioned risk factors, EIB often occurs in people whose occupations involve frequent contact with water. These lesions range from mild or asymptomatic to intensely erythematous and malodorous with maceration, fissures, desquamation, and ulceration.

## Differential Diagnosis

The differential diagnosis for intertrigo includes inverse psoriasis, tinea cruris, erythrasma, ACD, and seborrheic dermatitis.

- Inverse psoriasis (Fig. 5.1) is a variant of psoriasis that presents as well-demarcated, erythematous plaques, notably found in the intertriginous skin folds. Whereas classic psoriatic lesions often have micaceous or silvery scale, inverse psoriasis often lacks this because of the moist environment. The lesions may also be more symptomatic with associated pruritus and discomfort from fissuring and maceration. CI often has pathognomonic satellite papules and pustules, which are not seen in inverse psoriasis. A potassium hydroxide (KOH) preparation of skin scrapings will be negative for hyphae in inverse psoriasis. Lesions improve with topical calcipotriene, tacrolimus, and mild nonfluorinated topical steroids (for a limited time only to prevent skin atrophy).
- Tinea cruris is a dermatophyte infection that is commonly known as "jock itch." It is characterized by well-defined erythematous plaques in the skin folds of the groin or medial thighs and most commonly affects young men. A KOH preparation will show the presence of hyphae. Tinea cruris is treated with topical antifungal agents, but it often recurs.

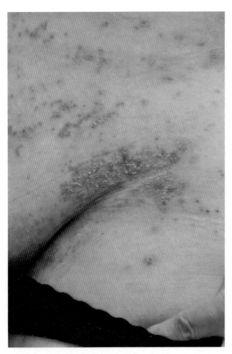

**Fig. 5.1 Inverse Psoriasis of the Groin.** Note the typical plaque psoriasis on the abdomen. (From the UConn Grand Rounds Collection.)

- Erythrasma is a bacterial infection characterized by symmetric, well-demarcated plaques in the groin, axilla, and interdigital web spaces. Erythrasma is diagnosed based on a physical examination and coral-red fluorescence with a Wood lamp test. It typically appears less inflammatory than intertrigo and can be treated with topical antibiotics (such as clindamycin solution or erythromycin cream).
- ACD sometimes occurs in association with intertrigo and presents with scaly, erythematous patches, occasionally with vesiculation, that can spread beyond the intertriginous skin. The physical examination findings, in combination with a positive exposure history, can help distinguish this from intertrigo. Treatment includes topical steroids and avoidance of the contactant agent.
- Seborrheic dermatitis can occur in association with intertrigo or in isolation. Sharply demarcated erythematous plaques can be seen in the skin folds of the axilla, groin, and inframammary region. When seborrheic dermatitis presents in a more classic distribution, such as on the scalp, face, and ears, the lesions

tend to have more yellowish, greasy scale. This may be less obvious, however, in the intertriginous areas because of the excess moisture. Diagnosis is usually made based on a physical examination, and the condition can be treated with ketoconazole cream.

## Work-Up

Intertrigo is a clinical diagnosis based on a physical examination and history. A skin biopsy may be done to exclude other potential conditions but is generally not indicated.
- A full skin examination is recommended to identify the involved areas.
- KOH can be used to confirm the presence of a superimposed infection. If pustules, crusting, abscesses, or vesicles are present, a culture from the affected areas should be done to identify the cause of secondary infection.
- A Wood lamp test can also be used to rule out erythrasma. The latter would show a bright coral red fluorescence when the lamp is shone over the affected area.
- A history of contactants, such as past creams, used to rule out a primary or secondary ACD is also recommended.

## Initial Steps in Management

The most important step in management is elimination of aggravating factors because this can alleviate the severity of the intertrigo and potentially prevent recurrences. It is important to counsel patients because they may be frustrated by the chronic nature of the condition and the multiple relapses.
- Recommend the use of gentle cleansers with thorough drying afterward. Patients can use a hair dryer on a low cool setting to minimize any excess moisture. The affected areas should be exposed to the air as much as possible.
- Antiperspirants and light, nonrestrictive cotton clothing are suggested to minimize sweating. Drying powders, such as aluminum sulfate, talcum, and calcium acetate, can be applied daily to help prevent recurrences. Gauze can be placed between the skin layers, if needed, to keep them dry and reduce friction.
- For those with hyperhidrosis, referral to dermatology is recommended to discuss treatments that may help decrease sweating, such as glycopyrrolate, topical aluminium chloride, and injections of botulinum toxin.

- Barrier creams that contain zinc oxide and/or petrolatum can be applied to affected areas to minimize frictional irritation and skin breakdown.
- For significant pruritus, a low-potency topical steroid cream (hydrocortisone 2.5%) may be applied twice daily for 10 to 14 days. Patients should be counseled on the potential side effects, such as skin atrophy, striae, and dyspigmentation. Combination antifungal and topical steroid formulations are not recommended because these contain higher potency steroids with an increased risk for cutaneous side effects.
- Management of common comorbidities, such as diabetes and obesity, can reduce the risk for recurrence.

CI or other associated fungal infections should be treated using topical antifungals. Creams are generally preferred for an active infection, whereas the powder may be useful as maintenance therapy to prevent recurrences.

- Azole treatments (ketoconazole, clotrimazole, miconazole, and econazole) can be applied twice daily for 2 to 4 weeks or until the infection resolves.
- Nystatin cream can be applied twice daily until resolution, but it is only effective in the treatment of intertrigo caused by *Candida* infection.
- Other antifungal treatment options include butenafine 1% cream, naftifine 2% cream, and terbinafine 1% cream, which can be applied once or twice daily.
- For resistant CI, oral fluconazole may be considered; however, a referral to dermatology is recommended to confirm the diagnosis.

Secondary bacterial infections should be treated promptly to avoid further complications.

- If a bacterial infection is a clinical consideration, a culture should be done to identify the offending agent and determine the appropriate treatment.
- Mild infections can be treated with topical antibacterials, such as mupirocin and erythromycin, depending on the pathogen.
- Oral antibiotics, such as first-generation cephalosporins, erythromycin, or penicillin may be prescribed depending on the severity of the infection and the bacterial species present.

If the treatment response is inadequate, reconsider the diagnosis and refer to dermatology for further evaluation.

## Warning Signs/Common Pitfalls

- Because this condition can be secondary or occur concurrently with other diseases, dermatology referral is important to establish the correct diagnosis.

- Secondary infection is a common occurrence in intertrigo. Patients should be referred to dermatology for management to minimize the risk for infection because this can progress to cellulitis or sepsis if untreated.
- Patients with intense pruritus can be prescribed a low-potency topical steroid cream. These agents should be used sparingly and for a limited time only because of potential cutaneous side effects.
- The use of topical agents may cause ACD, which can be alleviated by discontinuing the use of the offending agent.

## Counseling

You have a condition called intertrigo, which is caused by friction, moisture, and lack of ventilation in the folds of your skin. Maintaining proper hygiene and keeping the areas dry can alleviate your symptoms and prevent the risk for recurrent infection. Use gentle cleansers to keep the area clean and apply powder to keep the folds dry while exposing the skin to air as much as possible. Apply antiperspirants, wear loose-fitting cotton clothing, and avoid excessive heat to minimize irritation and sweating because these may exacerbate your condition. Creams containing zinc oxide can be used to create a physical barrier and reduce friction. If you have diabetes, maintaining tight control of your blood sugar can decrease the risk for intertrigo and secondary infection. In addition, maintaining a healthy weight can also be beneficial.

Contact your healthcare provider if the affected areas start to ooze or develop a foul smell because these are potentially signs of a superimposed infection that may need to be treated with antibiotics or topical creams.

# INVERSE PSORIASIS (SEE CHAPTER 3, "PSORIASIS")

# TINEA CRURIS (SEE CHAPTER 3, "TINEA CORPORIS")

# ERYTHRASMA

**Campbell Stewart**

## Clinical Features

Erythrasma is caused by the gram-positive bacillus *Corynebacterium minutissimum,* which infects the most superficial layer of the skin, the stratum corneum. *C. minutissimum* is a normal inhabitant of the skin; in the setting of excess heat and moisture, however, it can pervade the intertriginous sites of the body. Other contributing factors include obesity, diabetes, hyperhidrosis, lack of hygiene, and immunosuppression. Deeper/systemic infections by this bacterium are exceedingly rare outside of the setting of immunosuppression.

- The classic clinical feature is a well-demarcated, hyperpigmented or erythematous, reddish-brown patch. There may be accentuation of skin lines and some fine scale. The most commonly affected sites are the web spaces of the toes, the upper inner thighs, the inguinal folds, the scrotum/vulva, the axillae, and the gluteal cleft.
- Examination in a dark room with a Wood lamp demonstrates coral pink changes at the sites of erythrasma.
- The infection can last for years if left untreated. Although it can be itchy, it is normally asymptomatic.

## Differential Diagnosis

The main clinical differential diagnoses are tinea corporis/pedis/cruris, intertrigo, cutaneous candidiasis, tinea versicolor, and seborrheic dermatitis. Complicating matters, the bacterial and fungal diseases can coexist, as will be discussed in a later section. Inverse psoriasis is also in the differential.

- Tinea corporis normally presents with an annular, elevated, scaly border with central clearing. Erythrasma normally does not have an annular appearance. A skin scraping stained with KOH should be positive in the setting of tinea, and a Wood lamp examination should not show the coral pink changes.
- Tinea versicolor normally presents as a disseminated hyperpigmented or hypopigmented macular eruption with minimal scale on the trunk, which may involve the intertriginous sites as well. A KOH test will also be positive in this setting.
- Candidiasis normally presents with a deeper red plaque with satellite lesions and pustules. A KOH can be performed to detect yeast forms. Routine culture is also useful. Erythrasma normally is not deep red in color and lacks the satellite lesions/pustules.
- Seborrheic dermatitis can also involve the groin folds; however, it would typically present with significantly more scale that is waxy as opposed to fine. The red patches would typically be present on the head and neck, the axillae, and the central chest.
- Inverse psoriasis presents with well-demarcated red plaques with wet, macerated scale in intertriginous sites. Fissuring can occur. The scale in erythrasma is

much finer and typically not macerated. Completing a family history of psoriasis, inquiring about joint pains, and performing a complete examination to look for other signs, such as extensor surface plaques, scalp involvement, and nail changes, can be useful.

## Work-Up

A thorough physical examination that focuses on the aforementioned sites is recommended. Other corynebacterial diseases, such as pitted keratolysis, can be present in patients with erythrasma.

A Wood lamp examination of the lesions will reveal the characteristic coral pink (red) hue from the organism releasing porphyrins. Nevertheless, this test may be falsely negative if the patient recently washed the area.

A KOH test will be negative for yeast and hyphae. A Gram stain can be performed; however, the yield is poor and it is not generally recommended.

Concomitant infections of erythrasma and tinea corporis/pedis/cruris, as well as tinea versicolor, can occur and are common, so a combination of the aforementioned techniques is important for guiding diagnosis and treatment.

A biopsy can be performed; however, it should not be needed unless there is a failure of treatment that calls the clinical diagnosis into question. Of note, the histopathologic features of erythrasma are subtle, and the bacteria can be easily missed in the stratum corneum by a pathologist. Therefore the clinical concern should be stated on the pathology requisition to help guide interpretation.

There is no role for blood work unless recurrent widespread erythrasma is present, in which case screening tests for diabetes should be considered.

## Initial Steps in Management
### General Management Comments

Keeping the area dry and cool is essential. Any exposure to warm and wet environments will likely cause a recurrence of the infection.

### Recommended Initial Regimen

Topical erythromycin and clindamycin are the mainstays of therapy. Miconazole cream has also been used.

### Partial but Inadequate Response

If there is a partial but inadequate response after a 4-week trial of twice-daily topical antimicrobial treatment, question the diagnosis.

- Consider repeating a KOH test, Wood lamp examination, and/or a full skin examination. There may be a concomitant fungal infection or other disease present.
- Oral antibiotic therapy with a course of oral erythromycin, single-dose clarithromycin, or single dose amoxicillin-clavulanate should be trialed.

### Continued Inadequate Response

If the response continues to be inadequate, a biopsy could be considered at this time, particularly if the Wood lamp examination has been persistently negative and there has been no response to topical and oral treatment of both potential bacterial and fungal causes.

### Other Treatment Options

Fusidic acid cream is an effective therapy; however, it is not available in the United States. Photodynamic therapy has been tried but is not recommended.

### Warning Signs/Common Pitfalls

There can be postinflammatory pigment alteration after many intertriginous dermatoses. The hyperpigmentation from these disorders can mimic erythrasma and vice versa. Because it is asymptomatic and can look like postinflammatory pigment change, erythrasma can be dismissed as a resolved issue, leading to a delay in diagnosis and treatment.

Obese patients or physically impaired patients may be unaware of the infection, particularly because of the lack of symptoms. Examining folds thoroughly, especially ones that patients cannot examine themselves, is important.

Groin rashes are often empirically treated as fungal infections without consideration for this common bacterial infection. The previously described work-up should be used, especially if a patient has failed empiric topical and/or oral antifungal agents.

### Counseling

You have a superficial bacterial infection of the skin that is known as "erythrasma." Unless you have an impaired immune system, this infection is not serious or life threatening. The bacteria like to grow in dark, warm, moist areas on your body. The infection can be easily treated by keeping these areas dry and cool and using topical antibiotics, such as erythromycin or clindamycin.

Recurrences of erythrasma are very common, particularly in warmer, wetter climates, or if there is a lack of access to proper hygiene. If you have frequent recurrences, we should screen you for diabetes. If you do not improve after initial treatment, oral antibiotics, such as erythromycin, clarithromycin, or amoxicillin-clavulanate, can be used to treat your condition.

# LICHEN SCLEROSUS

### Campbell Stewart

### Clinical Features

Lichen sclerosus (LS) is an inflammatory disorder of the skin that presents in children and adults, primarily affecting the anogenital skin of females and males (Fig. 5.2). Females are more often affected than males. LS can present less commonly with widespread extragenital lesions (Fig. 5.3). The cause of LS is unknown. In the early inflammatory stage, the lesions may lack characteristic features, but there are certain classic features to note in general.

- The classic lesion shows a white (ivory to porcelain) macule/papule or patch/plaque, sometimes with scattered central petechiae/purpura and a slightly hyperpigmented border. The lesions may be flush with the skin, slightly elevated, or, in the chronic stage, atrophic. They often have a parchment paper–like appearance. The atrophy often feels superficial, with underlying induration, particularly in long-standing lesions.
- Plugging of hair follicles and/or sweat glands may occur, causing a textured, rather than smooth, appearance.

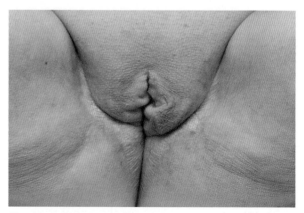

**Fig. 5.2 Genital Lichen Sclerosus.** Note the figure-8 distribution and cigarette paper–quality of the skin. (From the UConn Grand Rounds Collection.)

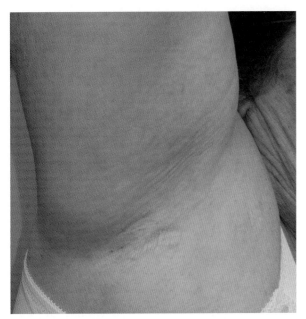

**Fig. 5.3** Extragenital Lichen Sclerosus. Note the cigarette paper–quality of the skin. (Courtesy Justin Finch, MD.)

- Maceration, erosions, bullae, and purpura are often seen. Vulvar lesions can take on a thickened (hyperkeratotic) appearance.
- Chronic, untreated lesions can scar, inducing fusion of the labia and shrinking of the vaginal introitus in women, and phimosis in uncircumcised men. Scarring of the urethral meatus can also occur.
- The lesions may be asymptomatic; however, pain and pruritus are commonly described, particularly in genital sites. There can be associated dyspareunia and dysuria. In uncircumcised males, balanitis can occur.
- Urinary retention secondary to scarring of the urethral meatus can also result in pyelonephritis.
- Patients with chronic genital lesions have up to a 5% increased risk for developing squamous cell carcinoma (SCC). SCC in extragenital LS is rare.
- LS often waxes and wanes; however, it can resolve spontaneously, particularly in younger patients with limited genital involvement. The extragenital variant can be more challenging and persistent in its course.

## Differential Diagnosis

The main clinical differential diagnoses for LS are lichen planus, morphea, vitiligo, sexual abuse/trauma, extramammary Paget disease (EMP), and SCC in situ/invasive SCC.

### Lichen Planus

Lichen planus normally presents with pruritic, purple, polygonal papules or plaques on the extremities and trunk. It can involve multiple sites and mucosal (genital and oral) involvement. Mucosal lesions can have erosive features, and there is a risk for SCC. Genital mucosal lichen planus can extend past the vaginal introitus, whereas LS never involves mucosa past the introitus (Chapter 6, "Lichen Planus").

### Morphea

This condition can overlap with LS. Typically, the lesions are more bound down and smooth, without the overlying parchment paper like change. A punch biopsy may be useful; however, these conditions can often have overlapping histologic features.

### Vitiligo

Vitiligo is common on acral sites and genitals and can present in similar age groups; normally, it lacks the atrophic features/induration and the associated petechiae/purpura (Chapter 8, "Vitiligo").

### Sexual Abuse/Trauma

See the later section on "Warning Signs/Common Pitfalls" for further commentary.

### Extramammary Paget Disease

EMP usually presents as slow-growing, erythematous, often scaling, well-demarcated plaques that are unresponsive to treatment. Over time, they may become erosive or ulcerated. Biopsy establishes the diagnosis.

### Squamous Cell Carcinoma in Situ/Invasive Squamous Cell Carcinoma

SCC in situ, or Bowen disease, can look very similar to an inflammatory persistent red scaling papule or plaque. Biopsy establishes the diagnosis.

### Other Conditions

Extragenital LS shows clinical features similar to forms of anetoderma, atrophoderma, metabolic diseases, atrophie blanche, idiopathic guttate hypomelanosis, and connective tissue diseases (i.e., lupus).

## Work-Up

A full-body skin examination is recommended to assess the scope of LS and see if there are any lesions more clinically consistent with morphea or LS–morphea overlap. A careful history is essential, particularly in children, to assess for any possibility of sexual trauma or abuse.

Blood work is not typically recommended, unless a thorough history and physical examination raises clinical concern for an associated connective tissue disease.

A punch biopsy is normally not necessary. The procedure can be performed in certain scenarios where the diagnosis is not clinically apparent.

- A punch biopsy of the most established lesion (whitest, most indurated), rather than newest (pink/red, not clinically well defined), is preferred for diagnostic accuracy.
- Biopsies are more often needed in extragenital LS, which is less common, and can raise a broader clinical differential.
- Any thickened, macerated, nonhealing/eroded site, particularly of the genitals, should be biopsied to rule out SCC.

## Initial Steps in Management

### Recommended Initial Regimen

Super-potent topical steroids (e.g., 0.05% clobetasol propionate cream or ointment) are the cornerstone of successful management of LS. The super-potent steroids should be initiated immediately after diagnosis to avoid long-term complications.

- Dosing should be once to twice daily for up to 3 months; however, frequency of application can decrease if there is a resolution of symptoms (which may include pain, pruritus, dysuria, or dyspareunia). Slowly reducing the application down to one to three times per week can be done once symptoms are under control and there is no evidence of disease progression. Other topical agents can be used for maintenance. Medium-potency and low-potency topical steroids are not recommended, even as part of a wean/taper.
- Careful and regular monitoring of the sites for improvement, disease progression, and any possible complications of high-potency steroid use is recommended.

### Partial but Inadequate Response

If there is a partial but inadequate response after a trial of super-potent topical corticosteroid monotherapy, topical calcineurin inhibitors (such as pimecrolimus or tacrolimus) can also be used with fairly good results.

- These agents can also be used to spare certain sites from steroid-induced atrophy. In challenging cases, high-potency steroids, such as clobetasol propionate, can be used twice daily for up to 2 to 3 weeks, with a spacer of twice-daily topical tacrolimus for at least 1 week, and then resumption of the topical steroid if symptoms flare or the disease progresses.

Hormonal agents (oral and topical) have no efficacy in treating LS and should not be used.

### Continued Inadequate Response

If the response continues to be inadequate, oral agents that can be used include hydroxychloroquine (5–6.5 mg/kg/day using ideal body weight), methotrexate (generally 10–15 mg weekly), cyclosporine, and oral retinoids.

- If there is resistance to treatment, if there is evidence of disease progression, or if the clinical picture is not clear, a punch biopsy should be considered to confirm diagnosis. Referral to a dermatologist should be made. If there is labial/urethral scarring, gynecology/urology should be consulted. In uncircumcised men with phimosis, circumcision can be helpful. Outside of that scenario, surgery is not recommended unless there is a biopsy-proven malignancy.

## Warning Signs/Common Pitfalls

Because of the commonly associated features of petechiae/purpura in LS, there can be clinical concern for child abuse and sexual trauma. This clinical differential must be explored carefully by the healthcare provider using both physical examination skills and history taking to avoid any underdetection or overdetection of abuse.

A lack of strong topical steroid use in the treatment of LS (i.e., the use of low-potency steroids, such as hydrocortisone 1%–2.5%) is a common pitfall. This undertreatment is usually because of concerns about stronger steroids causing atrophy/telangiectasias on the genitals/sensitive sites, particularly in younger patients. This action can result in a devastatingly progressive disease with long-term complications, such as narrowing of the vaginal introitus, labial fusion, phimosis, and SCC. It should be noted that the mucous membranes of the vagina and non-hairbearing sites of the vulva are resistant to steroid-induced changes; however, the remaining perineal sites can atrophy with longer term (greater than 3 weeks) super-potent topical steroid use.

LS can be associated with morphea in an overlap syndrome, which may require systemic therapies or light-based treatment. Prompt referral to dermatologist should be made if such a scenario is considered.

## Counseling

You have a condition known as "lichen sclerosus" that is caused by inflammation in your skin. There is no known cause, and it is highly unlikely that anything you (or your child) did caused this to occur.

Lichen sclerosus can be treated using a regular application of a super-potent topical steroid cream to the affected sites. We have to treat the area to avoid potential problems, including pain, itch, and permanent scarring. The scars cannot be reversed once they are present, so immediate and regular therapy is necessary. Scarring can result in vaginal/penile pain, difficulty urinating, and painful sexual intercourse. Untreated areas also have the potential to become cancerous.

You should be monitored every few months to make sure you are not having any of the aforementioned complications. In some cases, this condition fades over time, but recurrences can happen later in life. If your condition is not responsive to steroids or if it progresses, there are other topical creams that can be tried. Additionally, there are systemic agents (pills) that can be taken to reduce the inflammation in your body. We may need to involve other healthcare providers in your care if your condition does not improve or if scarring is present.

# RED SCROTUM SYNDROME

**Campbell Stewart**

## Clinical Features

Red scrotum syndrome (RSS), also known colloquially as "the angry red scrotum" or called "male genital dysesthesia," is an uncommon condition that affects older males. The cause is unknown; however, there is an association with chronic topical steroid use. RSS is defined by an intense burning sensation and pain. It is generally not pruritic, unlike many other scrotal dermatoses. There may be a relationship to erythromelalgia.

- RSS is clinically characterized by a sharply demarcated confluent patch of bright red erythema, involving mostly the anterior portion of the scrotum.
- There should be no associated scale, lichenification, or evidence of excoriation.

- The patch in RSS does not extend past the scrotum, unlike other groin and genital dermatoses.

## Differential Diagnosis

The clinical differential diagnosis includes contact dermatitis, psoriasis, tinea cruris, syphilis, and Langerhans cell histiocytosis.

### Contact Dermatitis

Contact dermatitis can be either irritant or allergic in nature. Common allergens include cosmetic products, dyes, elastic fibers in clothing/incontinence pads, and other chemicals. The lesions are less well demarcated, tend to be geometric, and may correspond to specific exposures. Contact dermatitis can be acute or chronic. The primary symptom is intense itch in contrast to the burning and pain of RSS. The lesions are often thickened, with features of excoriations and, in chronic cases, lichenification. If itch is the primary symptom, AD can affect the scrotum as well.

### Psoriasis

Psoriasis can be purely inverse in nature but rarely involves only the scrotum without involvement of the penis or other parts of the gluteal fold/perineum. There is normally scale and maceration, and the lesions can be sharply demarcated or less well defined. Fissures may also be present. Psoriasis can be painful or itchy but normally does not burn intensely the way that RSS does.

### Tinea Cruris

Caused by dermatophyte fungi (most commonly *Trichophyton rubrum*), and normally presents with widespread involvement of the inguinal folds. There is scaling, and a thickened annular (ring like) border, with central clearing. This diagnosis can be confirmed with a scraping of the scale and then a KOH preparation of the scale from the outer rim of the lesion.

### Syphilis

A careful sexual history should be taken and a rapid plasma reagin (RPR)/venereal disease research laboratory (VDRL) test as indicated.

### Langerhans Cell Histiocytosis

This diagnosis is less common than those previously mentioned, especially in the older demographic of men typically affected by RSS. Nevertheless, a punch biopsy of the site would be needed to exclude this from the clinical differential if there is concern.

## Work-Up

There is no defined method for creating a work-up for RSS, except to exclude other causes of scrotal rash. A careful history and physical examination should be performed to evaluate for other scrotal dermatoses such as those previously mentioned. A biopsy of RSS often shows dilated superficial blood vessels without inflammation and is therefore nondiagnostic. Biopsy should only be performed if there is suspicion of an inflammatory or neoplastic process. There is no role for blood work or imaging studies.

## Initial Steps in Management

### General Management Comments

RSS is a challenging condition to treat. The condition is rare, and treatment options are not well defined in the literature. Patients often have persistent symptoms and recurrences after periods of clearance or improvement. Counseling patients that there is no well-defined cause can be frustrating for both the healthcare provider and the patient. Encouraging patients to stop topical steroids can also be a challenge.

### Recommended Initial Regimen

Cessation of all topical steroids, even over-the-counter (OTC) hydrocortisone 1% cream, is essential.

Topical calcineurin inhibitors (such as tacrolimus or pimecrolimus) should be applied twice daily to the affected area for at least 4 weeks. Regular use of these topicals may be needed for long-term control. Occasionally, patients can have a burning sensation with the application of topical calcineurin inhibitors (particularly tacrolimus). This reaction normally subsides with repeated use, but if it does not, try changing to pimecrolimus or stopping these agents altogether.

### Partial but Inadequate Response

If there is a partial but inadequate response after a 4-week trial of topical calcineurin inhibitor monotherapy, some authors initiate doxycycline 100 mg twice daily for its antiinflammatory effects. If no response is noted at 3 months, doxycycline should be discontinued.

### Continued Inadequate Response

If the response continues to be inadequate, gabapentin and pregabalin have both been used with reports of success.

## Other Treatment Options

Oral carvedilol has also been used to treat refractory cases.

## Warning Signs/Common Pitfalls

A warning sign that a patient has RSS is a complaint of burning and pain, not itch, restricted to the scrotum. If the patient presents with those complaints and has a sharply demarcated bright red area that does not involve the rest of the perineum, RSS should be strongly considered. Other potential causes should be excluded as previously described because there is no confirmatory test for RSS.

The most common pitfall is misdiagnosis and treatment of chronic rashes in the groin/scrotum with topical steroids, which can make RSS worse and prolong the course.

## Counseling

You have a rash that involves your scrotum, which is characterized by burning pain and sensitivity. It is called the "red scrotum syndrome." There is no defined cause for this condition. This condition can be very frustrating and persistent, so please try to be patient as we trial different therapies to improve your symptoms. It is most important that you stop any topical steroids to the area, including over-the-counter products, because these can make the condition worse and harder to treat over time, even if they provide temporary relief.

You can be treated with a course of alternative topical agents, such as tacrolimus and/or pimecrolimus. These topicals decrease inflammation in the skin but are not steroids. Occasionally, these medications can cause some discomfort when they are first used, but after consistent use, this sensation should pass.

If the topical agents do not work, an oral antibiotic called "doxycycline" can be used. The antibiotic works by decreasing inflammation in your skin, not because this condition is an infection. Improvement can take months.

If these options do not work, there is a pill called "gabapentin" that modulates nerves to decrease pain. Some patients have responded well to this medication. Lastly, we can consider treating you with a low-dose blood pressure medication, such as carvedilol. We would need to make sure you do not have any cardiac issues and might need to check an electrocardiogram before starting this medication.

# FIXED DRUG ERUPTION

**Campbell Stewart**

## Clinical Features

Fixed drug eruption (FDE) is a skin-limited inflammatory reaction to a drug exposure. FDE is characterized by repeated flares at the same anatomic location with each exposure. Initial drug exposure may not cause an issue for up to 2 weeks; however, upon reexposure to the offending agent, the reaction is rapid, often occurring within 8 hours.

FDE is most commonly caused by:

- Trimethoprim-sulfamethoxazole
- Nonsteroidal antiinflammatory agents, such as ibuprofen and naproxen
- Anticonvulsant agents
- Other antibiotics
  - Tetracycline class, sulfonamide, metronidazole, and nystatin
    - Sulfa-based drugs can cross-react if the patient is allergic to sulfonamides.
- Phenothiazines
- Sildenafil
- Oral contraceptive agents
- Salicylates
- Quinine
- Laxatives (although phenolphthalein is no longer used)
- Foods, such as cashews and licorice, and food coloring

The classic clinical appearance is a solitary, well-demarcated, red to purple, sometimes dusky or violaceous, blanching patch or plaque, with or without an associated bulla or erosion (Fig. 5.4). The lesions can be annular, round, oval, or polycyclic. Solitary lesions can grow to alarming sizes (around 20 cm), especially with repeated exposure to the responsible drug.

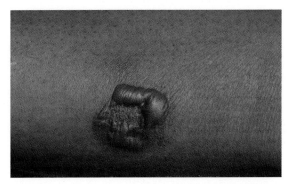

**Fig. 5.4 Fixed Drug Eruption.** Penile involvement is common.

Lesions can be multiple. They can cluster in a single anatomic site or can be generalized. Lesions can also progress to other sites with repeated exposure to the allergen.

The most common site is the genitalia, but FDE is not restricted and can occur on any skin site, including the oral and ocular mucosae.

Most lesions are asymptomatic, even when large, expanding, and bullous. Patients may complain of itch, pain, or burning.

## Differential Diagnosis

The clinical differential diagnosis includes genital/oral herpes simplex (HSV 1/2), impetigo, Stevens-Johnson syndrome (SJS)/toxic epidermal necrolysis (TEN), erythema multiforme, and aphthous stomatitis.

## Work-Up

A full physical examination is essential and inquiring about the involvement of oral and genital sites is important. Patients may not willingly share that they have lesions in these areas. The full examination is also necessary in the setting of widespread lesions because the clinical differential includes SJS/TEN, a spectrum of life-threatening severe cutaneous drug reactions.

A very careful history regarding ingested oral agents must be taken. Even when asked directly, patients will often not recall their use of OTC pain killers, laxatives, and health supplements. Even simple commercial food dyes and tonic water containing quinine can trigger a flare.

Remind the patient that a single exposure can cause a flare within 8 to 24 hours so that they can consider possible causes more carefully going forward. Also remind them that the lesions can persist for up to 8 weeks after exposure, with significant postinflammatory pigmentation.

If no oral agent is identified, consider intravenous agents or any agent that might be introduced to the vaginal/anal mucosa.

Viral culture/polymerase chain reaction (PCR) of recurrent lesions to evaluate for oral/genital HSV should be performed if there is clinical concern. Bacterial culture to rule out suspected impetigo should be accomplished if that is a clinical consideration.

Biopsy (preferably a punch) can be performed. This will differentiate the process from infectious causes, but erythema multiforme and SJS may show similar histopathologic features.

## Initial Steps in Management
### General Management Comments

Only a single reexposure can cause a flare. Identifying the responsible agent is essential for clearance. The longer the drug is continued, the more established the reaction is, and this can lead to long standing postinflammatory pigment changes. Educating patients about similar medications that can cause flares is necessary to avoid recurrence.

### Recommended Initial Regimen

The recommended initial regimen involves the cessation of the responsible oral agent. Once stopped, the reaction typically resolves within weeks.

Topical corticosteroids applied twice daily for 2 to 3 weeks will likely result in improvement. Topical calcineurin inhibitors, such as tacrolimus or pimecrolimus, may be used, especially in delicate sites such as the genitals, eyelids, or other parts of the face.

### Partial but Inadequate Response

If there is a partial, but inadequate response after a 2- to 3-week trial of topical corticosteroid/topical calcineurin inhibitor monotherapy, consider other agents that could be responsible for the eruption. Repeat a history with the patient.

### Continued Inadequate Response

If the response continues to be inadequate, a viral culture, bacterial cultures, and/or skin biopsy should be done to confirm diagnosis, if they have not already been performed at a previous encounter.

### Other Treatment Options

Systemic steroids can be used. Oral prednisone starting at 1 mg/kg and tapered over a 2- to 3-week period is effective, particularly if there is widespread involvement. Oral cyclosporine can also be used in severe widespread cases.

## Warning Signs/Common Pitfalls

A patient with a recurrent localized rash should raise the possibility of an FDE. Not considering HSV as a cause is a potential pitfall.

## Counseling

Your skin rash is called a "fixed drug eruption." This is a focal inflammatory skin reaction to a certain chemical or compound that you are taking by mouth. The most common causes are pills that are available over the counter, including pain killers. Prescription medications, including antibiotics, antiseizure medications, pain medications, and blood pressure medications, can be responsible. Even simple food products, such as items with food coloring and tonic water, can be causes. If we cannot determine a potential cause, you should track any flares you have in the future and think about everything you have ingested or been exposed to in the previous 8 to 24 hours.

Without stopping the responsible agent, the rash will persist. It can rarely spread to other parts of the body.

We can treat your active skin areas with prescription topical steroids or topical medications, such as pimecrolimus or tacrolimus. These can be applied twice daily to the affected sites for 2 to 3 weeks and should improve your symptoms. The discoloration at the site can take many months to fade. Regular use of moisturizing creams or ointments and sun protection can shorten the amount of time needed to even out your skin tone.

# HIDRADENITIS SUPPURATIVA

# HAILEY-HAILEY DISEASE

**Campbell Stewart**

## Clinical Features

Hailey-Hailey disease, also known as "familial benign pemphigus," is an autosomal dominant genodermatosis caused by a mutation in *ATP2C1*, the gene that encodes a calcium pump protein essential for intercellular attachment. This mutation results in loose attachments between the keratinocytes within the epidermis (acantholysis), causing fragility and fragmentation of the most superficial layer of skin.

The disease affects males and females in equal numbers and is relatively rare, affecting approximately 1 in 50,000 people.

Lesions of Hailey-Hailey typically involve the axillae, neck, inframammary chest, inguinal folds, and sometimes the scrotum/vulva (Figs. 5.5 and 5.6). Rarely, other body sites can be involved. Secondary infection with *Staphylococcus aureus* and *Candida* species is common and regularly complicates the course of Hailey-Hailey.

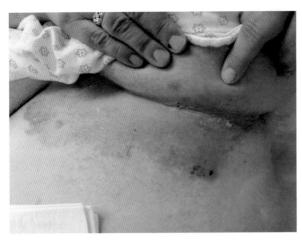

**Fig. 5.5** Inframammary Hailey-Hailey Disease.

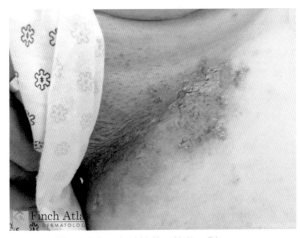

**Fig. 5.6** Inguinal Hailey-Hailey Disease.

Although genetic in nature, the onset of symptoms is often delayed until puberty or later and can start even in the fourth or fifth decade of life. The frequency and severity of the flares can wane in older patients.

- The classic lesion of Hailey-Hailey is an intertriginous, well-demarcated, macerated, fissured and often eroded, weeping plaque.
- The lesions can show secondary features of crust, particularly if they are impetiginized.
- Vegetative plaques can occur in chronic, poorly controlled disease.

- The lesions tend to wax and wane and are exacerbated by mechanical and shear forces, heat, perspiration, stress, secondary infections, and other factors.
- Sites heal without scarring, but there can be significant postinflammatory pigment change.

## Differential Diagnosis

The clinical differential diagnosis for Hailey-Hailey includes intertrigo, candidiasis, inverse psoriasis, and Darier disease.

### Intertrigo

These lesions can look identical to milder Hailey-Hailey disease. A diagnosis of Hailey-Hailey should be considered in those with refractory lesions in intertriginous sites, in cases where multiple body sites are involved, and in cases with neck involvement without significant affecting the tissue folds. A family history of other immediate family members with similar lesions can raise the suspicion of Hailey-Hailey.

### Candidiasis

Typically, this infection presents with a deeper red plaque with satellite lesions and pustules. Because Hailey-Hailey can be secondarily infected with *Candida* species, a positive routine culture does not exclude Hailey-Hailey from the clinical differential.

### Inverse Psoriasis

The plaques of inverse psoriasis can also be well demarcated but normally do not become crusted/secondarily infected. Although fissures and erosions may occur, it is not to the same degree as seen in Hailey-Hailey. Completing a family history of psoriasis, inquiring about joint pains, and performing a complete examination to look for other signs, such as extensor surface plaques, scalp involvement, and nail changes, can be useful. A skin biopsy can differentiate between the two diseases in challenging cases.

### Darier Disease

Darier disease is caused by a similar autosomal dominant mutation in a separate calcium transporter and is a close relative of Hailey-Hailey. The two have overlapping clinical features; however, the lesions of Darier disease more commonly involve the trunk, scalp, and neck than the lesions of Hailey-Hailey do. Nonetheless, there can be intertriginous involvement in Darier disease

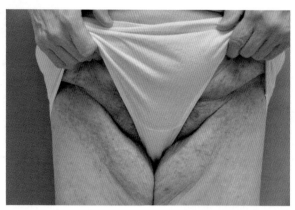

**Fig. 5.7** Inguinal Darier Disease.

(Fig. 5.7). Patients with Darier disease can have acral papules on their hands and feet, V-shaped nicking of the distal nails, and red-and-white striping (in a candy cane pattern) of the nails. These features are not seen in Hailey-Hailey.

## Work-Up

A punch biopsy is recommended if Hailey-Hailey is a clinical consideration. The features of suprabasilar acantholysis with minimal dyskeratosis are supportive. Immunofluorescence testing and serologic autoantibody tests are negative in Hailey-Hailey.

The lesions should be cultured to evaluate for active secondary bacterial, fungal, and viral infections, particularly in refractory lesions. Sensitivity studies are also useful, particularly because patients can be exposed to multiple topical and systemic antimicrobial agents throughout their lifetimes.

Remember that a positive culture for any of these infections does not exclude a diagnosis of Hailey-Hailey.

There is no defined role for blood work or imaging studies in Hailey-Hailey.

## Initial Steps in Management
### General Management Comments

There is no cure for Hailey-Hailey. Patient education about the chronic waxing and waning nature of the disease is essential to increasing patient-driven maintenance of the condition.

Minimizing triggers, such as friction, heat, and sweat, is important to disease control.

### Recommended Initial Regimen

The use of an antibacterial wash in the affected areas, such as chlorhexidine 4%, which should be allowed to sit on the skin for 2 minutes and then carefully rinsed, can reduce secondary infections. Avoidance of exposure to eyes and ears is essential.

Topical clindamycin and erythromycin are useful; however, gel- and alcohol-based solutions of these agents should be avoided because they can be highly painful to the fissured, macerated lesions.

Topical steroids, given at the lowest potency needed to control disease, can help clear flares. Because of the intertriginous nature of the disease, class V and class VI steroids applied twice daily directly to lesions over a period of 2 to 3 weeks are normally sufficient. Rarely, some cases may require super-potent steroids (class I) for clearance. Short courses of 2 to 3 weeks are unlikely to cause steroid-induced atrophy and telangiectasias, but these super-potent topicals should be prescribed with caution and for temporary use only.

Topical calcineurin inhibitors, such as pimecrolimus and tacrolimus, are beneficial. These are effective steroid-sparing options and work for prolonged maintenance of clearance. Some patients find these agents to be too irritating for regular use, however.

### Partial but Inadequate Response

If there is a partial but inadequate response after a 2- to 3-week trial of topical corticosteroid or topical calcineurin inhibitor use, a routine culture for bacteria and fungus from the most clinically impressive site is recommended (especially if there is malodor).

- A viral culture or PCR may also be obtained if there is clinical concern for secondary herpetic infection.
- Oral antibiotic therapy should also be initiated. Oral doxycycline 100 mg twice daily for 14 to 21 days in combination with the aforementioned topical care is recommended. Oral erythromycin can also be used.
- If yeast is cultured and positive, treatment with a topical azole antifungal agent, such as ketoconazole 2%, twice daily for 4 weeks should be sufficient. Oral fluconazole may also be used.
- Treatments focusing on the minimization of sweating can also be tried. Both intralesional botulinum toxin and oral glycopyrrolate (dosed as 1–3 mg twice daily, based on patient tolerance of anticholinergic effects) have been used with success.

## Continued Inadequate Response

If the response continues to be inadequate, there is increasing data that oral naltrexone is an effective, inexpensive maintenance therapy.

- Although naltrexone is only manufactured in 50-mg tablets, many experts recommend compounding naltrexone in solution and having patients take 3 to 5 mg nightly.
- There is no well-defined data to support the use of other agents in Hailey-Hailey; however, many different options have been reported. A referral to a dermatologist is recommended to discuss treatment options at this point in the patient's care.
- Oral dapsone, methotrexate, cyclosporine, retinoids, and prednisone have been tried with reported varying success.

## Other Treatment Options

Patients who are averse to taking pills by mouth can also consider interventional therapies. A fully ablative $CO_2$ laser applied to affected areas is frequently well tolerated and can lead to durable remissions. Unfortunately, it is often very costly for patients.

Other physical modalities mostly include dermabrasion and photodynamic therapy. These techniques have been reported with good response rates.

## Warning Signs/Common Pitfalls

The clinical feature of diffuse fissuring and/or crusting in intertriginous plaques should be a clue that the patient may have Hailey-Hailey. Intertriginous vegetative lesions are also a warning sign.

In mild disease, Hailey-Hailey can be easily confused with intertrigo and candida, or even psoriasis, all of which are far more common. The diagnosis of Hailey-Hailey should be considered in a patient with a family history of similar lesions, multiple intertriginous sites that are regularly involved, and lesions that are refractory to topical treatment.

## Counseling

You have a genetic condition called "Hailey-Hailey disease." This is an inherited disease that has a high likelihood of being passed on to any children you might have. A biopsy of the skin can be performed to confirm your diagnosis. The disease is caused by fragility in your skin, made worse by friction, heat, and sweat, and it primarily affects the folds of your body. The areas that are affected can become very painful or itchy, can drain fluid, and can ruin clothing. Odor can also be an issue. Although this is not an infection, your skin is fragile and is very susceptible to infections, particularly from bacteria and yeast.

There is no cure for Hailey-Hailey, and it will come and go. You can help decrease the frequency and severity of flares by wearing loose-fitting, breathable clothing, washing the areas with antimicrobial washes, and applying topical antibiotics. During flares, prescription topical steroids can also be prescribed. These should be applied twice daily for the best results. If your sites are not improved after 2 to 3 weeks of topical steroid use, other prescription topical antiinflammatory agents can be used. If you have persistent disease, we may need to culture your lesions and try a course of oral antibiotics. If the oral antibiotics are not effective, you should see a dermatologist to help you with your disease.

# Red and Purple Bumps

# 6

# Bumpy Rashes

## CHAPTER OUTLINE

# ARTHROPOD BITES

**Campbell Stewart**

## Clinical Features

Arthropods are responsible for many dermatologic complaints, including bites, stings, and infestations. They can also be vectors for numerous systemic and life-threatening diseases. The clinical manifestations of arthropod bites vary greatly depending on which arthropod is responsible. Because of the scope of this chapter and book, several arthropod reactions will not be covered, including hymenoptera (bees, wasps, hornets), centipedes, millipedes, caterpillars/moths, scorpions, scabies, chiggers, and lice.

Mosquitoes, midges, flies, bed bugs, and fleas are all insects that can cause papular urticaria. These lesions present as discrete, well-demarcated, pink-red, blanching papules at the site of the bite. The usually pruritic papules can last for several days and may not appear until 24 hours after a bite occurred. Occasionally, these lesions can appear papulovesicular or bullous. Often, a central punctum can be identified.

Mosquitoes, midges, and flies tend only to bite exposed sites. Flies (such as the horse fly, deer fly, and greenheads) mostly cause painless bites at first, followed by intense pain. The remaining lesions are often more painful than itchy. Fleas jump and therefore commonly affect the lower legs. Bed bugs tend to bite in groups or lines (the so-called "breakfast, lunch, and dinner" sign).

Mosquitoes can transmit numerous infections, most commonly malaria, worldwide. In the United States, West Nile, Eastern Equine, and Western Equine encephalitis, as well as Zika and chikungunya, are all relevant mosquito borne diseases. Flies do not tend to transmit disease in the United States but can cause myiasis, filariasis, and onchocerciasis elsewhere in the world.

Bed bugs can be a vector for Chagas disease (trypanosomiasis) where the disease is endemic. They may also transmit hepatitis B.

Fleas are vectors for murine typhus, tularemia, bubonic plaque, and tungiasis.

## Differential Diagnosis

The differential diagnosis for bites from the aforementioned insects includes allergic contact dermatitis (ACD), scabies infestation, lice infestation, and bullous pemphigoid (BP).

- ACD can present with papules; however, this phase tends to result in smaller papules that persist for weeks, as opposed to the 24 to 48 hours these last in bites. The papules in ACD tend to be arranged in a geometric manner and may coalesce into a plaque, unlike papular urticaria, which does not. Patch testing can be performed if there is consideration for ACD. A skin biopsy may be able to distinguish these two entities; however, they have overlapping features.
- Scabies presents as diffuse, whole-body itching from the neck down, often concentrated in the genitals, axillae, and umbilicus, with scaling, crusting, and burrows most often found on the hands. Papules similar to papular urticaria from arthropod bites may be seen in scabies. Scabietic papules, however, tend to cluster in areas like the genitalia, which are rarely involved in arthropod bites. A mineral oil prep of a burrow from the aforementioned anatomic sites could help in the diagnosis of scabies. A skin biopsy may look identical to an arthropod bite, unless a mite or mite eggs or excrement is captured (which is uncommon).
- Lice (pediculosis) can infest the body, scalp, and pubic region, causing diffuse pruritus. They cause lesions identical to the aforementioned arthropods. Unlike the limited nature of those bites, however, lice infestation results in diffuse pruritus, eczematous changes, lichen simplex chronicus, and occasionally crusting related to secondary infection. Finding lice on the body can be challenging and in pediculosis corporis should be looked for in the seams of the clothing. In pediculosis pubis and capitis, on the other hand, nits are usually identified along the hair shafts, and a louse comb may be employed. Skin biopsy would not reliably distinguish lice-induced skin changes from other biting insects.

- BP is an autoimmune pruritic blistering disorder that primarily affects the elderly. In the earliest stages, the eruption can present with small urticarial papules. Tense bullae develop later in the course. Both the initial lesions and bullae in BP can mimic arthropod bites clinically and histopathologically. Therefore referral to a dermatologist for direct immunofluorescence (DIF) testing and other work-up is recommended if there is concern for an autoimmune blistering disease.
- Spiders can bite with a similar reaction to those of the arthropods previously mentioned. Most bites will cause a solitary pruritic or painful red papulo-nodule that will resolve in days. The brown recluse and black widow spiders, however, do have significant cutaneous and systemic adverse effects. The brown recluse causes a painful swollen bite with hemorrhagic changes, central vesiculation, and resulting necrosis. Systemic reactions include fever, chills, disseminated rashes, hemolysis/disseminated intravascular coagulation, seizures and coma. The black widow bite causes autonomic dysfunction with urinary retention, abdominal pain, diaphoresis, hypertension, and, rarely, death. The clinical differential diagnosis for a brown recluse spider bite includes a methicillin-resistant *Staphylococcus aureus* (MRSA) abscess/cellulitis, pyoderma gangrenosum, and ischemia/vascular insufficiency.
- MRSA and other infections usually present as solitary, hot, red painful sites on the body. These tend to evolve from cellulitic plaques to abscesses that require drainage. Although brown recluse bites can cause necrosis, they are not commonly purulent. MRSA infections tend to lack the hemorrhagic appearance of brown recluse spider bites. A tissue or routine wound culture can aid in diagnosis. Other bacterial and viral infections can cause a similar picture but normally in the setting of immune compromise or a disseminated infection.

- Pyoderma gangrenosum (PG) is a neutrophilic dermatosis commonly associated with inflammatory bowel disease, rheumatoid arthritis, and hematologic malignancies. It presents as a painful ulcerated plaque with gray, undermined, irregular borders and often has a cribriform appearance. The clinical presentation can be identical to brown recluse spider bites; therefore a careful clinical history is essential. PG is a diagnosis of exclusion and can only be ruled on once infectious causes of ulceration have been excluded.
- Vascular causes of tissue necrosis include thromboembolism, chronic vascular insufficiency, small to medium and large vessel vasculitides, and calciphylaxis. Typically, patients will present with multiple lesions in these scenarios and will have a health history and other physical examination findings suggestive of a systemic process. A skin biopsy may be helpful in the setting of calciphylaxis and possibly vasculitis; however, all of these diseases may have overlapping features histopathologically. Therefore a careful history and comprehensive physical examination will be essential in differentiating them.
- Ticks bite and attach themselves to feed on humans and other animals. Their bite is painless. They can remain attached for days and may be found in an engorged state attached to the skin at presentation. The patient might ask about their new "mole." Initially, tick bites tend to be red papules. The bites may expand into a patch or plaque of erythema several centimeters large. Necrosis and granuloma formation are less commonly seen. If bitten by an *Ixodes* tick, there is a risk for Lyme borreliosis. Localized Lyme presents as erythema migrans, which is a red annular plaque that can evolve to the classic target-like lesion that enlarges to be 4 cm in diameter or more. Systemic symptoms, including fever and joint pains, may be present. This eruption may fade without treatment. Nonetheless, treatment is necessary to prevent disseminated Lyme and its complications. Persistent tick bite reactions can form large, purple papulonodules caused by cutaneous lymphoid hyperplasia or pseudolymphoma. These are benign reactions that mimic forms of cutaneous B-cell lymphoma. Other tick-borne diseases include Rocky Mountain spotted fever, ehrlichiosis, and anaplasmosis. The clinical differential diagnosis for tick bites includes gyrate erythema, erythema multiforme (EM), and granuloma annulare (GA).

- Gyrate erythema encompasses a group of inflammatory skin reactions that present as red, blanching, variably scaly annular or arcuate plaques on the extremities or trunk. They can be solitary or multiple. The exact cause is not known; however, infections, drugs, malignancy, and liver disease have been associated with them. The lesions in gyrate erythema tend to be more arcuate than targetoid and have defined central clearing, whereas erythema migrans normally retains central erythema. The lesions may have a classic trailing scale behind the annular edge. Nevertheless, scale may be absent in deeper variants. A skin biopsy, particularly if there is no scale, can have overlapping features with erythema migrans and therefore may not be fully diagnostic. A careful physical examination and clinical history is essential for differentiating these two entities.
- EM is a type IV hypersensitivity reaction caused by drugs or herpes simplex virus (HSV) infection. In contrast to the classic solitary appearance of erythema migrans, EM presents as numerous smaller, red papules that evolve into targetoid plaques that may coalesce. The border tends to be more indurated and urticarial than erythema migrans and lacks significant scale. The central lesion is normally vesicular or bullous. Mucosae may be involved as well. Skin biopsy can differentiate EM from a tick bite/erythema migrans.
- GA is an idiopathic inflammatory reaction pattern in the skin that presents with annular plaques without scale. Normally, the plaques are multiple in nature. The color of the lesions is more purplish-brown as opposed to the bright red seen in erythema migrans. Skin biopsy can differentiate these two entities when a clinical examination is not sufficient.

## Work-Up
## Initial Steps in Management
### General Management Comments

Most arthropod bites resolve without intervention. Determining the cause of the bites can be challenging if the practitioner does not ask about outdoor exposure, pet exposures, work, travel, and living arrangements.

### Recommended Initial Regimen

A thorough history is recommended to identify the most likely cause of the bites. If there is a clear history of outdoor exposure, counsel the patient regarding protective measures. These can include limiting outdoor time at twilight, avoiding stagnant water, and wearing long-sleeve shirts and pants. Insect repellents can be applied directly to skin (DEET or picaridin), and permethrin can be sprayed directly onto clothing and allowed to fully dry (not applied to skin).

If there is no clear history of outdoor exposure, then it is essential to take a travel history for the patient and anyone in the home. An infestation of the home by bed bugs or fleas is possible. An exterminator is essential because there is no clear way to determine the type of insect responsible based on the bites alone, unless the patient brings one in to be examined.

A mid-potency topical steroid, such as triamcinolone 0.1% cream, should be applied twice daily for up to 7 days.

For spider bites, referral to an emergency room may be needed for pain control and if there are systemic signs and symptoms. For brown recluse bites, light compression/immobilization and cooling of the sites may help. Patients may need supportive care and/or administration of antivenom if it is available. A tissue culture may be needed in the setting of necrosis to evaluate for infectious causes. Skin necrosis from brown recluse bites may require debridement and skin grafting. Black widow bites should be treated with pain management, including opioids, antihistamines, and benzodiazepines if needed.

If there is suspicion for tick exposure, even if no tick is found, treatment for Lyme disease is recommended in endemic areas. Normally, this includes treatment with oral doxycycline or amoxicillin.

### Partial but Inadequate Response

If there is a partial, but inadequate response after a 1-week trial of a mid-potency topical corticosteroid monotherapy, a higher potency steroid, such as a clobetasol 0.05% cream or ointment, may be applied twice daily for up to 7 days to the lesions of papular urticaria.

### Continued Inadequate Response

If the response continues to be inadequate, reconsider the diagnosis. A biopsy may be indicated. In a patient with lesions that continue to appear in new locations on the body, consider the possibility of an untreated infestation.

### Other Treatment Options

Topical calcineurin inhibitors, such as tacrolimus and pimecrolimus, may also be used for symptom relief.

## Warning Signs/Common Pitfalls

A common pitfall is not taking an adequate history. Asking specific questions about exposures will yield the correct causative type of arthropod most of the time.

Another pitfall is not counseling the patient appropriately about risks and procedures in the setting of home infestations. Many patients are concerned about added costs and are reluctant to pursue veterinary or exterminator appointments as needed.

## Counseling

Your skin lesions are small inflammatory reactions to the bite of an insect. These bites are usually very itchy. They can persist for several days or, rarely, weeks. You may not recall being bitten, and bites can take 1 to 2 days to appear. Most insect bites are caused by insects that live outside, such as mosquitoes, flies, or midges. These can be prevented by wearing clothing and applying insect repellent sprays. Most bite more frequently at twilight, so it is best to move indoors at that time. Avoid areas of standing water because these are places where most of them breed.

If you do not recall being outside at a time of year when insect bites are common, then you may have been exposed to insects that can live inside.

Fleas are common causes of insect bites and can infest pets and humans. They live in your home and are small insects that can be pulled from your involved pet's coat. They tend to cause bites on the lower legs.

Bed bugs can also cause bites. These insects infest homes and are extremely hard to detect except by trained professional exterminators. They live in walls, floorboards, bed frames, and other areas. They can be acquired by staying in an infested home or hotel room and may travel in your luggage. They only feed during a brief period in the night and leave small pinpoint bloodstains on the sheets. Without an exterminator, the infestation will persist.

These types of insect bites can be easily treated with topical steroids applied twice daily for 5 to 7 days.

If you notice blistering at your bite site, or if there is persistent pain or skin breakdown, you may have been bitten by a spider. You may need to have your home investigated for an infestation.

If you have pulled an insect off of you that seemed attached to your skin, it was almost certainly a tick. These bites can cause red target like rashes on the skin. We may need to treat you with an oral antibiotic for several weeks to treat any potential Lyme disease.

# GROVER DISEASE

**Shivani Sinha, Gloria Lin, and Katalin Ferenczi**

## Clinical Features

Grover disease (GD), also known as "transient acantholytic dermatosis," is an acquired condition usually seen in middle-aged Caucasian men. The etiology is poorly understood, but GD has been associated with heat, sweating, sun exposure, radiation, and certain medications. Although benign and potentially self-resolving, the rash may become chronic with fluctuating symptoms that can last for several months or even years.

- Patients who complain about their lesions often endorse a history of intense pruritus in the affected areas; however, GD may also be asymptomatic, in which case it is frequently identified with a full-body skin examination.
- It typically presents as pruritic, erythematous, scaly papules on the trunk with occasional vesicles, crusting, and erosions (Fig. 6.1).
- Factors that increase sweating, such as fever, heat, sun exposure, or prolonged immobility, may predispose patients to the development of GD-related pruritus.

## Differential Diagnosis

The differential diagnoses for GD are folliculitis, including pityrosporum folliculitis, acne, miliaria, morbilliform drug eruption, Darier disease (DD), and pemphigus foliaceus (PF).

- Folliculitis refers to inflammation of the hair follicles and presents with erythematous follicular-based papules and pustules. GD can typically be distinguished from folliculitis because the primary morphology of GD is scaled papules/plaques, whereas folliculitis is acneiform (looks like a pimple). Additionally, distribution is distinguishing because folliculitis can present in areas other than the abdomen and lower trunk, such as the face, scalp, and extremities. Finally, folliculitis will typically improve with a trial of treatment with topical or oral antibiotics, whereas GD will not.

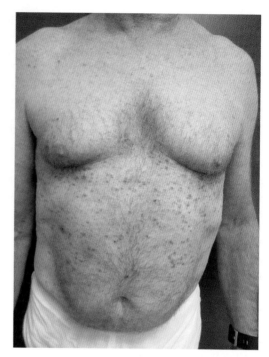

**Fig. 6.1 Grover Disease.** (From the University of Connecticut Department of Dermatology Grand Rounds Collection.)

- Pityrosporum folliculitis presents as intensely pruritic erythematous papules and pustules that are typically located on the trunk. These lesions are acneiform (typically pustular) and monomorphous, whereas GD lesions are papulosquamous (erythematous papules with overlying scale). Most patients with pityrosporum folliculitis are younger (15–35), whereas GD is almost exclusively a disease of late adulthood (with most patients over the age of 45). If a potassium hydroxide (KOH) examination is available, an examination of pityrosporum folliculitis pustular contents will reveal the classic, so-called "spaghetti and meatballs" appearance of the causative *Malassezia sp.* Similarly, if treated with topical and/or oral antifungals, pityrosporum folliculitis will typically respond.
- Acne, although typically seen in younger populations, can affect older patients. Acne of the lower trunk is frequently occlusive acne and is especially common in individuals with occupations that require prolonged sitting (e.g., truck drivers). Again, the primary morphology of acne is acneiform papulopustules and comedones, whereas GD is papulosquamous. Distribution can also distinguish acne

from GD because most patients with acne vulgaris have involvement of their face with or without involvement of the chest and upper back.

- Miliaria, also known as "heat rash," is a condition caused by blocked sweat ducts and is induced by heat and humidity. It presents as red papules that most often involve the trunk in a similar distribution to GD. Unlike GD, lesions of miliaria are frequently transient and episodic and lack overlying scale. Cooling the skin and avoiding heat exposure usually leads to resolution of the condition.
- Morbilliform drug eruptions can be challenging for nondermatologists to distinguish from GD because they can present as pruritic erythematous macules and papules on the trunk. Nevertheless, a history of new drug exposure (typically 7–14 days prior) and the presence of a rash on other areas besides the trunk may be helpful clues to differentiate these two conditions. Similarly, morbilliform drug eruptions are acute with rapid onset, whereas GD is a chronic condition with insidious presentation
- DD is an inherited acantholytic disorder that generally presents in early adolescence or young adulthood. It is characterized by greasy, yellow, keratotic papules in a seborrheic distribution with characteristic erythronychia and V-shaped notching of the nails. Although there are many histologic and clinical similarities, DD can be differentiated because many patients report a family history because it is a genetic condition with autosomal dominant transmission. Additionally, DD almost always presents by late adolescence, whereas GD is a disease of older adults. Finally, DD typically affects multiple seborrheic areas (e.g., the scalp and chest), whereas GD typically only affects the abdomen and lower back.
- PF is an autoimmune disorder characterized by blisters and crusted erosions with a cornflake like scale in a seborrheic distribution involving the head and trunk. Distribution is a key differentiator from GD. Lesions may have a positive Nikolsky sign where the superficial layer of skin dislodges from the deeper layers when pressure is applied. They are also often painful rather than pruritic. Biopsy can reliably differentiate between these two conditions.

## Work-Up

GD is typically a clinical diagnosis based on the findings of a pruritic papulosquamous eruption on the abdomen and lower back of an older adult. Clues in the patient history, such as symptomatic exacerbation with sweating/overheating, can be helpful in securing the diagnosis. Rarely, a punch biopsy of lesional skin is required to confirm the diagnosis.

## Initial Steps in Management

There are no disease-specific therapies for GD, and treatment is directed toward symptom management.

- Patients should avoid excessive heat and sun exposure because this may exacerbate the condition.
- Moisturizers and emollients containing camphor or menthol can be applied to help reduce pruritus and prevent xerosis, which may worsen the condition. These can be stored in the refrigerator to further enhance the cooling sensation when applied to the skin.
- Mid-potency topical steroid creams or ointments (such as triamcinolone 0.1%) can be applied twice daily for up to 2 weeks to the affected areas to alleviate pruritus. Patients should be counseled on the risk for skin atrophy, striae, and dyspigmentation associated with the long-term use of steroids.
- Calcipotriene 0.005% (a vitamin D analog) cream applied twice daily to affected areas can help manage symptoms and function as a steroid-sparing agent.
- Oral antihistamines (diphenhydramine 25–50 mg every 6 hours as needed, cetirizine 5–10 mg daily as needed, or hydroxyzine 10–25 mg every 6 hours as needed) can provide temporary symptomatic relief.

For GD that is refractory to topical steroids and supportive therapies, other treatment options may be considered.

- Narrowband ultraviolet B (NBUVB) radiation has been shown to improve GD but may initially exacerbate the condition before an improvement is seen.
- Systemic medications, such as oral retinoids (acitretin or isotretinoin) and methotrexate, may also be prescribed for severe and recalcitrant GD; however, these should only be prescribed by practitioners experienced with these medications because of the risk for potential side effects and the need for close monitoring.

## Inadequate Treatment Response

If treatment response is inadequate, reconsider the diagnosis and refer the patient to dermatology for further evaluation.

## Warning Signs/Common Pitfalls

- A high degree of suspicion should be maintained for GD in any mature patient with a chronic, pruritic papulosquamous eruption on the abdomen and lower back because this condition is very bothersome to many individuals.
- Many patients have symptoms out of proportion to their physical examination findings. These patients, who frequently have sleep disturbances, require aggressive management with systemic medications to achieve satisfactory disease control.

## Counseling

You have a condition called Grover disease, which is not dangerous to your health but can be challenging to treat. It is important to avoid any known triggers, such as excessive heat, sweating, and sun exposure, because these can exacerbate the rash.

The course of the condition can be unpredictable with fluctuating symptoms, and it may last anywhere between a few weeks to a few years. There is no cure for your condition, but certain over-the-counter (OTC) and prescription medications can help reduce your symptoms. Moisturizers, topical steroids, and antihistamines can help alleviate the itching and may be used as instructed by your physician. Other systemic medications and therapies can be prescribed if your rash is persistent. These medications can be discussed if your symptoms do not improve with the use of creams.

The itching you experience may become severe. Let your physician know if it begins to negatively affect your quality of life so that your treatment plan can be adjusted accordingly.

## PRURIGO NODULARIS

**Shivani Sinha, Gloria Lin, and Katalin Ferenczi**

### Clinical Features

Prurigo nodularis (PN) is a chronic skin condition caused by repetitive scratching, rubbing, or picking (Fig. 6.2). It is more commonly seen in middle-aged women, who often have an underlying condition that may be dermatologic or psychiatric. Less commonly, it can be seen in the pediatric population secondary to concomitant atopic dermatitis (AD). Early recognition is important to halt this cosmetically disfiguring process, which can be extremely distressing

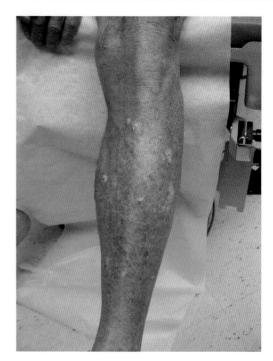

**Fig. 6.2** Prurigo nodularis. (Courtesy Justin Finch, MD.)

for the patient, and to address any underlying conditions that may be contributing to this disease.

- Patients are often unaware of or unwilling to admit that they are scratching or picking. The most common complaint is pruritus, which may be exacerbated by heat, sweating, or irritation from friction. Nevertheless, the patients may insist that the areas are asymptomatic, which can confuse the clinical picture.
- On examination, lesions often appear as multiple, firm, dome-shaped papules or nodules that can be hyperpigmented. The lesions may have overlying central scale or crust with an erosion or ulcer from manipulation of the area. These nodules are usually symmetrically distributed on the extensor surfaces of the extremities with classic sparing of the midback, which is known as the "butterfly sign" because patients are not able to reach that area. These lesions are rarely found on the face, palms, or soles. Although the pathophysiology is similar to lichen simplex chronicus, lichenification of the lesions is not usually present.
- Underlying conditions, such as xerosis, AD, chronic kidney or liver disease, thyroid issues, HIV infection,

psychiatric conditions, parasitic infestations, and malignancy may be present because these can be associated with pruritus.

- PN is often associated with sleep disturbances, anxiety, and depression, leading to a decreased quality of life for the patient.

## Differential Diagnosis

The differential diagnosis for PN includes keloids, acquired perforating dermatoses, pemphigoid nodularis, nodular scabies, hypertrophic lichen planus (LP), multiple keratoacanthomas, and epidermolysis bullosa pruriginosa.

- Keloids can be difficult to distinguish from PN because they can also present as pruritic, firm, hyperpigmented papules or plaques. History may be helpful in this case because the patient often relates a history of trauma or inflammation (i.e., acne) in those areas. Keloids are typically treated with topical or intralesional steroids for symptomatic relief.
- Acquired perforating dermatoses can be associated with chronic renal failure and diabetes. They usually present as multiple, flesh-colored papules with a central keratotic plug at trauma-prone sites, such as the hands and knees. These lesions often regress spontaneously; however, treatment of the underlying disease is important.
- Pemphigoid nodularis is a rare variant of BP, an autoimmune blistering disorder. It is classically seen more frequently in the elderly population. The lesions typically present as pruritic hyperkeratotic nodules that clinically resemble those found in PN. These two conditions may be distinguished through skin biopsy and DIF analysis. Pemphigoid nodularis often requires systemic treatment with steroids or immunomodulators.
- Nodular scabies is most commonly localized to the groin, buttocks, and axillae, with increased nighttime pruritus. More characteristic signs such as linear burrows, excoriations, and interdigital web space involvement may also be present on physical exam, which can help with the diagnosis. Microscopic examination of a burrow's contents may reveal the mites, eggs, or feces. Nodular scabies is typically treated with permethrin or oral ivermectin.
- Hypertrophic LP is characterized by pruritic, pink to purple hyperkeratotic or verrucous plaques that are usually localized to the anterior lower extremities. This can be a challenging diagnosis to make, and a referral to a dermatologist is recommended because a biopsy may need to be performed to establish a diagnosis.
- Keratoacanthomas, a well-differentiated subtype of squamous cell carcinoma (SCC), can also present as flesh-colored, dome-shaped nodules with a central keratotic plug on the extremities. Significant tenderness, a history of bleeding, ulceration, recurrence, or a history of immunosuppression should raise the clinical suspicion for a malignancy.
- Epidermolysis bullosa pruriginosa is a rare subtype of dystrophic epidermolysis bullosa. It can present as chronic pruritic hypertrophic plaques, usually on the lower extremities with sparing of the face. They are often lichenified with a linear configuration, which can help distinguish them from PN. Treatment can be challenging, but topical and intralesional steroids are often used, with more refractory disease requiring systemic therapy.

## Work-Up

Patients with suspected PN should be referred to a dermatologist for further evaluation and treatment. PN is usually a clinical diagnosis made by the dermatologist based on the patient's history and physical examination.

- If the history and clinical findings do not clearly indicate a diagnosis of PN, then the dermatologist can perform a skin biopsy for further evaluation.
- Diagnostic testing to identify systemic diseases that may precipitate pruritus should be considered, including a complete blood count (CBC), liver function test (LFT), basic metabolic panel (BMP), thyroid-stimulating hormone (TSH), HIV testing, urinalysis, and stool examination for ova or parasites.
- If there is any uncertainty in the diagnosis, the patient should be referred to a dermatologist.

## Initial Steps in Management

The most important step in management is to communicate expectations with the patient because PN can be a challenging condition to treat. The patients are often anxious and become easily frustrated by the lack of improvement. Helping to control the pruritus and urge to scratch or pick at the areas is of the utmost importance to stop the repetitive itch-scratch cycle. Based on the complexity and possible reactions to the treatments, a referral to dermatology is advised.

- Recommend that the patient maintain short nails, wear gloves when sleeping, and cover the lesions with bandages to reduce further injury from scratching.
- Gentle skin care, including the use of fragrance-free soaps and emollients, may help because xerosis is a common cause of pruritus.
- Recommend OTC soothing lotions that may be applied to the skin as needed. These include creams containing calamine, menthol, or camphor, which can be stored in the fridge, because this can further enhance the cooling sensation when applied. Topical capsaicin cream is also available over the counter and can be used to help with pruritus, but some patients may not be able to tolerate the burning sensation initially felt when the cream is applied.
- If the lesions look secondarily infected, a course of antibiotics may be warranted.

## Antihistamines

- Antihistamines can provide short-term relief from the pruritus and help improve sleep quality.
- Diphenhydramine 25 to 50 mg can be taken nightly or every 6 hours as needed.
- Cetirizine 5 to 10 mg per day can be taken as needed.
- Hydroxyzine 10 to 25 mg can be taken every 6 hours as needed.
- Patients should be counseled on potential side effects, including sedation, because they should not operate heavy machinery or drive.

## Steroids

- High-potency topical steroids (clobetasol 0.05%, betamethasone dipropionate 0.05%, or halobetasol 0.05%) can be applied twice daily to the affected areas to help alleviate pruritus. An occlusive dressing can increase the penetration of the steroid and protect the skin from further injury. Given the risk for potential side effects, including skin atrophy, a steroid-sparing agent such as calcipotriene or tacrolimus 0.1% ointment can be used in between steroid use to limit steroid exposure.
- Intralesional Kenalog to the individual lesions can be helpful, especially for those refractory to the topical steroids. Depending on the thickness and size of the lesions, different concentrations can be

used. Given the variability in response and dosing schedules, this medication is best administered by a dermatologist.

## Other Medications

- Oral naltrexone (25–150 mg/day), which is thought to act on opioid receptors, may help with symptomatic relief.
- Gabapentin (300–900 mg/day) and pregabalin (75 mg/day) may be effective in decreasing pruritus.
- If there is a suspected underlying psychiatric condition, a referral to a psychiatrist is recommended. Antidepressants (selective serotonin reuptake inhibitors [SSRIs] and tricyclic antidepressants), anxiolytics, psychotherapy, or behavioral therapy can be helpful adjuncts to reduce scratching behaviors and any psychological distress that the patient may be experiencing.
- The patient should be referred to a dermatologist if there is widespread, recalcitrant disease because other treatment modalities may need to be considered.

## Phototherapy

- NBUVB may be recommended by the dermatologist in combination with topical steroids and continued supportive treatment. For patients with multiple comorbidities that require polypharmacy, this option may be safe and efficacious.

## Cryotherapy

- Cryotherapy can be used on each lesion; however, the patient should be counseled that the liquid nitrogen may cause discomfort, erythema, edema, potential blistering, and possible permanent dyspigmentation or scar. A correct diagnosis is crucial before using this treatment modality.

## Immunomodulators

- Medications, such as methotrexate, azathioprine, and thalidomide, have shown benefit in this condition. Referral to a dermatologist is recommended to evaluate the patient before starting treatment because of the risk for potential side effects.
- Dupilumab, an interleukin (IL)-4 receptor inhibitor, which is approved for the treatment of AD, has shown promise in this condition. Referral to a dermatologist is recommended to decide if this is the best treatment modality.

### Biopsy

- A biopsy should be considered when there is a high clinical suspicion for a malignancy, there are recurrent lesions that have failed to respond to previous treatment, there is significant or larger-size hyperkeratosis or ulceration, or the patient is experiencing pain or bleeding.
- Given the risk for cutaneous malignancy in the immunosuppressed or immunocompromised population, there should be a lower threshold for potential biopsy if areas do not respond appropriately to treatment.
- If a biopsy is warranted, a referral to a dermatologist is recommended because incorrect sampling can lead to false negatives and a delay in diagnosis.

### Inadequate Treatment Response

If treatment response is inadequate, reconsider the diagnosis and refer to dermatology for further evaluation.

### Warning Signs/Common Pitfalls

- There should be a low threshold for referral to a dermatologist because this condition can mimic other diseases, and there is a wide differential that has to be considered. In addition, the early involvement of a dermatologist can be helpful to guide management.
- Work-up for underlying systemic diseases, including CBC, LFT, BMP, TSH, HIV testing, urinalysis, and a stool sample, should be considered when clinically indicated.
- Patients should be routinely screened for anxiety, depression, and psychological distress so that supportive therapy can be provided.

### Counseling

You have a condition called "prurigo nodularis," which refers to nodules (bumps) on your skin that are the result of long-term scratching, rubbing, or picking. They are often itchy, which can lead to a vicious itch-scratch cycle that may worsen your condition. The main treatment goal is to control this itching and prevent further injury to the skin. We recommend keeping your nails short, wearing gloves to bed, and keeping the areas covered with bandages to reduce further damage. You should avoid excessive heat exposure and tight garments because sweating and skin irritation from clothing may exacerbate your itching. We recommend gentle cleansers and emollients to keep the skin moisturized while avoiding any harsh scrubs or cleansing agents. Treatment of this condition depends on the number and severity of the lesions. Antihistamines and topical steroids can be helpful in this condition. For severe cases, other treatments, such as phototherapy, steroid injections, or immunomodulators, may be considered. In some cases, a biopsy (skin sample) may be necessary to determine a diagnosis.

Inform your physician if you are experiencing any stress, anxiety, depression, or sleepless nights. Psychological support and/or medication to manage these symptoms can be offered to you if appropriate.

## RENAL (UREMIC) PRURITUS

**Christian Gronbeck and Diane Whitaker-Worth**

### Clinical Features

Renal pruritus develops in patients with end-stage renal disease (ESRD) who are undergoing hemodialysis, with a prevalence of 20% to 60% in this population. Although the exact cause of renal pruritus is not known, it is potentially caused by stimulation of itch neurons from (1) a build-up of poorly dialyzed metabolic toxins, (2) opioid receptor derangements, and (3) systemic inflammation. As expected, dialysis patients are more likely to develop pruritus after inadequate dialysis and in cases where they have persistently elevated serum calcium, phosphorus, and magnesium levels.

Importantly, the majority of patients with ESRD develop comorbid xerosis (Chapter 3, Body Dermatitis section "Dry Skin"). Xerosis contributes to itch in these patients and also should be addressed. Renal pruritus has been identified as a key research priority by patients with ESRD because of its distressing impact and potential association with poor sleep quality, worsened quality of life, and depression. Renal pruritus typically exhibits a chronic course and, once present, generally remains for months to years and can often remain indefinitely.

Renal pruritus is characterized by the development of intense, generalized pruritus in the absence of primary skin lesions.

- The itch most frequently occurs on the back, arms, head, and abdomen, but it can also be widespread across the body.
- Only secondary skin changes, such as excoriations, and prurigo nodules are seen on examination.

- Pruritus can be constant or intermittent, but it is generally worse during the evening hours and frequently impedes adequate sleep.
- Patients may demonstrate elevated serum blood urea nitrogen (BUN), phosphate, calcium, magnesium, and parathyroid hormone (PTH) levels; however, these findings are not needed to make the diagnosis nor are they specific for the diagnosis because they are also present in many patients with ESRD who lack renal pruritus.

## Differential Diagnosis

In a patient with suspected renal pruritus with secondary skin changes, the main differential diagnosis is an acquired perforating dermatosis (APD).

- The development of secondary skin changes in renal pruritus, such as excoriations, erosions, and prurigo nodules, can be confused with APD (e.g., acquired reactive perforating collagenosis, acquired perforating folliculitis), especially because these conditions are all common in patients with ESRD and are incited in part by epidermal irritation. Nevertheless, prurigo nodules in renal pruritus are more often dome-shaped, firm, and flesh-colored, whereas the hallmark of APD is umbilicated papules with a hyperkeratotic central plug.
  - In clinical practice, renal pruritus with prurigo nodules can be difficult to distinguish from APD and, regardless of the exact diagnosis, antipruritic therapies are indicated for improvement of both classes of disorders.

In the absence of skin findings, generalized causes of isolated pruritus, such as primary biliary cholangitis, lymphoma, and polycythemia vera, should be considered.

- Patients with primary biliary cholangitis may also demonstrate significant pruritus in the absence of skin findings; however, they are likely to further exhibit jaundice and fatigue, and laboratory findings will be significant for elevated serum liver enzyme and bilirubin levels.
- Several lymphoma subtypes, including Hodgkin lymphoma and mycosis fungoides, commonly present with pruritus that may precede the development of other symptoms.
  - In the case of Hodgkin lymphoma, pruritus is generally localized to the lower extremities, and patients may have associated so-called "B symptoms" (e.g., fevers, night sweats, weight loss).

- Although it can be isolated, pruritus from mycosis fungoides is more likely to occur in association with numerous scaly skin plaques and diffuse erythroderma.
- Pruritus from polycythemia vera is typically elicited by contact with water (aquagenic pruritus) and is further associated with tingling or burning sensations.

## Work-Up

The diagnosis of renal pruritus is relatively straightforward given the high likelihood in a patient undergoing hemodialysis. As always, a careful evaluation of patient history and clinical examination is essential in solidifying the diagnosis.

- When considering patient history, it is important to assess for the temporal relationship between dialysis onset/significant decline in renal function and symptom presentation.
- A full-body skin examination is warranted to rule out the presence of a primary dermatosis that can have associated pruritus (e.g., ACD or irritant contact dermatitis, psoriasis).
  - If skin lesions are identified, they should be carefully evaluated because they may represent either prurigo nodules in the context of renal pruritus or a perforating disorder.
- Laboratory testing that indicates elevated calcium, phosphate, magnesium, BUN, or PTH levels is further supportive of a diagnosis of renal pruritus.

## Initial Steps in Management
### General Management Comments

- There is no cure for renal pruritus, nor are there any specific treatments, other than adjustment of dialysis, that target the pathogenesis of the condition. All other recommended therapies are itch-directed to help with symptom control.
- All patients with renal pruritus should have their nephrologists notified so that their nephrologist can determine whether adjustment of dialysis settings might help.
- Treatment of comorbid conditions that contribute to renal pruritus, such as hyperparathyroidism and xerosis, should also be implemented for all patients.

Initial symptomatic treatments consist of dry skin care (e.g., emollients, bathing modifications), topical pramoxine, oral gabapentin, and naltrexone.

- Topical pramoxine is available in multiple OTC anti-itch medications.

- These medications should be stored in the refrigerator and then applied as needed to itchy areas. They are often soothing; however, they do not decrease baseline itch and therefore are often not sufficient as a monotherapy.
- A first-line oral therapy for renal pruritus is oral gabapentin. It may be prescribed after dialysis sessions.
  - We generally recommend starting with a low dose of 100 mg, potentially increasing to 300 mg if it is well tolerated.
  - Pregabalin can also be used as an alternative to gabapentin should tolerance of gabapentin be poor.
- Oral naltrexone 50 mg oral daily is another consideration in reducing itch in select patients; however, it is not appropriate for patients currently using opioid analgesic agents because it can precipitate withdrawal.
- Patients often report a benefit from the use of sedating antihistamines (e.g., diphenhydramine) because it helps them fall asleep. Ideally, patients should be provided with other sleeping aids in place of antihistamines because use of these medications is associated with undesirable side effects, such as sedation and increased risk for falls, and these should be weighed against the potential clinical benefit.
  - Additionally, histamine is not a major mediator of itch in renal pruritus and therefore antihistamines are unlikely to improve pruritus.

## Unresponsive Case Management

In patients who are unresponsive or intolerant of oral therapy, NBUVB (i.e., phototherapy) can be very effective for renal pruritus; however, it is very time intensive (requiring three office visits each week).

- Patients who desire phototherapy can be referred to a dermatology office that has an NBUVB unit.

## Warning Signs/Common Pitfalls

- It is important to consider and address the day-to-day implications of renal pruritus on patients' lives. Pruritus can become particularly severe at night, which can adversely affect a patient's sleep. In these cases, treatments targeted at promoting sleep, such as melatonin, may be considered.
- In a patient not currently undergoing dialysis therapy (especially those with stages 1 to 3 of chronic kidney disease), renal pruritus is a very unlikely cause of pruritus and other potential differential diagnoses should be considered.
- Antiinflammatory medications, such as corticosteroids and tacrolimus, have not been shown to benefit individuals with renal pruritus and are typically not considered as potential treatments.

## Counseling

Your skin itching is because of a condition called "renal pruritus." This condition is very common in patients who are receiving dialysis treatments because you are more likely to build up certain chemicals in your blood that can cause your immune system to become more reactive than normal. Although this condition is not life-threatening, it can be very bothersome. Unfortunately, this is a chronic condition, meaning we do not have specific treatments that can make it go away completely. Nevertheless, we are able to use medications to manage the symptoms so that you are more comfortable.

To best treat you, we need to first ensure that your dialysis is working correctly. To assess this, we will ask you to get some blood tests so that we can look at a few chemicals in your blood. If necessary, we may work with your nephrologist to make any dialysis adjustments that we need to. In the meantime, I am recommending two over-the-counter skin creams to help with your symptoms. The first is a topical cream called "pramoxine." Two widely available products that contain pramoxine are Sarna Anti-Itch Lotion and CeraVe Itch Relief. You should store this cream in your refrigerator and apply it to itchy areas as needed. This cream should soothe the skin shortly after application. You should also be using a thick moisturizer to hydrate dry skin. This will help with your itch over time. You should apply this twice a day to your entire body.

# KERATOSIS PILARIS

## Clinical Features

Keratosis pilaris (KP) is a very common skin condition that results from abnormal keratin build-up in the hair follicles, leading to perifollicular keratosis and erythema. Most cases are felt to be the result of defective keratinization in the hair follicle, leading to a keratinous follicular plug. The authors view KP as a nonpathologic normal skin variant; however, KP is commonly associated with ichthyosis vulgaris and atopic diathesis.

KP most commonly presents during childhood or the teenage years, typically becoming less severe as patients age. In many cases, it is an incidental finding that is noticed on physical examination. KP is more commonly seen in the winter months because dry skin and subsequent keratin plugging of follicles is more common during this time.

### Geographic Morphology

- KP is characterized by highly symmetric clusters of hyperkeratotic follicular papules distributed over the extensor surfaces of the upper arms, cheeks, thighs, and buttocks.
- Multiple monomorphous flesh-colored to hyperpigmented follicular keratotic 1- to 2-mm papules tend to cluster over involved areas.
- There is often a sandpaper like quality to the skin in affected areas.
- Hairs may exhibit a twisted or corkscrew appearance in involved follicles.
- Keratin cysts in some follicular openings can mimic pustules.
- It is not uncommon for erythema or hyperpigmentation to surround many of the affected follicles.
- KP rubra (KPR) is a benign clinical variant that demonstrates increased erythema and more widespread involvement, classically on the bilateral cheeks.

### Differential Diagnosis

The differential diagnosis for KP includes other conditions that cause perifollicular keratinization, such as acne vulgaris, lichen spinulosus, ichthyosis vulgaris, and keratosis follicularis.

- Acne vulgaris is also a common skin condition affecting teenagers; however, by definition, it presents with open and closed comedones (blackheads and whiteheads) and can have true inflammatory papules, pustules, and cystic lesions. It typically affects the face, chest, and back, and spares other areas. KP of the face tends to improve at puberty, just when early acne starts to emerge.
- Lichen spinulosus affects a similar demographic to KP and looks very similar to KP. Lichen spinulosus can be differentiated from KP because it presents with discrete rather than generalized patches of spiny papules along the elbows, knees, and trunk. Lichen spinulosus is also associated with atopy. Importantly, both are benign and self-limited and treated similarly.
- Ichthyosis vulgaris is an inherited genetic condition characterized by extensive polygonal plaques that resemble fish scales. These lesions are not follicular-based and are not raised papules.
- Keratosis follicularis (DD) is an uncommon genetic condition that creates keratotic follicular lesions. The lesions of Darier, however, tend to favor seborrheic areas and are usually more widespread and larger with a warty, greasy, and/or crusted texture. Characteristic nail and oral changes may be present as well.

KP should also be distinguished from a less common variant known as "KP atrophicans."

- KP atrophicans also involves abnormal follicular keratinization but leads to follicular depressed scarring and alopecia in the areas affected. It is most commonly seen on the lateral eyebrows and cheeks.

KPR may sometimes mimic viral exanthems in younger children.

- A chronic course of localized and stable skin involvement (greater than several weeks) in the absence of systemic signs (e.g., fever, chills, aches, headache) is supportive of KP rubra as opposed to a viral etiology.

### Work-Up

The diagnosis of KP is supported by a patient history and skin examination.

- Supportive features in the patient history include a chronic, asymptomatic, stable skin disorder starting in childhood or the teenage years, possible worsening during the winter months, and a family history of KP or atopy.
- KP is a clinical diagnosis based on the characteristic lesions seen on the skin exam.
- Labs and skin biopsy are not typically needed to make the diagnosis.

### Initial Steps in Management
#### General Management Comments

- Few treatments offer significant benefit in KP; therefore, patient education regarding the chronic and persistent but benign nature is an important part of the visit.
- KP may be an incidental finding in some patients; the choice of treatment is best dictated by patient preference.

#### Recommended Initial Treatment

- All patients should receive dry skin care instruction. This includes the use of mild soaps, or no soap, in these areas and the application of simple emollients (e.g., CeraVe, Aquaphor) at least daily.

- If patients are significantly bothered by the roughness of the papules, the addition of keratolytics, such as ammonium lactate, urea, or salicylic acid creams, can be helpful.
- Exfoliation is sometimes recommended but should be gentle if attempted because irritation is common with overzealous efforts to scrub the scale off.
- If there is notable inflammation, brief courses of medium-potency topical steroids (triamcinolone acetonide 0.1% cream) may be applied twice daily in addition to emollient use.
- When hyperpigmentation is the primary complaint, hydroquinone 4% cream can be applied twice daily for several weeks to the affected skin regions.

### Partial but Inadequate Response

If there is a partial but inadequate response after a 4-week trial of topical emollient/keratolytic therapy, the treatment of KP can involve the application of several creams; therefore, reviewing what and how the patient is using the topicals is an important but often overlooked step.

- In patients demonstrating good compliance, intermittent courses of topical retinoids, applied daily to weekly depending on tolerance, may expedite exfoliation.
- An emerging treatment option is topical diclofenac gel applied daily to affected areas; however, it is often very expensive and not frequently covered by insurance for this indication.

### Warning Signs/Common Pitfalls

Although KP can be an incidental finding in certain patients, extensive involvement can cause emotional distress and reduced self-image, particularly if it occurs during the teenage years. As such, we advise questioning patients regarding the impact of the disease on their daily life to guide multidisciplinary treatment approaches (e.g., counseling efforts).

Patients diagnosed with KP should be evaluated at follow-up visits for significant inflammation, follicular atrophy, or hair loss (especially the eyebrows) because these signs may suggest a diagnosis of KP atrophicans.

- For optimal management, patients with this more severe variant are best referred to a dermatologist because they are often poorly responsive to typical emollient and keratolytic therapies.

- UV protection is particularly important in these individuals because sunlight is known to exacerbate follicular atrophy.

Although topical vitamin D derivatives are helpful in minimizing scale in psoriasis, they have not been effective in treating KP and are best avoided.

In children with KP rubra of the face, topical corticosteroid use is best limited to a shorter duration (e.g., 2 weeks) and only very low-potency steroids or topical calcineurin inhibitors should be used.

### Counseling

The small bumps on your skin are caused by a condition called "keratosis pilaris." In most patients, this is a genetic condition, meaning that you have inherited the tendency to have it from your mother or father. Although the skin condition is often mild and harmless, the rough patches can become bothersome to some people. Therefore the treatment that we recommend will depend on how irritating the skin condition is to you.

We advise all patients with this condition to keep their skin moisturized. This can be achieved by using mild soaps in the shower or by using soap-free cleansers on the affected regions. Some patients like to use an exfoliating scrubbing sponge in the shower to remove excess dry skin and make the bumps less rough; however, this should only be done gently. If it causes irritation, it should be discontinued. After getting out of the shower, we recommend you use a moisturizing cream, such as AmLactin or Gold Bond Rough & Bumpy. You can apply this cream multiple times per day. Sometimes another prescription topical cream can be tried if that is not effective enough.

With these treatment efforts, most patients notice that their rash becomes less rough and irritating. Unfortunately, however, we do not have perfect treatments that can make the rash disappear completely. Luckily, most people notice that the rash becomes less noticeable as they age.

## LICHEN NITIDUS

**Campbell Stewart**

### Clinical Features

Lichen nitidus (LN) is a relatively rare, chronic inflammatory disorder of the skin that can appear in any age, gender, or race. Children and young adults appear to be more commonly affected, and widespread LN appears to be more prevalent in women.

LN may be related to LP; however, this connection has not been clearly established. Features of both diseases can be present in individual patients. LN does not have an impact on long-term health and tends to resolve spontaneously in a matter of years.

LN presents classically with several features.

- It has groups and clusters of 1- to 3-mm, sharply demarcated, monomorphic, flat-topped papules, typically without scale.
- It is mostly distributed on the extensor arms, hands, trunk, groin/genitals, and occasionally the legs. Oral mucosal, facial, and nail involvement are less common.
- Lines of papules can be seen, normally induced by scratching (Koebner phenomenon).
- There can be significant variation in the color of the papules ranging from skin-colored to erythematous or even yellowish. The lesions can be hypopigmented or, rarely, hyperpigmented, regardless of background skin type.
- LN is normally asymptomatic but can be pruritic.

## Differential Diagnosis

The clinical differential diagnosis includes LP, lichen striatus, flat warts (verruca plana), and folliculotropic (papular) eczema.

### Lichen Planus
#### Gloria Lin and Katalin Ferenczi

- LP typically presents with purple, pruritic, polygonal papules and plaques, mostly on flexural sites. The lesions are typically larger and less well grouped. Oral involvement and genital involvement are common. Lesions tend to have Wickham striae. Both LP and LN can koebnerize. Usually LN and LP can be differentiated clinically and histologically. Occasionally, however, patients with LP can have overlapping features of LN both clinically and histopathologically.

### Lichen Striatus

- Lichen striatus normally presents with a linear arrangement of red to hypopigmented, grouped, fine papules extending along a single extremity. It can involve the nail unit with resulting dystrophy, which is less common in LN. Generally, it is asymptomatic

like LN, but it can also be very itchy. Early cases that have not progressed can be challenging to distinguish from LN; however, a punch biopsy can be useful for diagnosis.

### Flat Warts (Verruca Plana)

- These lesions are typically hyperpigmented as opposed to hypopigmented. They can be challenging to differentiate; however, a biopsy can easily distinguish the two.

### Folliculotropic (Papular) Eczema

- This variant is more common in patients with darker skin (types V–VI), is chronic as opposed to acute in onset, and is pruritic. The lesions tend to be more widespread and involve the trunk. A biopsy can differentiate it from LN.

If there is genital involvement, there can also be consideration for genital human papilloma virus (condyloma acuminata). Lesions greater than 3 mm are unlikely to represent LN. Finally, secondary syphilis should also be considered, especially in the setting of more widespread, asymptomatic papular eruptions.

## Work-Up

A complete history and physical exam, including of the oral and genital mucosa, is necessary to help exclude other diagnoses. If there is genital involvement, a thorough sexual history should be taken to exclude sexually transmitted infections (STIs) with any further blood work guided from there.

A biopsy is useful if there is clinical uncertainty; however, histopathology may not always reliably distinguish the condition from LP.

## Initial Steps in Management
### General Management Comments

LN does not need to be actively managed if the patient is asymptomatic and not concerned from a cosmetic perspective. The patient can be counseled about the expected duration of 1 year or several years before spontaneous resolution.

### Recommended Initial Regimen

There is no specific clinical trial to reference because the disease is uncommon and resolves without intervention. Nevertheless, most sources list topical steroids as first-line therapy. Topical calcineurin inhibitors can also be used. These should be applied twice daily for at least 2 to 4 weeks. Recurrences after treatment are not uncommon, and flares can be re-treated as previously described.

### Partial But Inadequate Response

If there is a partial but inadequate response after a 4-week trial of topical corticosteroid or topical calcineurin monotherapy, and pruritus remains a concern, oral minimally sedating antihistamines, such as cetirizine 10 mg taken daily for at least 4 to 6 weeks, can be added to the previously described topical regimen.

### Continued Inadequate Response

If the response continues to be inadequate, phototherapy can be used and is particularly useful in the setting of diffuse LN. NBUVB and UVA enhanced with oral psoralen have been reported. UVA treatments can only be used for a limited period of time because of the increased risk for skin malignancies.

If these therapies are not effective, the clinician should reconsider the diagnosis and further explore those listed in the aforementioned differential. A punch biopsy to confirm diagnosis should be performed if it has not been done already.

### Other Treatment Options

Other systemic treatment options, including oral retinoids, oral cyclosporine, oral itraconazole, and oral levamisole, have been reported; however, the data supporting their use are limited to case reports.

### Warning Signs/Common Pitfalls

A common pitfall is not performing a full-body skin exam. Skipping this step can result in missing a diagnosis of LP or another differential condition. LP of the genital and oral mucosae can be painful, particularly if it is erosive. Patients may not volunteer this information and may not connect their skin and mucosal eruptions. Although LN can have oral lesions, these tend to be subtle and asymptomatic. Wickham striae are absent from lesions of LN, which is a helpful clinical clue.

### Counseling

You have a condition called "lichen nitidus." The exact cause is not known, but it is the result of inflammation in your skin. The good news is that this condition does not affect your long-term health. If you have no symptoms and are not bothered by the appearance, there is a high chance the spots will clear on their own, so there is no need to treat them.

If you are itchy, applying topical steroids twice daily for at least 2 weeks during flares can be helpful. There are nonsteroid-based antiinflammatory creams called "tacrolimus" and "pimecrolimus" that can be applied similarly with improvement. Oral antihistamines can also help with the itching.

If your condition becomes more widespread, or if your itching is not controlled, then regular in-office light therapy, called narrowband ultraviolet B light, can be used.

## Lichen Planus
### Clinical Features

LP is an inflammatory condition that affects the skin (Fig. 6.3), nails (Fig. 6.4), and mucous membranes (Fig. 6.5), most commonly in middle-aged adults. There are multiple clinical variants, which can make the diagnosis challenging to recognize; therefore a skin biopsy may be required for histopathologic confirmation. In addition, close monitoring is recommended because of the small risk for the appearance of potential malignancies in LP lesions. The etiology of this condition is not well elucidated; however, there are multiple factors, including genetics, environment, and immune dysregulation, that may play a role in the pathophysiology.
- Patients may relate a history of a pruritic rash, odynophagia (painful swallowing), nail dystrophy, or

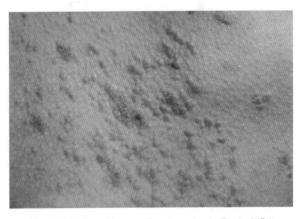

**Fig. 6.3** Lichen Planus. (Courtesy Justin Finch, MD.)

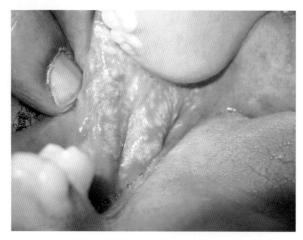

**Fig. 6.4** Oral lichen planus. (Courtesy Justin Finch, MD.)

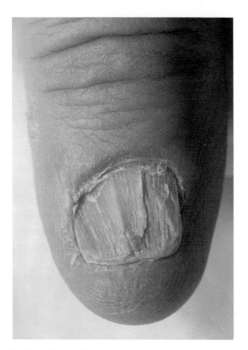

**Fig. 6.5 Nail Lichen Planus.** The photographed findings are the result of permanent scarring and will not resolve with therapy. (Courtesy Justin Finch, MD.)

ventral wrists, dorsal hands, shins, and genitalia. In darker-skinned individuals, the lesions often appear more purple or brown in color. Often, there are overlying Wickham striae, described as a reticulated lacelike pattern of scale. Koebnerization can also occur in which the condition appears at sites of cutaneous injury, thereby forming a linear configuration. The lesions can resolve with resulting hyperpigmented macules.

- Hypertrophic LP can present with violaceous to hyperpigmented verrucous plaques on the pretibial shins. Other variants of LP include annular, linear, actinic, bullous, and pigmented types. Biopsy may be needed to confirm the diagnosis because these variants can be clinical mimickers of other conditions.

- Oral LP can present in isolation, without cutaneous involvement, as a reticulated, lacy patch on the buccal mucosa. Rarely, recurrent painful ulcers and erosions, along with desquamative gingivitis, may be seen. Hepatitis C screening should be considered because this is a known associated risk factor for oral LP. A similar lacelike scaly pattern and erosions can be seen in genital LP. These variants are typically more refractory to treatment.

- LP can cause longitudinal ridging, splitting of the nails, and dorsal pterygium (overgrowth of proximal nail fold onto nail bed) formation. This may lead to trachyonychia that presents with abnormalities of all twenty nails. These changes seen in LP that involve the nails can become permanent and disfiguring.

- Lichen planopilaris is LP that involves hair-bearing areas and can cause scarring alopecia.

## Differential Diagnosis

The main differential diagnoses for LP and its variants are lichenoid drug eruption, GA, lichen amyloidosis, chronic graft versus host disease (GVHD), cicatricial pemphigoid (CP), and pemphigus vulgaris (PV).

- Lichenoid drug eruption can present with widespread, pruritic, scaly, violaceous papules and plaques. In contrast with classic LP, the anatomic distribution often favors more photoexposed areas. Multiple medications can be potential triggers for this condition, including angiotensin-converting

genital erosions. Associated triggers can include the hepatitis B vaccine; hepatitis C; contact allergens, such as metal fillings; and other viral infections.

- Classically, LP presents with pruritic, pink to purple, polygonal, flat-topped papules, usually seen on the enzyme (ACE) inhibitors, thiazide diuretics, beta blockers, gold, lithium, antimalarials, and tumor necrosis factor–alpha inhibitors. Even after discontinuation of the offending agent, the lesions may persist for months. Histologically, lichenoid drug eruptions demonstrate a more mixed inflammatory infiltrate than classic lichen planus.

- GA presents as pink to brown papules or plaques, often in an annular configuration on the hands, elbows, and feet. It is caused by granulomatous inflammation in the dermis or subcutis, which typically resolves spontaneously but may persist for several years. Symptomatic treatment includes topical or intralesional steroids, phototherapy, and, in generalized cases, systemic treatment.

- Lichen amyloidosis occurs because of amyloid deposition and is characterized by pruritic hyperpigmented papules that coalesce into plaques on the extensor surfaces. Like hypertrophic LP, it has a predilection for the anterior shins, so the two conditions can be easily confused. Symptomatic treatment includes topical steroids, phototherapy, and possible systemic agents.

- Chronic GHVD can have a presentation similar to LP; however, the history of transplant or blood transfusion can help differentiate these diseases. There is an increased risk for cutaneous malignancies associated with this condition, so the patient should be referred to a dermatologist for monitoring. Sun avoidance is essential because chronic GHVD can be exacerbated by ultraviolet light.

- CP, also known as mucous membrane pemphigoid, is an autoimmune blistering condition. Mucosal erosions and ulcers can be seen with rare intact blisters and desquamative gingivitis, making it a clinical mimicker of oral LP. This condition, however, lacks Wickham striae on the buccal mucosa. Topical steroids and systemic immunosuppressive agents can be used as treatment.

- PV can present with erosions and vesicles of the skin and mucosal surfaces. Classically, the cutaneous blisters will have a positive Nikolsky sign (superficial layers of the skin will spread with pressure leading to flaccid bullae) and a positive Asboe-Hansen sign (pressure to an intact bulla leads to spreading of the fluid laterally), which are not seen in LP. Treatment includes systemic steroids and immunosuppressive agents.

## Work-Up

LP is usually a clinical diagnosis made by the dermatologist with the aid of a physical examination; however, a biopsy may be necessary for confirmation.

- A complete physical examination, including the oral cavity and nails, is important because this can help establish the extent of the disease.
- Patients should provide a complete medication list because there are many cutaneous manifestations caused by prescriptions and OTC medications that can mimic LP.
- For oral LP, hepatitis C testing should be considered because of its known association with this condition.

## Initial Steps in Management

Although many forms of LP will resolve in 1 to 2 years, treatment should be initiated to help with symptomatic relief because the pruritus can be challenging to manage.

### Cutaneous Lichen Planus

- Antihistamines (diphenhydramine 25–50 mg nightly or every 6 hours as needed, cetirizine 5–10 mg daily, loratadine 10 mg daily, or hydroxyzine 12.5–25 mg every 6 hours as needed) can be used to help temporarily control the pruritus. Patients should be counseled on the possible sedating effects and advised against using heavy machinery or driving.
- Moisturizers and emollients containing camphor or menthol can be applied to help reduce pruritus. These can be stored in the refrigerator to further enhance the cooling sensation when applied to the skin.
- Mid- to high-potency topical steroids can be applied twice daily to the affected areas. Patients should be counseled on the risk for skin atrophy, striae, and dyspigmentation. A steroid-sparing agent, such as a topical calcineurin inhibitor, can be used in between courses of topical steroids.
- For localized areas or hypertrophic lesions, intralesional Kenalog injections can be considered. Given the variability in dosing and the injection schedule, this medication is best administered by a dermatologist.
- Phototherapy (including NBUVB) can be considered for diffuse involvement. Patients may prefer this modality based on the side effect profile; however, the required time commitment can be a deterrent.
- Other systemic agents, including methotrexate, mycophenolate mofetil, and retinoids, have shown some

benefit; however, given the potential risk for side effects, the patients should be referred to a dermatologist for management.

## Oral Lichen Planus

- Topical steroids or rinse formulations ("swish and spit") can be used to decrease inflammation in the affected areas.
- Anesthetic agents, such as viscous lidocaine, can be used for symptomatic relief before meals.
- Severe cases may require systemic therapy. These are best prescribed by a dermatologist, so a referral should be made for further management.
- Some cases are secondary to amalgam fillings and may improve or resolve with replacement or removal.
- Careful monitoring of the involved areas is required because there is a potential risk for transformation to SCC.
- If an oral biopsy is required, a referral to oral pathology can be considered.

## Nail Lichen Planus

- Although the nail manifestations are typically asymptomatic, the cosmetic appearance can be distressing for the patient. Severe cases can lead to permanent disfigurement. This variant can be challenging to treat, so it is important to counsel patients on the unpredictable success rates.
- Topical and intralesional corticosteroids have been used with some success. Calcineurin inhibitors (such as tacrolimus 0.1% ointment) can be used in between courses of topical steroids to decrease the potential risk for side effects.
- Systemic immunosuppressants may also help with nail involvement.

## Lichen Planopilaris

- This is a very difficult condition to treat and often results in permanent scarring hair loss. Referral to a dermatologist is recommended.
- Treatments that might be tried include hydroxychloroquine, retinoids, methotrexate, mycophenolate mofetil, oral cyclosporine, rituximab, and pioglitazone.

## Biopsy

- A biopsy should be considered if there is ambiguity regarding the diagnosis.

- In addition, there is a small risk for a malignancy to arise in long-standing cutaneous lesions and oral LP. For the immunosuppressed or immunocompromised population, there should be a lower threshold for potential biopsy if lesions do not respond appropriately to treatment.
- If a biopsy is warranted, a referral to a dermatologist is recommended because incorrect sampling can lead to false negatives and a delay in diagnosis.

## Inadequate Treatment Response

If treatment response is inadequate, reconsider the diagnosis and refer the patient to dermatology for further evaluation.

## Warning Signs/Common Pitfalls

- LP can mimic other diseases, and there is a wide differential that has to be considered; therefore there should be a low threshold for referral to a dermatologist.
- Given the risk of malignancy in certain types of LP, the patient should be followed closely for skin cancer monitoring.

## Counseling

You have a condition called "lichen planus," which has multiple different variants that can affect the skin, nails, mucosal surfaces, and hair-bearing skin like the scalp. In some cases, a biopsy (skin sample) may be necessary to determine the diagnosis. You should avoid any trauma to the skin because this can worsen the condition. If you have oral lesions, then your healthcare provider should consider testing for hepatitis C because that can be associated with this variant. In addition, amalgam fillings may also result in oral lesions that may resolve if these are replaced. Some medications may cause an eruption that can appear similar to lichen planus, so it is important to provide a complete medication list.

Although this condition may spontaneously clear after a few years, there are cases where it has continued to persist beyond that. Treatment may provide symptomatic relief but does not always significantly improve the appearance of the lesions. When the lesions resolve, they often leave dark spots that may take a long time to resolve. Antihistamines, topical or intralesional steroids, phototherapy, and systemic immunosuppressants may be used. Let your physician know if your symptoms begin to negatively affect your quality of life so that your treatment plan can be adjusted accordingly.

For chronic lesions, there is a small risk for malignancy in that area. It is important to see a dermatologist for skin cancer monitoring.

# WARTS

**Payal Shah, Nikita Lakdawala, and Jane Grant-Kels**

## Clinical Features

- Common warts occur most commonly on the dorsal hands, distal fingers, feet, and knees (Fig. 6.6).
- Plantar warts occur most commonly at pressure points such as the heel or ball of the foot.
- Genital warts occur most commonly at sites of sexual intercourse.
- Morphologically, common warts appear as 2- to 6-mm, skin-colored, hyperkeratotic papules, often with tiny black dots on the surface (which represent thrombosed capillaries).
- Plantar warts can have a similar morphology but may also appear as a plaque because of the merging of many smaller warts. They may have an overlying callus or can also be inverted because of the pressure-bearing location.
- Genital warts can be either solitary or in clusters with coalescing plaques. The morphology of genital warts is known to be very heterogeneous, including a flat, dome-shaped, pedunculated, cauliflower-shaped, filiform, fungating, cerebriform, smooth, or verrucous appearance. The color ranges from white to skin-colored, violaceous, erythematous, or brown.

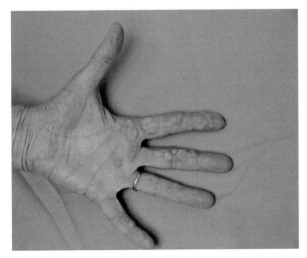

**Fig. 6.6 Palmar Warts.** (From the University of Connecticut Department of Dermatology Grand Rounds Collection.)

The size of individual warts ranges from 1 mm to more than several centimeters in diameter.
- Warts may be pruritic. Clinical evidence of this can be found on an examination as a linear distribution of lesions from scratching near the lesion because of autoinoculation.
- Plantar warts in particular may cause pain with walking on pressure points.
- Genital warts are typically asymptomatic but may additionally cause bleeding and dyspareunia.
- Common and plantar warts are common in children, young adults, and the elderly.
- Plantar warts are especially common in females; genital warts are particularly common in young, sexually active females.
  - Pregnant women in particular may have rapid growth of condyloma acuminata with a small risk for fetal transmission (estimated near 1:1500) and a higher association with Cesarean sections.
- Common warts are particularly common in Hispanic individuals, often presenting as multiple lesions.
- A diagnostic pearl for common and plantar warts is interruption of normal skin lines.

## Differential Diagnosis

The main differential for warts (depending on subtype) includes seborrheic keratosis, corns, molluscum contagiosum, and SCC.
- Seborrheic keratosis can have a waxy, stuck-on appearance.
- Corns lack thrombosed capillaries and retain skin lines. These occur at areas of repeated friction/pressure.
- Molluscum contagiosum can have a smooth, dome-shaped papular morphology with central umbilication.
- SCC can arise from prior warts. Malignant transformation should be considered in warts now recalcitrant to treatment and in the immunosuppressed population.

## Work-Up

- Based on the patient's history and the distribution of the warts, the subtype should be assessed as common, plantar, or genital because the predominate human papillomavirus (HPV) subtypes that cause disease are different.
  - Common and plantar warts are most often caused by HPV types 1, 2, and 4.

- Genital warts can have multiple HPV subtypes involved, which are further classified as low risk or high risk based on their association with cutaneous carcinomas. High-risk subtypes include 16, 18, 31, 33, and 35. Low-risk subtypes include 6 and 11.
- Persistent common warts that are also large lesions (up to 8 cm), that occur in multiples, or that are diffusely present may be a sign of immunocompromise. Additionally, coalescing genital warts may be a sign of immunocompromise. If other clinical signs of immunocompromise are also present, an additional immunologic work-up may be needed.
- Patients with genital warts should have a thorough physical examination.
  - In uncircumcised patients, the glans penis, coronal sulcus, frenulum, and inner foreskin should all be examined for lesions.
  - The penile shaft should be examined in circumcised individuals.
  - All patients should be examined at the urinary meatus and perianal area.
  - Women should be examined at the pubis, perineum, labia majora, labia minora, clitoris, urethra meatus, perianal area, and introitus.
  - A more detailed examination of the anal canal can be enabled with proctoscopy. A more detailed examination of the vagina and ectocervix can be enabled by a cervical exam.
- Warts are a clinical diagnosis; routine histologic confirmation is not indicated but may be considered if clinical doubt is present.
- Warts with recalcitrance, warts that appear visually atypical, or warts in immunocompromised individuals are recommended for biopsy to rule out SCC.
- Surgical removal in patients with poor wound healing, such as those with moderate to severe vascular disease or diabetes, should be avoided to mitigate the risk for poor healing/scarring.
- Medical treatments used for pregnant patients with warts should be verified for fetal risk.

## Initial Steps in Management
### General Management Comments
- Warts can self-remit over several months to years. Nevertheless, treatment can also be considered to improve cosmetics; treat symptoms of pain, discomfort, or functional impairment; prevent spread to others or self-inoculation; or provide a safety net if the patient is known to be immunocompromised.
- If self-remission is chosen for management, pain alleviation for plantar warts can occur with corn pads to alleviate pressure at the site of the wart.
- Condyloma acuminata that develop in pregnant women will likely be refractory to treatment.
- Because HPV infection is known to be associated with smokers, smoking cessation is encouraged in those with genital warts.
  - A sexual health history should be taken to evaluate risk for other STIs.
  - Condom use is recommended in those with genital warts to prevent transmission to sexual partners.
  - Current sexual partners and those of the past 6 months should be notified to enable early treatment and prevent further viral transmission.
  - Anal and urinary meatus warts may require further treatment by urologists and gastroenterologists to improve access for local treatment.
- The HPV vaccine covers 9 viral subtypes (6, 11, 16, 18, 31, 33, 45, 52, and 58).
  - Two doses are recommended for children 9 to 14 years of age; three doses are recommended for those 15 to 26 years of age.
- Patients with darker skin types may have hyperpigmentation or hypopigmentation in response to treatment options to warts. These pigmentary changes may be present for 1 to 2 years and at times can be permanent.

## Recommended Initial Regimen for Warts
- All warts should ideally be pared down with a file (or similar appliance) between applications of therapeutic methods to improve the chance of success.
- Common or plantar warts can be treated first line with a daily application of 17% to 40% salicylic acid and occlusion with duct tape (or similar) adhesive for 2 to 4 days.
  - Silver nitrate 6% with citric acid 9% can also be considered.
  - Trichloroacetic acid (TCA) 80% to 90% solution and monochloroacetic acid can also be used along with occlusion for 48 to 72 hours.
- Cryotherapy with liquid nitrogen for 5 seconds in 1 to 3 freeze/thaw cycles is frequently used for treatment of all types of warts. Residual warts can be treated in intervals of 2 to 4 weeks.

## Inadequate Response

If there is an inadequate response to a trial of the previously mentioned therapy (i.e., no clinical response by 3 weeks of treatment or residual disease remains at 6–12 weeks of treatment), other topical medications or therapies can be tried.

- Other topical medications include 5-fluorouracil (1 or 5% cream) daily or twice daily; imiquimod 5% cream three to five times per week for 6 weeks or longer; tretinoin 0.1% cream or gel daily or twice daily. Occlusion may be used with all of these to improve efficacy.
  - Genital warts can also be specifically treated with topical podophyllotoxin (0.15% cream or 0.5% solution) for 3 days on and 4 days off for 6 weeks or sinecatechins (10% ointment) until cleared.
- Intralesional therapies may also be considered. These include topical diphenylcyclopropenone, topical squaric acid, intralesional Candida antigen, mumps antigen, and trichophyton antigens to help sequester the immune system to the local sites of HPV infection.
- Rarely, intralesional chemotherapy with bleomycin 0.5U/mL can be used, with up to 3 mL used at once. This therapy may cause side effects of scarring and neuropathy.
- Combination therapies may also be tried, such as imiquimod with TCA or intralesional interferon and TCA.

## Continued Inadequate Response

If the response continues to be inadequate, severe disease in immunocompromised patients may be treated with intravenous cidofovir or oral acitretin or isotretinoin.

- Treatment with electrosurgery or carbon dioxide and pulsed-dye lasers with local anesthesia can also be considered. Surgical masks and smoke evacuators should be used to prevent occupational hazards of viral transmission to the provider.
- Surgical excision with general anesthesia may also be considered for bulky lesions or anal involvement.

## Warning Signs/Common Pitfalls

- Warts are transmissible to others and to self by skin and fomite contact.
- Patients with condyloma acuminata may experience significant psychological distress. Appropriate psychological support should be offered to these patients.

- Precautions should be taken to prevent transmission.
  - Autoinoculation is also extremely common after scratching near the site of the lesion and subsequent skin contact in an unaffected area. Scratching near the lesion should be avoided. For patients with pruritis, lesion occlusion may help prevent autoinoculation.
  - Plantar wart transmission is most typical from exposure to locker room floors, public showers, and pool areas. Use of shower shoes is encouraged to prevent transmission.
  - Condom protection for preventing transmission of genital warts may not be effective if warts are found at the base of the penis.
- Resolution of visible warts does not equate with eradication of the underlying HPV infection. Recurrence in warts after resolution from therapy is very common and should be expected. Plantar warts are especially known to recur. Although exact recurrence rates are unknown, local inflammation, mechanical irritation, and systemic immunosuppression increase the chance of recurrence.
  - Successful treatment on initial therapy is also likely to be successful with recurrent disease.
  - The HPV vaccine does not treat existing lesions but rather assists prevention of primary infection acquisition and is ideally administered before the first sexual encounter.

## Counseling

You (or your child) have been diagnosed with warts. Warts are benign skin proliferations that are caused by human papillomavirus (HPV), which is a double-stranded DNA virus that belongs to the *Papillomaviridae* family. The incubation period of HPV can be from 2 months to a year. Warts are often a self-limited disease and do not always require treatment. Nevertheless, self-resolution may take several months to years. Recurrence is very common for warts and repeated medical encounters for treatment will likely be needed.

# MOLLUSCUM CONTAGIOSUM

Nikita Lakdawala and Jane Grant-Kels

## Clinical Features

- Molluscum contagiosum is a common, benign, viral infection caused by a double-stranded DNA virus in the poxvirus family.

- Molluscum contagiosum can be spread by direct viral transmission through skin contact, autoinoculation, or sexual transmission in adults.
- Molluscum contagiosum is common in children and patients with AD.
  - Patients in an immunocompromised state, such as HIV, are at greater risk for molluscum.
- Distribution is variable and lesions can be found on any part of the body, including the face, trunk, or extremities, with molluscum arising in any area of direct skin contact; in cases caused by sexual transmission, distribution around the genital region and buttocks is characteristic.
- Morphologically, it is characterized by umbilicated smooth, firm, monomorphic pink papules.
- Lesions may be asymptomatic or pruritic.
- During the clinical evolution of molluscum, lesions may become inflamed. Inflammation is associated with clinical improvement in lesions.
- An eczematous eruption with erythema and scale, known as "molluscum dermatitis," can also develop around molluscum.
- The incubation period for molluscum is approximately 2 to 6 weeks, but lesions may arise anywhere from 1 week to 6 months after exposure.
- A molluscum contagiosum infection can persist from between 1 to 2 months to as long as 2 years. In immunocompetent individuals, the infection is self-limited, resolving spontaneously. In those that are immunocompromised, infection may take a more chronic and severe course.

## Differential Diagnosis

The differential diagnosis includes HSV, flat warts (verruca plana), sebaceous hyperplasia, milia, nevi, and fungal infections.

- The presence of central umbilication can help distinguish molluscum from other lesions, including flat warts, milia, and nevi.
- HSV is typically vesicular, clustered, and localized, whereas molluscum may have broader distribution.
- Sebaceous hyperplasia may also have umbilication, but it is typically yellowish in color and lobulated and located predominantly on the head and neck.
- Other infectious etiologies, such as cryptococcosis, histoplasmosis and penicillium infection, can mimic molluscum contagiosum, especially in immunosuppressed patients (e.g. patients with AIDS). Biopsy or culture can help establish the correct diagnosis.

## Work-Up

- A diagnosis of molluscum contagiosum is clinical and can typically be made with a history and physical examination.
- History should include timing, onset and duration of lesions, and symptomatology (including pruritus).
- Risk factors should also be assessed, including contacts with similar eruption and behaviors that promote transmission (i.e., sharing towels or bathing together in the case of children).
- A medical history should include history of atopy and any conditions associated with an immunocompromised state.
- Physical examination should include an examination of morphology and distribution of lesions.
- Umbilication is characteristic of molluscum. Dermoscopy or simple magnification can aid in visualization.
- In cases where umbilication is not readily clinically evident, it can be more readily visualized after with liquid nitrogen application to a lesion with a cotton tip applicator or spray gun.
- In select rare cases, where clinical diagnosis cannot be made, histologic confirmation with skin biopsy can confirm diagnosis.
- A classification of the severity of disease as mild, moderate, or severe can aid in management.

## Initial Steps in Management
### General Management Comments

Because molluscum is a benign viral infection, options for management include nonintervention and active therapy.

- The decision to treat a molluscum infection is based on several factors.
  - The severity of the infection can influence the decision to treat. The presence of numerous lesions, facial lesions or genital lesions, or molluscum dermatitis may indicate greater severity.
  - Treatment can also be used to limit the duration of the condition or spread of the infection on the individual or to close contacts.
  - Parental preference in the case of children and psychosocial considerations (e.g., lesions on visible skin, presence of genital lesions in adults) should also be taken into account.

- Counseling about the etiology, benign nature, and natural history of molluscum is essential.
  - As previously mentioned, molluscum can be present from 1 to 2 months to up to 2 years.
  - Most molluscum lesions resolve without sequelae, but scarring may occur.
  - Because molluscum is contagious through direct skin contact, it is important to review precautions to prevent spread of infection. This includes avoiding scratching or picking at the lesions, sharing clothing or towels with others, and bathing with siblings.
  - Because molluscum is not harmful to health, children should not be withheld from school.
- Treatment options for molluscum contagiosum include at-home treatments and office-based treatments.
  - At-home treatments include topical retinoids (OTC tretinoin .025 cream or gel; differin 0.1% gel) and salicylic acid 17%.
  - Other treatments, including naturopathic remedies with tea tree oil (e.g., ZymaDerm), MolluscumRx, ingenol mebutate, and imiquimod, have been used, but strong supportive scientific data is not present.
  - Office based interventions include cantharidin, cryotherapy, and curettage.
  - Other office-based interventions include podophyllotoxin and Candida antigen. Podophyllotoxin use can be limited by skin irritation. Candida antigen may be implemented for management of numerous lesions, although the pain associated with the injections often limits its use in children.
- Treatment should include management of sequelae of molluscum, including molluscum dermatitis.
  - Gentle skin care using a daily fragrance-free emollient is recommended to minimize pruritus and maintain the skin barrier.
  - Topical corticosteroids, such as hydrocortisone 2.5% (cream, ointment), represent the mainstay of treatment of molluscum dermatitis; twice-daily application to eczematous patches is generally recommended for up to 1 week on the face or 2 weeks on the body.

## Initial Steps in Management

- If observation is elected, counseling should include a recommendation for repeat evaluation if lesions worsen or become symptomatic. Transmission to others by skin contact should be reviewed.
- If at-home therapy is elected, topical retinoids may be initiated every other day and increased to daily or twice daily. It is important to recommend applying the retinoids only at the sites of molluscum and to caution the patient regarding the risk for skin irritation.
  - Topical salicylic acid may be applied to lesions every other day and increased to daily. Reviewing the risk for skin irritation is essential.
- If an office-based approach is elected, cantharidin, cryotherapy, or curettage may be employed.
  - Cantharidin is a painless topical that causes blistering; it is applied with the blunt tip of a cotton tip applicator over the molluscum lesions. Lesions are then allowed to dry, followed by washing areas where the topical was applied in approximately 2 to 6 hours. Washing off cantharidin limits the intensity of inflammation and blister formation; the treatment may be repeated in 2 to 4 weeks. Most common side effects include local skin irritation, blistering, discomfort, and postinflammatory pigment alteration. Areas such as the facial and genital skin should not be treated because of the risk for irritation.
  - Cryotherapy with liquid nitrogen may be performed on the molluscum; the swab of a cotton-tipped applicator is placed in liquid nitrogen and may be applied to molluscum lesions for approximately 5 to 10 seconds. Treatment may be repeated in approximately 4 weeks. Risks for treatment include discomfort with treatment and temporary or permanent pigment alteration after treatment. In general, darker skin types have a higher risk for skin discoloration.
  - Curettage may be performed to molluscum lesions; this has shown to be an effective procedure in management. Risks include discomfort, minor bleeding, and scarring at the sites of treatment.

## Inadequate Treatment Response

If the response with treatment is inadequate, other treatments may be tried.

- If at-home therapy is initially elected, treatment options can include transitioning to an alternate topical agent or using a combination therapy of at-home topical treatments and office-based interventions.

- If office-based therapy is elected, treatment options include transitioning to an alternate office-based approach or using a combination therapy of at-home topical treatments and office-based treatments.

## Warning Signs/Common Pitfalls

- Although molluscum contagiosum is a benign viral skin infection, it can be a significant source of emotional distress for patients and families. Care must be taken to counsel about the natural history and expectations for resolution, the benign nature of the skin condition, and potential therapeutic options. Gentle skin care and tactics to minimize spread of infection should also be reviewed.

## Counseling

Your doctor has diagnosed you (or your child) with molluscum contagiosum. This is a benign skin infection that results from a virus. It is very common and can occur in healthy individuals, including children. No treatment is necessary because the skin condition resolves on its own. It can last from between 1 to 2 months to up to 1 to 2 years. The course varies for each individual. It can spread through skin-to-skin contact, so others in your home (or at your child's school) may contract the infection.

If you desire treatment, there are potential treatments you may use at home and there are office-based therapeutic options as well. Some of the treatments are limited by side effects of skin irritation. Please review the options with your doctor and decide which, if any, would be appropriate for you (or your child).

## GENITAL HERPES SIMPLEX

### Clinical Features

- Genital herpes is an STI that is more often caused by HSV 2 than HSV 1.
  - It is spread from person to person by oral, vaginal, and/or anal intercourse.
    - Asymptomatic shedding of the virus is common and allows for the virus to be transmitted even in the absence of clinical disease.
- Classically, genital herpes presents as crops of vesicles overlying an erythematous base; however, it quickly evolves into eroded or ulcerated papules that may coalesce into plaques with overlying crusting.
  - Genital herpetic lesions may affect the penis, vaginal labia, urethra, vaginal canal, mons pubis, anus, buttocks, and mouth.

- Atypical presentations of genital HSV are not uncommon, especially in immunocompromised individuals.
  - HSV frequently presents as a large, nonhealing genital or perianal ulcer in patients with poorly controlled HIV.
- Severity of disease is highly variable, with initial infections and infections in immunocompromised hosts tending to be the most severe.
  - Occasionally, genital HSV can present with noncutaneous symptoms, including urinary retention and meningism.
- Some patients experience systemic prodromal symptoms before each outbreak, characterized by malaise with or without the presence of fever.
- Patients frequently complain of localized cutaneous pruritus or, more commonly, pain, burning, soreness, or even tingling at the site hours to days before the appearance of the visible lesions.
- Frequency of recurrence of genital HSV is highly variable, with a minority of patients developing more than 6 recurrences per annum. Recurrences have a tendency to decrease in frequency over time.
- Patients with eczema may develop a herpes infection within their eczema plaques called "eczema herpeticum" that is characterized by the development of many punched-out ulcerations within established plaques, with or without a flu like illness. Eczema herpeticum typically arises from orolabial HSV; however, it can arise from genital HSV as well. In cases where lesions disseminate to the entire body, eczema herpeticum can be fatal; therefore it should be treated as a medical emergency requiring hospitalization, intravenous antivirals, and supportive care.

### Differential Diagnosis

The differential for genital HSV includes gonorrhea, chlamydia, primary syphilis, fixed drug eruption, ulcerative LP, Zoon balanitis, and Behcet disease.

- Gonorrhea and chlamydia do not typically present with skin lesions; however, they can cause dysuria. Similarly, genital HSV may present without cutaneous herpetic lesions and instead may only present with dysuria with or without urinary retention. The presence of characteristic herpetic lesions is diagnostic of genital HSV.
- Primary syphilis presents with an ulcerated genital lesion called a "chancre." Unlike herpetic lesions, these do not initially present as vesicles, are typically

painless, are solitary, are larger than most herpetic lesions, and have heaped-up borders.

- Fixed-drug eruption frequently presents with isolated genital involvement and can blister like HSV. The presence of a solitary lesion, history of a medication exposure, characteristic post fixed-drug eruption hyperpigmentation, and biopsy can distinguish between the two entities.
- Ulcerative LP can present with painful ulcerations of the glans penis or the labia. These lesions are typically larger and more persistent than herpetic lesions and may be associated with oral and/or cutaneous LP.
- Zoon balanitis presents with maceration of the glans penis, predominantly in uncircumcised men. Chronicity; lack of involvement of other areas; and a shiny, macerated appearance distinguish it from HSV.
- Behcet disease presents with recurrent oral and genital ulcers plus uveitis. The painful genital ulcers of Behcet disease are almost always initially misdiagnosed as HSV. Polymerase chain reaction (PCR) and biopsy can help distinguish between the two.

## Work-Up

Patients with suspected active genital HSV that present for initial evaluation should undergo confirmatory testing.

- Viral PCR is now the confirmatory test of choice for genital HSV because it is fast, sensitive, and specific. To perform viral PCR, a cotton swab applicator should be brushed against the base of a denuded vesicle. Patients presenting with only active vesicles should have a vesicle deroofed with a sterile needle before obtaining a sample.
  - In scenarios in which viral PCR is unavailable, viral culture is the next best confirmatory test.
  - Direct fluorescence antibody (DFA) testing and Tzanck smear are now outdated and should only be performed in resource-poor environments that do not have access to viral PCR or cultures.
- All patients with genital HSV should be tested for concomitant STIs, including HIV, chlamydia, gonorrhea, syphilis, and trichomonas.
- HSV serologies may be performed in symptomatic patients in whom culture and/or PCR have not been diagnostic.
  - Both the U.S. Centers for Disease Control and Prevention (CDC) and U.S. Preventive Services Taskforce (USPTF) recommend against screening asymptomatic individuals with HSV serologies

because of the high false-positive rate and lack of clinical utility of the testing.
- Rarely, biopsy is necessary to confirm the diagnosis of genital HSV in atypical cases.

## Initial Steps in Management

Acute initial outbreaks of orolabial genital herpes should be managed with valacyclovir 500 mg by mouth twice daily for 10 days, if possible within 48 hours of symptom onset.

- Some patients, especially those with HIV or who are otherwise immunosuppressed, may require higher doses of valacyclovir. Patients who are not demonstrating clinical improvement within 5 days of valacyclovir initiation should have their dose of valacyclovir increased to 1 gram twice daily.
  - Resistance to valacyclovir is relatively rare in the immunocompetent population; however, it should be considered in immunosuppressed patients who are not responding appropriately to high-dose valacyclovir.
    - Switching between antivirals with the same mechanism of action (e.g., acyclovir, penciclovir) is not effective in cases of antiviral resistance because the resistance affects all agents within the class.
    - Patients resistant to valacyclovir should be evaluated by an infectious diseases specialist because they likely require treatment with foscarnet.
- Topical antiviral therapy (e.g., topical acyclovir) is generally not recommended for genital HSV because it is not particularly effective and frequently promotes antiviral resistance.
- Topical docosanol (Abreva) is not recommended for genital HSV.
- Severely symptomatic lesions can be managed with adjunctive topical corticosteroids (e.g., hydrocortisone 2.5% ointment).

Patients with infrequent flares (fewer than 6 a year) can be provided with extra valacyclovir to take as previously described at the first sign of a flare (valacyclovir 500 mg twice daily for 3 days).

- Patients who flare more than 6 times a year or who desire suppressive therapy can take 500 mg of valacyclovir daily.
  - Immunosuppressed patients may require higher suppressive doses of valacyclovir, as previously mentioned.

Patients should be tested for concomitant STIs and treated appropriately for these infections.

## Warning Signs/Common Pitfalls

The biggest pitfall when managing genital HSV is failing to appropriately counsel patients about genital herpes because of its associated stigmatization. Patients must be told a few key facts:

- Genital HSV is sexually transmitted and sexual partners should be notified about the infection.
- Patients can acquire HSV from their partner years into a monogamous relationship.
- Female patients should notify their obstetrician about their HSV status should they become pregnant or consider becoming pregnant because HSV can spread to a baby in utero and during vaginal delivery. Resulting neonatal herpes infection may be fatal or confer extreme morbidity.
- Condoms can help prevent the transmission of HSV and HSV can be spread even when an infected individual is asymptomatic.

Pregnant women with a suspected flare or initial episode of genital HSV should be referred to an obstetrician urgently.

Patients who develop eczema herpeticum and are febrile and/or have disseminated lesions should be admitted to the hospital for intravenous antiviral therapy.

## Counseling

You have genital herpes, a type of viral infection within the herpes simplex virus (HSV) family. Around 15% of American adults are infected with this virus. It is a sexually transmitted infection that is spread from one person to another by oral, vaginal, and anal intercourse. You should notify your recent sexual partners about your infection so that they can seek appropriate medical care. Importantly, genital herpes can be acquired from a sexual partner years into a monogamous relationship.

Because genital herpes is a sexually transmitted infection, you have been tested for other sexually transmitted infections. You will be notified about the results of these tests and treated appropriately.

There is no cure for genital herpes, and it is frequently recurrent. Recurrences are triggered by stress, illness, and trauma. You may notice that you feel flu like symptoms or develop a fever before recurrent episodes. Many patients also note local pain, tingling, burning, or pruritus at the site before the appearance of the visible lesions. Even if you are completely asymptomatic, you may still be infectious to your sexual partners; therefore it is important that men use condoms during sex because condoms have been proven to decrease the likelihood of infecting someone else with HSV.

If you are a woman who is pregnant or who intends to become pregnant, it is important that you tell your obstetrician about your infection. Rarely, genital herpes can be transmitted to a baby during delivery. This infection can be fatal to babies. Your obstetrician will take special precautions to decrease the likelihood that your baby becomes infected during delivery.

Fortunately, there is a treatment for your infection. Your doctor has prescribed you valacyclovir. This medication comes in 500 mg tablets. You should take one of these every 12 hours for the number of days prescribed by your doctor. This will shorten the severity and duration of your outbreak and decrease the likelihood that you will spread the infection to someone else. Importantly, if you notice that your infection is not improving despite completing the course of antivirals, you should notify your doctor.

Additionally, if you are having frequent recurrences, you should ask your doctor about treatment to decrease the number of recurrences that you have.

## GRANULOMA ANNULARE

### Campbell Stewart

### Clinical Features

GA is a common, benign, inflammatory reaction in the skin. It can present in any age group, but women are more often affected. There is variety in both the clinical appearance and the distribution of GA. The cause is not known.

Variants include localized, generalized, subcutaneous, and perforating forms. The latter two are uncommon. Subcutaneous GA is usually located on the plantar/palmar surfaces, scalp, buttock or shins; it occurs mostly in the pediatric population and in young adults. Perforating GA presents on the dorsal surfaces of acral sites, also more commonly in children. Actinic granuloma may represent a variant of GA, but the relationship is unclear.

GA typically resolves without intervention over a period of 2 to 3 years. Some patients may have persistent or chronic relapsing-remitting lesions for decades.

The classic clinical lesion is a slightly blanching, annular (ringlike) plaque without scale. There is often central depression without associated induration (Fig. 6.7). The lesions are usually purplish-brown, red, or skin colored. Other clinical presentations include papules, polycyclic

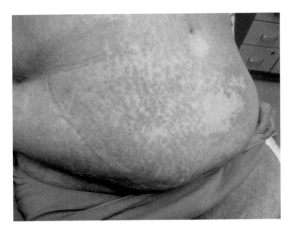

**Fig. 6.7 Granuloma Annulare.** Note the annular morphology. (From the University of Connecticut Department of Dermatology Grand Rounds Collection.)

plaques, deep dermal nodules (subcutaneous GA), or small, spiny papules coalescing into larger plaques with crust and ulceration (perforating GA).

Lesions are usually asymptomatic, but some patients complain of itch.

Sites that are commonly involved include the dorsal hands/feet (localized GA), the trunk and extremities (generalized GA), and the palms and soles (subcutaneous GA).

Generalized GA may be present in the setting of diabetes mellitus type 2 (and, rarely, 2). Thyroid disease has also been associated with forms of GA.

### Differential Diagnosis

The clinical differential diagnosis includes necrobiosis lipoidica, sarcoidosis, LP, Hansen disease (leprosy), rheumatoid nodules, and tinea corporis.

### Necrobiosis Lipoidica

Necrobiosis lipoidica may have overlapping features with GA and is significantly more challenging to treat. It shows a more yellowish coloration and telangiectasias and is most commonly located on the shins. It also heals with scarring in contrast to GA. Patients can have both disorders simultaneously, and some believe them to be part of a spectrum of disease.

### Sarcoidosis

A biopsy showing features of dermal granulomas without a significant inflammatory infiltrate can help differentiate sarcoidosis from GA. If a biopsy raises concern for sarcoidosis, a comprehensive work-up is encouraged because of the associated systemic complications.

### Lichen Planus

LP normally affects the flexor surfaces of the extremities and is typically pruritic. Lesions also show Wickham striae. Unlike GA, oral and genital involvement are also described. LP can be easily distinguished from GA by histopathology.

### Hansen Disease (Leprosy)

Hansen disease is not common in the United States and therefore can be missed. Plaques often have associated anesthesia. If there is clinical concern, a biopsy should be performed and a Fite stain should be requested from the pathologist. Slit-skin smears can also be submitted for pathology, but the sensitivity of this test is low.

### Rheumatoid Nodules

These lesions can look identical to GA on a biopsy. Obtaining other elements of the history and physical, inquiring about joint symptoms, and completing laboratory testing for rheumatoid factor are useful actions.

### Tinea Corporis

GA lacks the scale that is classic in tinea. Normally, a KOH test of the outer edge of an annular plaque shows hyphae. If negative, a biopsy with a periodic acid–Schiff stain can be performed to confirm the diagnosis.

## Work-Up

Performing a full-body skin examination and taking a careful history is essential. Patients may be unaware of more widespread involvement because of the normally asymptomatic nature of GA.

Generally, no systemic work-up is necessary. If a patient has generalized GA, screening for diabetes is recommended.

If clinical diagnosis is difficult, a punch biopsy of the lesion, preferably along a border of an indurated aspect, can be performed. Histopathology reveals areas of altered dermal collagen and mucin deposition palisaded by a lymphohistiocytic infiltrate, sometimes with necrobiosis and giant cell formation.

## Initial Steps in Management
### General Management Comments

If the lesions are asymptomatic and otherwise not bothersome to the patient, no treatment is required. Particularly in the localized form, lesions will likely resolve without intervention over a matter of years.

Generalized GA can be particularly frustrating for patients because it is often persistent and progressive.

Multiple treatment options can be tried before achieving a response in generalized GA.

## Recommended Initial Regimen

Topical corticosteroids, applied twice daily for up to 3 to 4 weeks, taking a break for a week, and then resuming, are effective. This treatment cycle can be repeated unless signs of atrophy appear. On acral sites, it is often necessary to use high-potency steroids (class I or II) to achieve the desired effect. Patients should be counseled to monitor for steroid atrophy and telangiectasias with prolonged, uninterrupted use.

Topical calcineurin inhibitors (e.g., tacrolimus, pimecrolimus) can also be applied twice daily. They do not carry the same adverse effects as topical corticosteroids; however, they may not be as effective as higher potency topical steroids. These can also be used during breaks from topical corticosteroids.

## Partial but Inadequate Response

If there is a partial but inadequate response after a 4-week trial of potent topical corticosteroid monotherapy, intralesional triamcinolone (normally 10 mg/mL), given in the office every 4 to 6 weeks, can improve the appearance of stubborn lesions.

- In more delicate sites, such as the face (rare in GA), a lower concentration such as 2.5 to 5 mg/mL is normally needed to avoid atrophy. Patients may avoid this option because of the pain associated with the injections.

## Continued Inadequate Response

If the response continues to be inadequate, NBUVB light can be used with a good response and is particularly useful in generalized GA. Psoralen-enhanced ultraviolet A (PUVA) has also been used in both localized hand/foot GA and generalized GA, but long-term use is contraindicated because of the increased risk for skin cancer from this treatment.

## Other Treatment Options

There are a few other treatment options.
- Pulsed-dye laser and Excimer are useful, particularly for stubborn disease.
- Cryotherapy is effective but is not generally recommended because of concerns for permanent pigment change and the risk for scarring.
- Generalized GA treatments are numerous because there is no defined agent of choice. If NBUVB is not

effective, one low-risk option is oral nicotinamide (500 mg three times daily) taken for 3 to 6 months. Nicotinamide can be used alone or in combination with light or other oral agents.
- Other oral options for generalized GA include isotretinoin; adalimumab; infliximab; combination minocycline, ofloxacin, and rifampin for 3 months; hydroxychloroquine and other antimalarials; methotrexate; cyclosporine; and dapsone.
- Referral to a dermatologist is recommended in the setting of diagnosed or suspected generalized GA.

## Warning Signs/Common Pitfalls

A sudden onset, asymptomatic, annular eruption without scale on the dorsal hands or feet is a common presentation for GA. If the rash is itching or scale is present, a KOH prep is recommended to exclude tinea.

If a rash worsens after empiric treatment with topical high-potency steroids or if the patient develops pustules, a biopsy should be performed to rule out tinea incognito.

Because of the persistence of GA over a period of months or years, patients are prone to topical steroid overuse and side effects. Regular office visits to reinforce appropriate steroid application and assess for side effects are useful.

## Counseling

You have a condition called "granuloma annulare." This rash is the result of inflammation in your skin that is not life-threatening. It can resolve without any treatment in a few years. If your lesions are bothersome or symptomatic, topical steroids can be tried to minimize their appearance. Recurrences after topical clearance are common and somewhat expected. A repeated course of topicals is often required. Steroids can also be injected into your skin lesions; however, these shots are painful.

If your rash does not improve or if it worsens, we should consider a biopsy of your rash to confirm your diagnosis.

Normally, the rash is contained to your hands and feet. Less commonly, it can spread to involve other parts of your body. If it does, you may need to have a consultation with a dermatologist. The treatment options for widespread disease include multiple oral medications and in-office, light-based treatments. Tanning bed use for widespread disease is neither recommended nor safe.

# Hyperpigmented and Hypopigmented Rashes

# 7

# Hyperpigmented Rashes

## MELASMA

**Casey Abrahams and Afton Chavez**

### Clinical Features

Melasma is also known as "chloasma" or, colloquially, the "mask of pregnancy." It is characterized by light to dark-brown or brown-gray patches with irregular borders that appear primarily on the face (Fig. 7.1) but also on the forearms (Fig. 7.2) and mid-upper chest.

- A centrofacial distribution on the forehead, cheeks, nose, upper lip (sparing the philtrum), and chin is the most common pattern.

- Melasma may also present in a malar (affecting the cheeks and nose) or mandibular (along the jawline) distribution.

- There is an increased prevalence of melasma in young to middle-aged women with darker skin types, such as those of Hispanic, Asian, or African descent.

- Exacerbating factors include ultraviolet (UV) and visible light and hyperestrogenic states, such as when pregnant or using oral contraceptives.
  - Patients frequently report a waxing and waning course with dramatic worsening in the summer months.

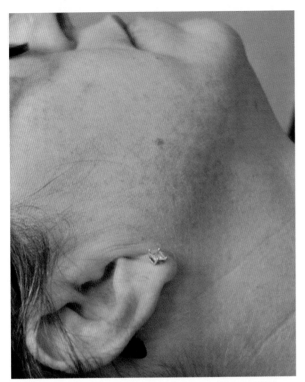

**Fig. 7.1** Melasma, Right Cheek. (From the UConn Grand Rounds Collection.)

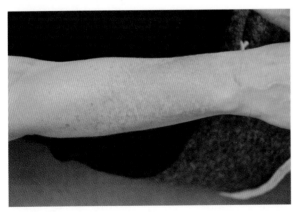

**Fig. 7.2** Melasma, Forearm. (From the UConn Grand Rounds Collection.)

## Differential Diagnosis

The primary differential for melasma includes drug-induced hyperpigmentation or discoloration, postinflammatory hyperpigmentation, pigmented contact dermatitis (Riehl melanosis), acquired bilateral nevus of Ota-like macules (Hori nevus), actinic lichen planus, lichen planus pigmentosus (LPP), erythema dyschromicum perstans (EDP), and exogenous ochronosis.

- Drug-induced hyperpigmentation may be differentiated from melasma based on history of exposure to commonly implicated medications, such as minocycline, chemotherapeutics, antimalarials, zidovudine, heavy metals, or clofazimine. Drug-induced hyperpigmentation may be localized or generalized. Unlike melasma, the oral mucosa and nails may also be affected in drug-induced hyperpigmentation.
- Postinflammatory hyperpigmentation can occur anywhere on the body and may be differentiated from melasma based on a history of prior inflammation, such as rashes or injury to the skin.
- Pigmented contact dermatitis occurs after exposure to certain chemicals typically found in cosmetic products, such as dyes or fragrances, and presents in the areas in which the product has been applied.
- Acquired bilateral nevus of Ota-like macules (Hori nevus) presents as multiple brown-gray-blue macules, primarily on the malar cheeks in Asian women in their fourth or fifth decade of life. If there is a question regarding the diagnosis, biopsy of Hori nevus shows dermal melanocytes.
- Actinic lichen planus, LPP, and EDP are all somewhat similar and may exist on a spectrum. Actinic lichen planus typically has fine scale overlying violaceous lesions. LPP usually starts on the temples/preauricular face and neck, and patients may have concomitant lichen planus. EDP tends to occur more on sun-protected areas (Fig. 7.3). Biopsy can help distinguish these conditions from melasma.
- Exogenous ochronosis may be differentiated from melasma based on a history of long-term use of hydroquinone. If there is a question regarding the diagnosis, histology reveals yellow to brown banana-shaped deposits in the papillary dermis.

## Work-Up

- The diagnosis may be made based on clinical appearance if history and distribution are suggestive.
- A thorough history of topical and systemic medications and UV exposure should be obtained in all patients to eliminate any exacerbating etiologies.

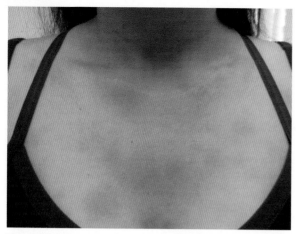

**Fig. 7.3 Erythema Dyschromicum Perstans.** Note the ashy appearance. (From the UConn Grand Rounds Collection.)

## Initial Steps in Management
### Prevention and Maintenance

- Patients should minimize UV exposure by avoiding tanning beds, wearing sun-protective hats and clothing, and using broad-spectrum sunscreen (ideally with an SPF greater than 30) daily.
- Emerging data suggests that blocking visible light with iron oxides and supplementing with oral antioxidants, such as polypodium leucotomos, may prove beneficial in minimizing melasma.
- Discontinue estrogen-containing oral contraceptives, if possible.

### Treatments

- Hydroquinone, alone or in triple combination with a retinoid and corticosteroid, may be used for periods of up to 3 to 6 months to avoid exogenous ochronosis.
- Other treatment options include azelaic acid (15%–20%); L-ascorbic acid (vitamin C; 10%–15%); kojic acid (1%–4%); topical or oral tranexamic acid (oral tranexamic acid must be used with caution given the risk for thrombogenicity); glycolic or salicylic acid peels; and targeted laser therapies.
- Patients can also use camouflaging makeup to minimize the appearance of the melasma.

### Warning Signs/Common Pitfalls

- Even small amounts of UV exposure can exacerbate melasma, so patients must practice strict adherence to sun protection.

- Extreme caution must be taken when treating melasma patients with peels or lasers. Only an experienced professional should perform these procedures on patients of darker skin types because, if conducted improperly or with the wrong laser, patients can have subsequent dyspigmentation and/or scarring.

### Counseling

You have melasma, a type of skin pigmentation disorder characterized by light to dark brown or brown-gray patches with irregular borders. You may notice these patches primarily on your face, but they can also be found on your forearms and mid-upper chest. If you are a young to middle-aged women with a darker skin type, you are at an increased risk for melasma.

There are many treatment and prevention options for melasma. The most important step is to minimize UV exposure by wearing sun-protective hats and clothing and applying broad-spectrum sunscreen (ideally with an SPF greater than 30) daily. Melasma is exacerbated by pregnancy and estrogen-containing oral contraceptives, so you may want to consider switching to an alternative nonestrogen-containing birth control if you are on one.

Your doctor may recommend as treatment the use of hydroquinone, azelaic acid, topical vitamin C, kojic acid, tranexamic acid, peels, or lasers. Topical hydroquinone should not be used for more than 3 to 6 months because of the risk for paradoxical worsening of the hyperpigmentation. Peels and lasers should only be performed by an experienced professional. If performed using an improper technique, hyperpigmentation can result.

## LENTIGINES

Gregory Cavanagh and Afton Chavez

## Clinical Features

Lentigines are also known as "liver spots," "age spots," "senile freckles," and "lentigo senilis." They are 0.2 cm to 2 cm, well-circumscribed, round, oval, or irregularly shaped macules that vary in color from tan to dark brown or black.

- Lighter lesions are typically homogenous, whereas darker ones may appear more mottled.
- Dermoscopic features include a diffuse light brown structureless area, sharply demarcated and/or moth-eaten borders, finger-printing, and a reticular pattern

with thin lines that are occasionally short and inter-
rupted.

- Because they are induced by UV radiation (UVR),
  lentigines typically occur on sun-exposed sites, such
  as the face, dorsal aspects of the hands and forearms,
  upper trunk, and shins.
- Lesions persist indefinitely but may fade slightly after
  cessation of UV exposure or may darken with increased UV exposure.

## Differential Diagnosis

The differential for solar lentigines includes ephelides
(freckles), PUVA (psoralen and UVA) lentigo, macular
seborrheic keratosis (SK), pigmented actinic keratosis
(AK), lentigo maligna, simple lentigo, junctional melanocytic nevus, and large cell acanthoma.

- Ephelides are typically 1 to 5 mm, light to medium
  brown macules. They tend to be smaller and lighter
  than lentigines. They often initially develop in childhood, unlike lentigines, which develop in individuals
  over the age of 25 and increase in incidence with increasing age. Both are oval-to-irregularly shaped
  macules with smooth or jagged edges and can be
  found on the face and arms. Unlike lentigines, however, ephelides rarely localize to the dorsal aspect of
  the hands.
- PUVA lentigines are well-defined, hyperpigmented
  macules that commonly develop in individuals
  undergoing long-term PUVA photochemotherapy.
  Compared with solar lentigines, PUVA lentigines
  are typically darker brown with a more stellate
  appearance.
- There is a continuum extending from solar lentigo to
  macular SK; however, demonstration of a keratotic
  surface with horn cysts is more consistent with an
  SK. SKs can develop anywhere, except mucous membranes, palms, and soles. SKs are tan to black in color
  and have a waxy, stuck-on appearance.
- In contrast to solar lentigines, pigmented AKs are
  more likely to have a scaly, rough surface. Pigmented
  AKs are considered precancerous, so additional follow-up and treatment is recommended if this is
  suspected. Most pigmented AKs display lateral
  growth, and irritation and pruritis may occur.
- Lentigo maligna often exhibits greater variation in
  pigmentation and irregularity of borders compared
  with solar lentigines (Fig. 7.4) and may stand out in
  comparison with other lentigines. Lentigo maligna

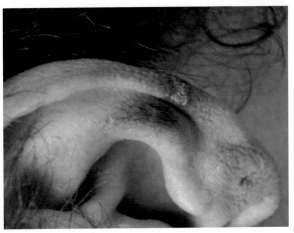

**Fig. 7.4 Lentigo Maligna.** Note the variegated colors. (From
the UConn Grand Rounds Collection.)

presents most commonly on the face. The spots grow
slowly over time. On dermoscopy, rhomboid structures and gray dots can be seen in lentigo maligna
lesions. These lesions should be biopsied because
they are a type of melanoma.

- Simple lentigines are often smaller and more heavily
  pigmented than solar lentigines. Additionally, they
  arise during childhood with less relationship to UVR
  exposure. Simple lentigines and solar lentigines are
  both brown to black in color, but simple lentigines
  are more symmetric and uniformly pigmented. Solar
  lentigines tend to arise on sun-exposed areas of the
  body, whereas simple lentigines can arise anywhere
  on the body, including the mucous membranes and
  palmoplantar skin. Simple lentigines present differently on mucous membranes, however; there, they
  frequently have irregular borders and mottled non-
  homogeneous pigmentation. In the case of both
  generalized and localized lentiginosis, simple lentigines may or may not be associated with an underlying
  disorder. In this particular case, further investigation
  and testing may be needed.
- Solar lentigines are typically less well defined and
  discreet than junctional melanocytic nevi but may be
  indistinguishable on a clinical examination.

## Work-Up

- Lentigines are typically diagnosed based on characteristic physical examination findings and a positive
  history of UV exposure.

- Lentigines are considered a marker of excessive UV exposure; therefore patients should be monitored with regular skin examinations to screen for cutaneous malignancies.
- Lesions should be monitored for growth or change. The ABCDE criteria (asymmetry, border irregularities, color variation, large diameter, and evolution of the lesion) should be implemented to screen for atypical lesions.
- If atypical features are noted on an examination a biopsy is recommended for definitive diagnosis.

## Initial Steps in Management

- Solar lentigines are benign lesions that are of cosmetic concern only, but patients might desire treatment.
  - Preventative measures include minimizing UV exposure through the use of sunscreen, sun-protective clothing, and sun avoidance during peak hours.
  - Cryotherapy, chemical peels, and laser surgery have been shown to be effective. Caution must be used to prevent posttreatment dyspigmentation.
  - Bleaching agents, such as hydroquinone, have been shown to be ineffective.
- Continued skin monitoring for cutaneous carcinomas is also indicated because solar lentigines are an indication of chronic UVR exposure.

## Warning Signs/Common Pitfalls

- Solar lentigines are benign lesions; however, it is important to distinguish them from lesions that present similarly, such as pigmented AKs, PUVA lentigines, lentigo maligna, or atypical junctional melanocytic nevi.
- Rarely, lentigines can be a part of genetic syndromes, such as xeroderma pigmentosa, Noonan syndrome with multiple lentigines, Peutz-Jeghers syndrome, or Bannayan-Riley-Ruvalcaba syndrome. The presence of multiple widespread lesions, onset at a young age, or presence in uncommon locations should merit further investigation.
- Solar lentigines are most common among Caucasian and elderly people; however, lentigines can occur in younger individuals, Asians, and lightly pigmented African Americans as a result of acute or chronic sun exposure. One pitfall is to rule out this diagnosis based on the demographics of the patient.

## Counseling

You have solar lentigines, which are also known as "sun spots." They are caused by ultraviolet radiation exposure, which can come from the sun or tanning beds. They are more common in older individuals. Lentigines are benign, but you should monitor them regularly. If you notice one is asymmetric, has an irregular border, is not uniform, is composed of multiple colors, has a large diameter, or is changing, you should contact your doctor to have it inspected and ensure it is not a skin cancer.

Although lentigines are benign, having them indicates that your skin has had excessive chronic sun exposure, which puts you at higher risk for developing melanoma and other skin cancers. Therefore you should have regular skin checks.

Lentigines and skin cancer can be prevented by using sunscreen, seeking shade, wearing sun-protective clothing, and avoiding peak sun exposure from 10 AM to 4 PM. No treatment is required for lentigines, but if you would like to have them removed for cosmetic reasons, they may be treated with cryotherapy, lasers, or chemical peels. Bleaching agents, such as hydroquinone, are not considered an effective treatment.

If you notice new, abnormal, or changing lesions, contact your doctor.

# TINEA VERSICOLOR

## Clinical Features

Tinea versicolor (TV; formerly known as "pityriasis versicolor") is a very common fungal infection caused by *Malassezia sp.*

- It presents with many scaly patches that are most commonly hypopigmented but sometimes hyperpigmented and occasionally erythematous. They appear most often on the trunk, followed by the neck and other upper extremities.
- Some patients are asymptomatic and others complain of pruritus.
- Although associated with an increased presence of *Malassezia*, this bacterium is a normal body organism and therefore TV is not contagious.
- This condition is diagnosed clinically because of its characteristic distribution and usual hypopigmentation and because it presents with scaly patches that seem to coalesce.

- This condition has a characteristic distribution because *Malassezia* is lipophilic and prefers sebaceous areas.
  - This also explains why this condition is almost exclusively seen after puberty.
- The condition is named "versicolor" because it can present with patches of variable colors (i.e., hypopigmented, hyperpigmented, pink).
- Scale is easier to appreciate when the skin is stretched (which is known as the "evoked scale sign").
- Pigmentary changes caused by TV take months to return to normal after successful treatment, and the condition has a tendency to recur.

## Differential Diagnosis

The differential for TV includes progressive macular hypomelanosis (PMH), pityriasis alba, idiopathic guttate hypomelanosis, vitiligo, confluent and reticulated papillomatosis (CARP), vitiligo, and postinflammatory pigmentary changes.

- PMH is the main mimicker of TV, although it is much less common than TV. Unlike TV, PMH lesions are frequently ill defined, cone shaped (nummular), and lacking in overlying scale. A Wood lamp examination, if available, can differentiate the two as PMH demonstrates diagnostic coral red perifollicular fluorescence because of the presence of *Propionibacterium acnes*. PMH should be considered in all patients with suspected TV who are unresponsive to two different topical antifungals.
- Pityriasis alba can be distinguished from TV because it predominantly affects the face, has ill-defined lesions, and occurs in individuals with a history of atopy.
- Idiopathic guttate hypomelanosis appears as asymptomatic white macules (usually less than 3 mm in diameter) without any scaling, most commonly on the sun-exposed extremities of older lighter-skinned individuals.
- Vitiligo presents with depigmented (complete absence of pigment), usually sharply circumscribed patches that may affect the trunk. Vitiligo is differentiated from TV by the depigmented nature of the lesions, which is notable on a Wood light examination (versus hypopigmented in TV), and the lack of overlying scale.
- CARP may be mistaken for hyperpigmented TV because the conditions have similar distributions;

however, CARP has palpable plaques rather than the patches seen in TV.
- Postinflammatory hyperpigmentation can mimic hyperpigmented TV because the hyperpigmentation in TV is a form of PIH. Nevertheless, non-TV–related PIH occurs in individuals with a history of an antecedent rash, as does postinflammatory hypopigmentation.

## Work-Up

If available, a potassium hydroxide (KOH) examination can be performed on scrapings of scale from lesional skin. The identification of *Malassezia* (which has a pattern colloquially known as "spaghetti and meatballs") on examination is diagnostic of TV.

If available, a Wood lamp examination can also be helpful for distinguishing TV from mimickers. TV will either not fluoresce or will fluoresce yellow-green, depending on the causative *Malassezia* species.

Biopsy should be performed in cases that are refractory to management or very atypical in appearance because some neoplastic conditions (such as a variant of the patch-stage cutaneous T cell lymphoma or mycosis fungoides) and other infectious conditions mimic TV in rare cases.

## Initial Steps in Management

Management of TV is divided into acute management and prevention of recurrence.

### Acute Management

- Antifungal shampoos (e.g., selenium sulfide, ketoconazole 2%, zinc pyrithone) used as a body wash are the first-line treatments for TV.
  - We typically start with ketoconazole 2% shampoo every other day, applied from the belt to the scalp and left in contact with the skin for 10 minutes before rinsing.
    - The reason it is used three times weekly is that ketoconazole binds to the hair shaft and remains present for 2 to 3 days.
    - The infection should typically be cured within 4 weeks of application, although the pigmentary alterations that TV causes persist for months.
      - Absence of scale overlying previously scaly lesions is suggestive of treatment response.
      - A KOH examination can be repeated to confirm a cure, if available.

- Switching between shampoos should be trialed for patients who do not seem to respond after 4 weeks.
- Oral azole antifungals can be considered in severe cases, in cases that are resistant to topical therapy, or in cases where topical therapy is not feasible (e.g., quadriplegic patients).
  - Itraconazole 200 mg by mouth daily for 7 days or fluconazole 200 mg by mouth weekly for 4 weeks are reasonable options.
    - Oral ketoconazole should not be used because of its risk for causing hepatotoxicity.
    - Griseofulvin and terbinafine are not effective against TV.

### Maintenance

Most patients require a maintenance strategy or they will see annual recurrence during humid months.

- Topical medicated shampoos can be used once weekly to prevent recurrence of TV. The importance of maintenance therapy should be stressed to all patients.
- Preventative therapy with oral antifungals is typically not recommended.

### Warning Signs/Common Pitfalls

The biggest pitfall when managing TV is failure to recognize dangerous mimickers. Although rare, neoplastic and other infectious conditions can mimic TV and should be considered in cases where patients are not responding to conventional therapy.

Failure to counsel patients about the delayed normalization of skin pigmentation after successful treatment of TV can prompt patient treatment dissatisfaction.

Many patients have frequent recurrences. Implementing maintenance strategies early can be helpful to limit patient frustrations. Some patients prefer over-the-counter shampoos for maintenance (e.g., selenium sulfide) because they feel these have less risk for side effects.

### Counseling

You have a fungal infection known as "tinea versicolor." This infection is very common, is not considered contagious, and is not dangerous to your overall health. The fungus that causes this infection, *Malassezia,* lives on the skin and does not get into your blood or your body. To eliminate your rash, your fungal infection must be treated.

Your doctor has prescribed you ketoconazole 2% shampoo. This shampoo should be applied from the belt line to the scalp every other day. You should leave the shampoo in contact with the skin for at least 10 minutes so it can be effective. You must do this for 4 weeks to cure your infection. Even once your infection is cured, it may take months for your skin color to return to normal.

Many people with tinea versicolor are prone to reinfections even after successful treatment. To prevent reinfection, you should continue to use the shampoo you were prescribed once per week after you have finished your initial treatment course.

## CONFLUENT AND RETICULATED PAPILLOMATOSIS

### Clinical Features

CARP is a disorder of keratinization that presents with asymptomatic, reticulated (configured in a net like pattern), warty papules coalescing into plaques that most commonly affect the trunk, then the axilla, and finally the neck.

- It affects both men and women and presents as early as adolescence.
- Characteristic lesions typically have overlying epidermal changes (i.e., scaling, flaking).
- It is typically responsive to antibiotics; however, it runs a chronic course and frequently recurs on treatment discontinuation.

The presence of certain criteria is suggestive of a diagnosis of CARP:

- It clinically presents with reticulated and papillomatous, scaly, brown macules/papules and patches/plaques.
- Characteristic lesions involve the trunk (typically above the umbilicus), neck, and/or flexural areas.
- Lesions are either negative for fungi on KOH examination or do not respond to an appropriate course of antifungals.
- Lesions are responsive to antibiotics.

### Differential Diagnosis

The differential for CARP is TV, acanthosis nigricans (AN), Darier disease, and other rarer disorders of keratinization that will be grouped together for the purposes of this chapter.

- Tinea versicolor is distinguished from CARP because the lesions are frequently hypopigmented and most

visible during summertime and look more fawn colored in the winter; the lesions are collections of scaly macules and patches that are not warty in appearance; a KOH staining of a skin scraping from TV lesions demonstrate *Malassezia sp.*; and lesions are responsive to topical and systemic azole antifungals.
- AN is more common than CARP and thus CARP is often initially misdiagnosed as AN.
  - CARP is distinguished from AN because CARP affects the trunk with or without the involvement of the axilla and neck, whereas AN typically spares the trunk and tends to involve body folds. Moreover, CARP is responsive to antibiotics. Histologic examination does not reliably distinguish between the two.
- Darier disease is a genetic condition characterized by the development of greasy, warty lesions in a seborrheic distribution. It can be distinguished from CARP based on family history (autosomal dominant inheritance); widespread distribution; lesional appearance (not reticulated in pattern/distribution, has overlying, greasy scale); and steroid responsiveness.
- There are other rare disorders of keratinization (Dowling-Degos disease, Galli-Galli) that can clinically mimic CARP and are typically considered in patients with a family history of these conditions or in patients diagnosed with CARP who fail to respond to multiple rounds of antibiotics and systemic retinoids.

## Work-Up

CARP is diagnosed clinically. No specific work-up is required to make a diagnosis of CARP. Similarly, because CARP is a skin-limited condition, no additional work-up is required once a diagnosis of CARP is made.

## Initial Steps in Management

Oral antibiotics are the treatment of choice for CARP. Their presumed mechanism of action is that they kill *Dietzia sp.*, the gram-positive bacteria pathogen implicated in CARP development.
- Minocycline 50 mg by mouth twice daily for 6 weeks is the initial treatment of choice. Many patients will respond in this time frame; however, they relapse after discontinuation is common.
  - Patients should be counseled about minocycline-associated risks, including drug hypersensitivity, drug-induced lupus, vestibular dysfunction, and dyspigmentation.

- Patients who fail on minocycline or who are intolerant/allergic to the tetracycline class can be started on azithromycin 500 mg three times weekly for 3 weeks.
- Patients who are antibiotic nonresponders or relapse quickly can be managed with systemic retinoids. Because isotretinoin is a federally regulated medication, patients who may benefit from it must be referred to a prescriber who is registered with iPledge, the program that regulates isotretinoin use.

## Warning Signs/Common Pitfalls

The biggest pitfall when managing CARP is failing to reconsider the diagnosis after patients have failed multiple rounds of antibiotics and/or systemic retinoids. Both AN and genetic disorders of keratinization clinically mimic CARP and should be considered when patients are nonresponders to conventional therapy.

Older literature suggests that CARP is fungal-mediated and recommends treatment with antifungals. This is no longer recommended and will result in treatment failure.

## Counseling

You have confluent and reticulated papillomatosis. This condition is caused by a bacterium that lives on the skin called "*Dietzia.*" This condition only affects your skin, and it is not an infection, meaning it is unlikely to be spread from person to person. Additionally, it is a chronic condition, which means that it frequently comes back despite being treated.

Your doctor has prescribed you an oral antibiotic called "minocycline." You should take this medication twice daily for the time period that your doctor has recommended. It may take weeks for you to notice that your skin is improving. Please let your doctor know if your skin is not improving after 2 months because this may suggest that you need a different treatment for your condition.

## ACANTHOSIS NIGRICANS

**Taylor Cole, Sarah Lonowski, and Preeti Jhorar**

## Clinical Features

- AN typically presents as asymptomatic, hyperpigmented patches or plaques with a velvetlike texture.
  - It is classically brown, black, or gray in color.
  - It may be pink or red in some patients with a lighter complexion.

- AN plaques typically appear within skin folds or on flexural surfaces and are often symmetric.
  - Common locations include the posterior neck, axilla, groin, and inframammary regions.
  - Less common locations include the popliteal fossa, nipples, umbilicus, perioral, and perianal areas.
  - Rarely, AN may also arise on the extensor or acral surfaces.
- Patients with AN frequently also have acrochordons (skin tags) within the affected region.

## Epidemiology

- AN is more prevalent in darker-skinned individuals.
  - It is more common in patients of Hispanic, African, and Native American descent.
  - Although less common, it can also affect lighter-skinned patients.
- It has equal incidence among males and females.
- It affects older patients more often than younger patients but can present at any age.
- It is associated with obesity and insulin resistance in both children and adults.
  - In children, the presence of AN is a particularly strong indicator of insulin resistance and/or diabetes mellitus (DM).
  - In obese women, a clinical triad of AN, hirsutism, and polycystic ovaries is often observed (called HAIR-AN for hyperandrogenism, insulin resistance, acanthosis nigricans).

## Clinical Classification

- The two common forms of AN are obesity-associated AN and endocrinopathy-associated AN.
  - Obesity-associated AN is the most common cause of AN overall. It can occur with or without a concurrent insulin resistance state.
  - Endocrinopathy-associated AN is most commonly associated with insulin resistance/DM. It may also occur in association with polycystic ovarian syndrome (PCOS) or thyroid disease.
    - The severity of AN often mirrors the severity of insulin resistance.
- More uncommon forms of AN include malignant/paraneoplastic AN, drug-induced AN, genetic/syndromic AN, and idiopathic AN.
  - Malignant/paraneoplastic AN is characterized by rapid onset and extensive distribution. It is more common in adults but has been reported in children. It may occur in the context of a known cancer diagnosis or be a presenting sign of an occult malignancy.
    - It is most frequently associated with gastric adenocarcinoma.
    - It has also been reported in the setting of other gastrointestinal malignancies and with genitourinary, hematologic, cutaneous, and endocrine cancers.
    - It may affect the classic flexural areas or may manifest in other locations, including extensor surfaces (i.e., knees, elbows, knuckles), the lips/oral mucosa, and the palms (a manifestation that is also known as "tripe palms").
    - Other occasional associated features include multiple new seborrheic keratoses (sign of Leser-Trélat) or skin tags, severe pruritis, and glossitis.
  - Drug-induced AN typically occurs with medications that promote hyperinsulinemia, including oral contraceptive pills, nicotinic acid, human growth hormone, protease inhibitors, and corticosteroids. The skin lesions typically resolve with discontinuation of the offending agent.
  - Genetic/syndromic AN occurs in association with autosomal dominant mutations in the fibroblast growth factor receptor (FGFR) gene and in certain lipodystrophy syndromes.
    - Patients typically present with extensive AN at a young age (birth or early childhood).
  - Idiopathic AN is an uncommon form of AN that occurs in healthy individuals with darker skin. It typically involves the dorsal hands and feet and may also involve extensor elbows and knees.

## Work-Up

- Diagnosis can typically be made by visual inspection alone. If the diagnosis is uncertain, a skin biopsy may be warranted for confirmation.
- A thorough skin examination is recommended for all patients with AN or suspected AN to evaluate the extent of involvement.
  - If AN is extensive and/or new onset, consider examining less frequently affected areas such as the eyelids, nipples, hands and feet, perianal area, lips/oral cavity, and palms.

- Obtain a relevant history, which may include the age of onset (birth/childhood vs. adulthood); timing of onset (abrupt vs. insidious); relevant past medical history, specifically history of obesity, insulin resistance/DM, or PCOS; and current medications (if drug-induced AN is suspected).
  - If the onset was abrupt, obtain an appropriate review of systems to evaluate for symptoms of occult malignancy, such as decreased appetite, unintentional weight loss, and fatigue.
- Also consider calculating the body mass index (BMI); screening for type 2 DM (i.e., fasting blood glucose, hemoglobin A1c); and, if clinically suspected, evaluating for PCOS.

## Management

- Assess patient goals and set proper expectations; most forms of AN pose no threat to the patient's health.
- The primary goal in treating patients with AN is to address the underlying cause(s).
  - Patients who are obese or overweight should be encouraged to lose weight.
    - AN may resolve completely with weight reduction.
  - Patients with DM will benefit from lifestyle changes and pharmacologic interventions, such as metformin, when appropriate.
  - Patients with drug-induced AN can consider discontinuing the implicated medication if medically feasible.
  - Patients with malignancy-associated AN typically have resolution after seeking treatment for the underlying cancer.
- Topical, oral, and procedural therapies for AN are of limited efficacy, but topical retinoids and/or keratolytics; bleaching creams (containing a combination of topical steroids, hydroquinone, and retinoids); oral isotretinoin; or laser therapy and chemical peels may be considered.
  - The combination of tretinoin cream and ammonium lactate cream has been found to be helpful for obese patients, but use them with caution because these agents may be irritating in the flexural areas.
  - Oral isotretinoin may have some efficacy, but this treatment modality is not widely used.
  - Laser therapy or chemical peels may be helpful for some patients.

## Counseling

You have a common skin condition called "acanthosis nigricans" (AN). This condition causes the skin to get thicker and darker. It commonly affects areas such as the back of the neck, armpits, and groin. This condition is more common in individuals with darker complexions and in those who are overweight or have diabetes.

### For Individuals with no Metabolic Disturbances or Malignancy

The form of AN that you have is completely harmless and poses no threat to your overall health. If you are interested in reducing the appearance of the lesion, however, I can refer you to a dermatologist for further discussion of treatment options.

### For Individuals who are Obese or have Diabetes

The form of AN that you have is related to excess weight gain and/or hormonal changes. As your weight increases, your body undergoes hormonal changes that make it less responsive to the sugars that you eat. It is important that we address some of the hormonal changes that may be occurring in your body.

*For patients with confirmed diabetes.* My recommendation is to start a medicine called "metformin." This medication will help your body to respond more appropriately to the food that you eat. We will also need to work on lifestyle changes, including exercise and dietary modification.

*For patients without diabetes.* My recommendation is to work on losing weight. The best way to start is by increasing the amount of exercise that you are doing and making some basic changes to your diet, such as consuming fewer processed foods and foods that are high in sugar and simple carbohydrates. If you are interested, I can also refer you to a licensed dietician.

### For Individuals with Suspected Malignancy

I am concerned that your AN could be a sign of something more dangerous going on in the rest of your body, such as cancer. To evaluate this further, I would like to do some basic tests and I may refer you to another physician who is more familiar with malignancies originating in other areas of the body.

# 8

# Hypopigmented Rashes

## CHAPTER OUTLINE

# PITYRIASIS ALBA

**Elizabeth Dupuy and Preeti Jhorar**

## Clinical Features

Pityriasis alba is a benign inflammatory skin condition that presents with poorly circumscribed hypopigmented oval or round macules, patches, or thin plaques.

- Pityriasis alba is generally asymptomatic; patients may seek medical attention because of the cosmetic appearance of the lesions.
- Occasionally, it is scaly and may cause mild pruritus.
- It affects children and adolescents more often than adults.
- It is more common, or at least more apparent, in patients with darker skin tones.
- Pityriasis alba is commonly located on the cheeks and proximal upper extremities.
- It frequently coexists with, and sometimes is considered to be a minor feature of, atopic dermatitis (AD).
- Pityriasis alba is seen more commonly during the summer or fall; sun exposure and tanning may accentuate the contrast between normal and hypopigmented skin.

## Differential Diagnosis

The important differential diagnoses include vitiligo, tinea versicolor, seborrheic dermatitis, nevus depigmentosus, nevus anemicus, postinflammatory hypopigmentation, mycosis fungoides, leprosy, and ash-leaf spots of tuberous sclerosis.

## Vitiligo

Vitiligo is well demarcated, with a chalky-white appearance and no skin surface change, such as scale. Vitiligo is completely depigmented, whereas pityriasis alba is hypopigmented.

## Tinea Versicolor

A KOH preparation will reveal hyphae and spores in the case of tinea versicolor. It is commonly located on the upper chest and back, unlike pityriasis alba, which almost exclusively affects the cheeks.

## Seborrheic Dermatitis

Especially in patients with darker skin tones, seborrheic dermatitis can present with hypopigmented macules or patches along the eyebrows, nasolabial folds, frontal hair line, and retroauricular skin. It may be associated with a greasy scale or scalp dandruff.

## Nevus Depigmentosus

Nevus depigmentosus is a congenital disorder of hypopigmentation that is present at birth or noticed shortly thereafter. It has an asymmetric distribution and is stable over time.

## Nevus Anemicus

Nevus anemicus is noticed at birth or in early childhood and presents as an irregular, hypopigmented patch. It is not truly a pigmentary disorder but is instead caused by vascular hypersensitivity that leads to vasoconstriction. It is typically a focal lesion. Pressing a glass slide onto the border of nevus anemicus will cause the hypopigmentation to expand out as the periphery blanches.

## Postinflammatory Hypopigmentation

Postinflammatory hypopigmentation can result from any inflammatory process on the skin, but there usually is a history of preceding rash.

## Mycosis Fungoides

Mycosis fungoides involves multiple hypopigmented macules, usually in photoprotected areas. Referral to dermatology should be considered if there is a more extensive distribution of pityriasis alba-like lesions, especially in darker skin patients.

## Leprosy

Leprosy presents with hypoesthetic patches and can be considered with appropriate clinical history and geographic risk factor.

### Ash-Leaf Spots of Tuberous Sclerosis

In tuberous sclerosis, lesions are typically present at birth, can be tear-drop or ash-leaf shaped, and accentuate with a Wood lamp examination. In older patients, lesions can be associated with other features of tuberous sclerosis, such as facial angiofibromas.

Referral to dermatology should be considered when there are doubts as to the diagnosis or if the clinical course is atypical.

## Work-Up

- The diagnosis of pityriasis alba is usually established clinically.
- Skin biopsy is generally not needed.
- A Wood lamp examination can help distinguish pityriasis alba from vitiligo.
  - Pityriasis alba will appear accentuated with poorly defined borders, whereas vitiligo will show milky-white fluorescence with sharply demarcated borders.
- A potassium hydroxide (KOH) preparation can help distinguish pityriasis alba from tinea versicolor.
  - Pityriasis alba will not show fungal hyphae or spores, which are seen in tinea versicolor.

## Initial Steps in Management

- Patients should be reassured of the benign nature of the condition.
- Treatment is usually not necessary.
- Sun protection can help minimize the demarcation between affected and nonaffected areas.
- Moisturizers can address scaling and potentially prevent the development of new lesions.
- Low-potency topical steroids, such as 1% or 2.5% hydrocortisone cream, or topical calcineurin inhibitors may be used if there is any erythema or pruritus.
  - Topical calcineurin inhibitors include tacrolimus ointment and pimecrolimus cream.
  - Tacrolimus is available in two strengths: 0.03% or 0.1% ointment.
  - Pimecrolimus is available as a 1% cream.
    - Topical calcineurin inhibitors have a U.S. Food and Drug Administration (FDA) black box warning associating their use with a theoretical risk for lymphoma because of the classification of systemic calcineurin inhibitors as immunosuppressive medications.

- Patients can be reassured that most dermatologists believe these medications are safe to use and several professional organizations, including the American Academy of Dermatology, do not agree with this warning.

## Warning Signs/Common Pitfalls

Pityriasis alba is included in the differential diagnosis of hypopigmented or depigmented patches. Patients and sometimes physicians may be concerned that these lesions represent a more ominous depigmenting condition or an infectious process.

## Counseling

The white spots on your skin are caused by a condition called "pityriasis alba." This is not an infection, and it is not contagious. The cause of this condition is unknown; however, some believe it is a feature of atopic dermatitis or eczema. This condition will improve over a period of a few months to years and gradually the skin will return to normal pigmentation. Treatment is not necessary but if your skin is itchy, or if you desire treatment, we can try to use a low-potency topical steroid. Topical steroids should not be used for extended periods of time because their use may lead to side effects, such as thinning of the skin. An alternative treatment is a nonsteroidal antiinflammatory called a "topical calcineurin inhibitor," such as tacrolimus ointment or pimecrolimus cream. Although these are labeled with an FDA black box warning regarding a theoretical increase in risk for lymphoma, most dermatologists believe they are safe to use, and studies have not shown any increased risk for cancer with topical use. Other interventions that may improve the appearance of skin are the use of sun protection and moisturizers.

# VITILIGO

**Regina Liu, Amy R. Vandiver, and Preeti Jhorar**

Vitiligo is a common acquired disorder of pigmentation that results from the loss of functional melanocytes.

## Epidemiology

Vitiligo affects approximately 0.5% to 2% of the population worldwide. The peak incidence is in the 10- to 30-year-old age group with an average age of onset of approximately 20 years, although it can manifest any time from shortly after birth to late adulthood.

## Clinical Features

- Vitiligo classically presents as milky-white or chalky-white, nonscaling macules or patches that are completely depigmented with no overlying skin changes.
  - At initial onset, involved areas may appear lighter in color rather than completely depigmented.
  - There is a variant of active vitiligo, known as "trichrome vitiligo," in which lesions can have an intermediate zone of hypochromia between normal and totally depigmented skin (Fig. 8.1).
- The primary macules are often round or ovoid and become confluent as they enlarge, often leading to patches with irregular but sharply demarcated borders surrounded by normal skin.
  - Lesions range from millimeters to centimeters in diameter.
- Lesions in vitiligo are usually asymptomatic but can present with mild pruritis and/or loss of pigment in associated hair.
- Lesions can be stable or undergo centrifugal expansion at varying rates.
  - A stable lesion is defined as one in which no change is detected by serial photography in a 12-month period.
- Vitiligo can affect any area of the skin and mucous membranes.
  - It has a predilection for the extensor surfaces of the extremities (backs of the hands, elbows, and knees) and the periorificial areas (around the mouth, eyes, rectum, and genitalia).

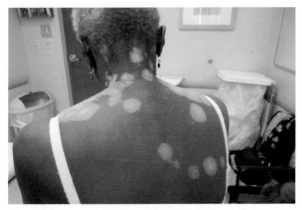

**Fig. 8.1 Trichrome Vitiligo.** This form of vitiligo is unstable and is likely to progress rapidly without immediate immunosuppression.

- The distribution of lesions can be localized or generalized.
  - Localized lesions can be focal, segmental, or mucosal.
    - Focal means that one or more macules are in a single area but are not in a segmental distribution.
    - Segmental indicates that the macules do not cross the midline and instead involve only one segment of the body.
    - Mucosal means that there is only involvement of the mucous membranes.
  - Generalized lesions can have vulgaris, acrofacial, mixed, or universal distributions.
    - Vulgaris is a very common distribution with scattered and widely distributed patches and macules.
    - Acrofacial is another very common distribution with involvement of the face and distal extremities.
    - A mixed distribution is a combination of segmental type with acrofacial and/or vulgaris type.
    - Universal distribution is rare and shows near complete depigmentation.
- The Koebner phenomenon has been observed in vitiligo when areas have been subjected to repeated trauma, pressure, or friction.

## Differential Diagnosis

Early vitiligo is often misdiagnosed as pityriasis versicolor or medication-induced or chemical-induced leukoderma.

### Pityriasis Versicolor

Pityriasis versicolor can be differentiated because it presents with dust like scales and an incomplete loss of pigment.

### Medication-Induced and Chemical-Induced Leukoderma

Leukoderma can only be distinguished from vitiligo based on a history of exposure to known culprits (e.g., imiquimod, tumor necrosis factor inhibitors, monobenzyl ether of hydroquinone, hair dyes such as paraphenylenediamine).
- Lesions are otherwise clinically and histologically indistinguishable from vitiligo.

Another common mimicker of vitiligo is leukoderma of the penis from latex exposure.
- This diagnosis should also be considered when patients present with depigmented patches on the genitals.

## Work-Up
- Vitiligo is a clinical diagnosis. A full skin examination should be performed in all patients presenting with vitiligo.
- A Wood lamp examination can be particularly useful in visualizing vitiligo in individuals with lightly pigmented skin because the lesions usually emit a bright blue-white fluorescence and appear sharply demarcated.
- Laboratory studies are usually not helpful in diagnosing vitiligo.
- Biopsy is usually not necessary, but if performed, will show an absence of melanocytes with or without associated inflammation.
- Vitiligo is associated with various conditions, although this association is not strong enough to warrant empiric screening for every patient. Careful history taking should be performed for all patients with new-onset vitiligo, and further tests should be ordered if the history and review of systems suggest the patient is at higher risk.
  - If personal or family history is suggestive of autoimmune disease, screening of autoimmune antibodies and titers should be ordered.
  - If history is concerning for associated thyroid disease, screening should be performed with serum thyroid-stimulating hormone.
  - If the patient presents with symptoms of diabetes mellitus, fasting blood glucose should be obtained.

## Initial Steps in Management
There is no cure for vitiligo, but available treatment options can lead to satisfactory results. The goals of therapy are to stabilize depigmentation and induce repigmentation.
- Another important goal of therapy is to address the psychological needs of the patient.

Therapy for repigmentation is often prolonged and responses to treatment are variable. Therapy should be guided by the patient's age and skin type, the extent and location of the vitiligo, and patient preference.
- Patients can have partial repigmentation, full repigmentation, or no response to treatment.

- A period of 8 to 12 weeks is needed to gauge whether a particular treatment is effective. For phototherapy, a much longer period (at least 6 months) is required.

For localized areas of vitiligo, topical medications are often used as first-line therapy.
- The choice of topical medication will depend on the site of the lesion and age of the patient.
  - In adults, lesions on the body may be treated with ultrapotent or potent corticosteroids.
  - Lesions on the face, neck, and intertriginous areas should be treated with calcineurin inhibitors to avoid skin atrophy.
  - Ultrapotent and potent corticosteroids are also avoided in children in favor of mid-potency corticosteroids or calcineurin inhibitors.
- Long-term steroids should be started and monitored by a dermatologist because of the risk for adverse effects, such as skin atrophy, telangiectasia, and hypertrichosis.
- When using steroids long term, regimens often include daily or twice daily application in a cyclical fashion, alternating with calcineurin inhibitors or drug holiday to minimize the risk for adverse effects.

For generalized vitiligo, narrowband ultraviolet B (NB-UVB) phototherapy is the first-line treatment.
- Patients should be counseled that this option requires frequent in-office treatments, generally 2 to 3 times per week.
- Side effects range from pruritus and erythema to sunburn like reactions and possible reactivation of latent herpes simplex virus.

Treatment with tofacitinib, an oral Janus kinase inhibitor, has also been shown to be effective in treating generalized vitiligo. This medication should only be prescribed by a specialist, however.
- Other oral immunosuppressants, including pulsed oral corticosteroids, methotrexate, and cyclosporine, can be considered in patients who cannot obtain coverage for tofacitinib.

Treatment with an excimer laser is an alternative therapy for more localized lesions.

A variety of surgical repigmentation techniques have also been successful, including minigrafting and autologous suction blister grafts.
- Surgical repigmentation is typically reserved for vitiligo patients with recalcitrant disease that has failed to respond to medical therapy and whose disease has

remained stable for at least 6 months before surgical intervention.

- It is a good treatment option for segmental vitiligo, which is otherwise recalcitrant to medical treatments.

For patients with disseminated and widespread vitiligo, depigmentation of the remaining normally pigmented skin is an alternative option.

- Depigmentation is most commonly performed using 20% monobenzyl ether of hydroquinone applied once or twice daily for a minimum of 9 to 12 months.
  - Patients should be counseled that this treatment option will require strict and lifelong photoprotection.
    - Patients who cannot adhere to strict photoprotection should not undergo this treatment.

Therapy for vitiligo should also address how the condition affects the quality of life of the patient. Vitiligo can have devastating psychosocial effects on the patient, including low self-esteem. Patients can also suffer from social stigmatization. The impact of vitiligo on quality of life should be thoroughly assessed, and psychological support and therapy should be offered to patients.

It is important to establish expectations for treatment in patients early in the discussion. Realistic expectations about the length and efficacy of treatment are helpful in achieving patient satisfaction.

- Because response to treatment is slow, patients can also be counseled to use cover-up makeup, such as Dermablend, on the face and other cosmetically significant areas.

## Warning Signs/Common Pitfalls

Although the majority of patients with vitiligo are otherwise healthy, vitiligo can be associated with a number of autoimmune conditions. In particular, there is a well-established association between vitiligo and autoimmune thyroid diseases, such as Graves disease and Hashimoto thyroiditis. Other associated endocrinopathies include diabetes mellitus, lupus erythematous, alopecia areata, rheumatoid arthritis, pernicious anemia, and Addison disease. In rare cases, vitiligo can present in patients as part of a polyglandular autoimmune syndrome.

Ocular disease, including uveitis, has also been rarely associated with vitiligo. Careful history taking and review of systems should be performed in patients with new-onset vitiligo.

Vitiligo is generally a benign condition. Nevertheless, the depigmentation seen in vitiligo can also be caused by melanoma-associated leukoderma. Clinicians should be aware of the association between malignant melanoma and vitiligo-like depigmentation and should perform a total body inspection on suspected melanocytic lesions, especially in patients who present at an older age, and should refer the patients to a dermatologist when necessary.

## Counseling

You have a relatively common skin disorder called "vitiligo," in which there is a loss of the cells that provide color in the skin (melanocytes). It is not well understood why people develop vitiligo. It is a chronic condition and although there is currently not a cure, there are available treatments. It is important that you see a dermatologist to determine which treatment is right for you.

The goal of treatment is to stop the process that is destroying the cells that make color so that they can resume making color for the skin. It is important to understand that results can be highly variable and not all patients will have complete repigmentation. The treatment course is usually long, on the order of months, and will require you to be followed by a dermatologist to assess your response to treatment.

The depigmentation in vitiligo can be very distressing to patients. There are mental health resources and support groups available if you are interested. There are also resources available online through the National Vitiligo Foundation.

# IDIOPATHIC GUTTATE HYPOMELANOSIS

**Regina Liu, Amy R. Vandiver, and Preeti Jhorar**

Idiopathic guttate hypomelanosis (IGH) is a pigmentary disorder of sun-exposed skin that is commonly seen in older patients.

## Epidemiology

IGH is very common, with incidence increasing with age. The prevalence is up to 70% in patients in their 50s, and 80% in patients over the age of 70 years. IGH occurs in all races and skin types but is more easily observed in darkly pigmented skin. IGH occurs equally among females and males.

## Clinical Features

- IGH classically presents with confetti like, white macules symmetrically scattered over the extremities.
- The macules of IGH are well circumscribed, sharply defined, and lightly colored or porcelain white.
  - There is no textural change to the associated skin, and hairs within the lesions typically retain their pigment.
  - Lesions are not itchy or painful.
- The lesions are usually small, ranging from 0.5 mm to 6 mm, but can rarely be up to 2.5 cm in size.
  - After initial appearance, the lesions do not change in size or coalesce.
- The number of lesions in affected patient averages around 10 to 15, but some patients can develop over 100 lesions.
- The lesions typically localize to sun-exposed areas of the extremities.
  - The extensor forearms and shins are most commonly involved, but the remainder of the extremities can also be affected.
  - The face is rarely involved.

## Differential Diagnosis

Various conditions can mimic IGH, including vitiligo, pityriasis versicolor, and progressive macular hypomelanosis.

### Vitiligo

Vitiligo, especially early-stage confetti type, can be distinguished because vitiligo typically presents at younger ages and its lesions grow and coalesce and can affect the face and any other part of the body.

### Pityriasis Versicolor

In pityriasis versicolor, lesions have a fine scale and are frequently found in seborrheic distribution on the shoulders and upper trunk.

### Progressive Macular Hypomelanosis

With progressive macular hypomelanosis, lesions are coalescing and typically distributed on the trunk and only rarely extend to the extremities.

## Work-Up

The diagnosis of IGH is usually made clinically. Although rarely necessarily, a punch biopsy can be performed for definitive diagnosis.

## Initial Steps in Management

IGH is a benign condition that does not require referral to a dermatologist or further treatment.

- Avoidance of sun exposure and concomitant use of sunscreens and physical barriers should be recommended.
- Cosmetic concerns may motivate patients to seek medical care despite the benign course of the disease.
- There is currently no standard treatment for IGH.
  - Cryotherapy with liquid nitrogen is a possible therapy for focal lesions.
  - Variable success has also been achieved with topical steroids, retinoids, and calcineurin inhibitors.

## Warning Signs/Common Pitfalls

IGH is a common and benign condition but is often underrecognized among physicians. Early diagnosis and reassurance can help patients avoid an unnecessary work-up and undue emotional stress.

## Counseling

You have a very common skin condition called "idiopathic guttate hypomelanosis," or "IGH" for short. The exact cause of IGH is unknown, but it is thought to be a result of chronic sun exposure or even a part of the normal aging process. This condition is benign and does not require treatment. The lesions are generally permanent, and you may continue to develop more lesions as you age. Avoiding sun exposure whenever possible and using sunscreens is important in preventing more spots from developing in the future. Although the condition is benign, if you are concerned about the appearance of the spots, there are some treatments that have had some variable success.

# PROGRESSIVE MACULAR HYPOMELANOSIS

**Logan Thomas and Preeti Jhorar**

## Clinical Features

Progressive macular hypomelanosis (PMH) is an acquired pigmentary disorder of the skin that presents as poorly defined, circular macules (less than 1 cm in size) and small patches, mainly distributed on the trunk. These lesions can sometimes coalesce together to form bigger patches in the mid-trunk region (see Fig. 8.1).

- PMH occurs more commonly in woman than men, can occur in all age groups but is prevalent in the teenage population, is more common in people with darker skin than in people with lighter skin, and more often affects the trunk than the extremities and face.

- It is more prevalent in tropical climates.
- Typically, it is asymptomatic at onset and can be commonly misdiagnosed as residual or postinflammatory hypopigmentation from pityriasis versicolor.
- Lesions tend to resolve within 3 to 5 years but can persist longer and even increase in size. Spontaneous resolution normally occurs at around 40 years of age.

## Differential Diagnosis

It is important to rule out other common causes of hypopigmentation before making the diagnosis of PMH.

The differential for PMH includes hypopigmented pityriasis versicolor and postinflammatory hypopigmentation.

### Hypopigmented Pityriasis Versicolor

This typically has overlying fine dust like scales and show pseudohyphae (spaghetti) and spores (meatballs) on KOH preparation.

### Postinflammatory Hypopigmentation

Postinflammatory hypopigmentation can be secondary to any inflammatory conditions, such as eczema or psoriasis, and patients usually provide a history of antecedent rash.

### Other Differential Diagnoses

Other differential diagnoses to consider include idiopathic guttate hypomelanosis, which typically has a whiter appearance, is distributed centripetally, and is found in older populations; vitiligo, in which lesions are completely depigmented and appear milky-white in color; and leprosy, which causes depigmentation but also causes loss of sensation in the affected area. Patients typically are from endemic areas.

## Work-Up

- Diagnosis can be aided with the use of a Wood lamp examination, which will fluoresce hypopigmented spots and show nothing in nonaffected skin. Red follicular fluorescence may also be seen, demonstrating the presence of the microorganism *Cutibacterium acnes*, which is thought to play a role in the pathogenesis of PMH.

- Diagnosis of PMH is usually made clinically, but if a skin biopsy is performed, it will reveal reduced melanin in the affected skin and normal levels of melanocytes.

## Initial Steps in Management

PMH is a relatively benign condition but can be aesthetically displeasing to the patient. Pathogenesis of the condition has some association with *C. acnes,* so most therapies are similar to acne treatment.

### Initial Management

- A 1% clindamycin lotion can be used during the day, along with a 5% benzoyl peroxide gel at night with or without NBUVB light irradiation three times a week for a period of 12 weeks.
  - It is important to notify the patient that benzoyl peroxide can bleach towels and clothing, so the patient may want to use a white towel when washing and wear old clothing to bed.

### Other Management Therapies

Other management therapies include the use of doxycycline 100 mg twice a day for 2 to 3 months or psoralen plus UVA (PUVA). There are also a few reported cases of treatment with isotretinoin. There are mixed recurrence rates with these therapies.

## Warning Signs/Common Pitfalls

PMH is a clinical diagnosis. The biggest pitfall when addressing PMH is failing to keep it in the differential of hypopigmented macules in the first place.

If the lesion fails to resolve with therapy, referral to dermatology is warranted to rule out other diagnoses.

## Counseling

You have a common condition called "progressive macular hypomelanosis," or "PMH" for short. It is a benign condition that causes white spots to appear, mainly on your trunk. The progression is variable; some patients see complete resolution in 3 to 5 years, whereas others remain stable or worsen with eventual resolution around mid-life. Treatment consists of application of clindamycin 1% lotion during the day, benzoyl peroxide 5% gel at night, and light therapy with narrowband UVB three times a week. Benzoyl peroxide can bleach fabrics so it is recommended that you use a white towel and wear old clothing to sleep in. We will have you return to the clinic in 3 months to assess the treatment response and adjust treatment or refer you to a dermatologist as needed.

# NEVUS ANEMICUS

Michelle W. Cheng, and Preeti Jhorar

## Clinical Features

Nevus anemicus is a vascular birthmark that occurs because an area of the skin is persistently vasoconstricted.

- Nevus anemicus presents as a hypopigmented macule or patch present at birth.
  - Typically, it affects the upper trunk, but patches have also been reported on the face and extremities.
- These patches do not exhibit reactive erythema in response to usual triggers such as trauma, heat, or cold.
- Diascopy (i.e., pressing on the border with a glass side) can be helpful in diagnosis; the surrounding normal skin will blanch and become indistinguishable from the lesion, making it difficult to delineate the margins of the patch.
- A Wood lamp examination will not accentuate the hypopigmented patch of nevus anemicus, which can aid in distinguishing it from vitiligo, which can mimic nevus anemicus clinically.
- Nevus anemicus affects an estimated 1% to 2% of the population, but the true numbers are thought to be underreported because of its subtle presentation, particularly in lighter-skinned individuals.
- In most cases, nevus anemicus is not associated with systemic findings.
  - Rarely, it has been seen in patients with certain genodermatoses, such as neurofibromatosis and phakomatosis pigmentovascularis.

## Differential Diagnosis

The diascopic features of nevus anemicus are diagnostic and help differentiate it from common mimickers. Common differential diagnoses include nevus depigmentosus, vitiligo, postinflammatory hypopigmentation, and leprosy.

- Nevus depigmentosus lacks border obscuring with diascopy.
- Vitiligo shows a chalky-white fluorescence with a Wood lamp examination.
- Postinflammatory hypopigmentation lacks the stability of a congenital lesion, and patients usually have a history of a preceding rash.

- In leprosy, the hypopigmented patches are usually hypoesthetic.

## Work-Up

No further work-up is necessary.

## Initial Steps in Management

No further management is necessary.

- The patches can be camouflaged using makeup if the patient is bothered by the appearance.

## Warning Signs/Common Pitfalls

Nevus anemicus is usually easy to diagnose clinically.

- If other cutaneous findings are present, consider referring the patient to dermatology for an evaluation of rare genodermatoses.

## Counseling

You have a condition called "nevus anemicus," which is a benign birthmark of the skin. No further work-up is necessary. If the lesion is in a cosmetically concerning area, you can use makeup for camouflage. If this lesion starts to change or you begin developing additional similar lesions, contact your doctor for reevaluation.

# NEVUS DEPIGMENTOSUS

Michelle W. Cheng, and Preeti Jhorar

## Clinical Features

Nevus depigmentosus is an uncommon congenital skin lesion that presents as a hypopigmented macule or patch.

- It occurs in 1 in 50 to 75 individuals.
- The lesions are usually solitary and well demarcated with serrated borders and are notably hypomelanotic, not amelanotic.
- A Wood lamp examination can be of assistance in determining whether or not the lesion is hypomelanotic or amelanotic. The lesion will be off-white if hypomelanotic and a chalky-white color if amelanotic.
- The lesions are stable, do not demonstrate changes in sensation or morphology, and do not alter in distribution or number.

## Differential Diagnosis

The differential for nevus depigmentosus mainly includes nevus anemicus, vitiligo, postinflammatory hypopigmentation, and leprosy.

- Nevus depigmentosus can be distinguished from nevus anemicus because the borders of nevus depigmentosus will not blanch with pressure.
- Nevus depigmentosus can be differentiated from vitiligo because it presents with a solitary lesion; is hypopigmented not depigmented; and has serrated, not rounded borders.
- Postinflammatory hypopigmentation lacks the stability of a congenital lesion and usually has a history of a preceding rash.
- Leprosy has hypopigmented patches; however, these are usually hypoesthetic.

## Work-Up

No further work-up is necessary.

## Initial Steps in Management

No further management is necessary.
- The patches can be camouflaged using makeup if the patient is bothered by the appearance.

### Warning Signs/Common Pitfalls

If a suspected lesion is present with neurologic, ophthalmologic, orthopedic, or dental symptoms, consider a diagnosis of hypomelanosis of Ito, which usually has more extensive distribution clinically compared with nevus depigmentosus.

### Counseling

You have a condition called "nevus anemicus," which is a benign birthmark of the skin. No further work-up is necessary. If the lesion is in a cosmetically concerning area, you can use makeup for camouflage. If the lesion starts to change or you begin developing additional similar lesions, contact your doctor for reevaluation.

## STRIAE DISTENSAE

**Shivani Sinha, Gloria Lin, and Katalin Ferenczi**

### Clinical Features

Striae distensae (SD), commonly known as "stretch marks," are the result of dermal atrophy and elastic fiber fragmentation secondary to stretching of the skin. Although SD are typically asymptomatic, the cosmetic appearance can cause significant frustration and psychosocial distress for the patient. SD are often associated with periods of rapid growth, such as pregnancy; puberty; weight gain; rapid muscle growth as a result of excessive weight lifting; prolonged oral or topical corticosteroid use; and underlying conditions, such as Cushing syndrome. Striae from steroids are not because of tension on the skin but rather because of inhibition of fibroblasts, collagen synthesis, and hyaluronan synthase 3 enzyme.

- SD can be classified as striae rubra (SR) when the lesions are red and striae alba (SA) when they are white. The red linear striations seen in SR represent an early manifestation of SD. With time, these lesions gradually become hypopigmented or white in color, characteristic of SA. These depressed linear striations are most commonly distributed symmetrically on the abdomen, breasts, buttocks, and thighs. The long axis lies parallel to the direction of skin tension that resulted in their formation. Excessive stretching can rarely lead to tearing and ulceration of the lesions.
- When associated with pregnancy, SD is referred to as striae gravidarum (SG) and typically develops in the second or third trimesters on the abdomen and breasts.
- SD secondary to oral corticosteroids may be more widely distributed, in contrast to the localized striae seen at topical steroid application sites. The use of occlusive wraps that are sometimes recommended to enhance topical corticosteroid efficacy can increase the risk for SD. The presence of striae in uncommon locations, such as the face or axillae, is suggestive of prior use of topical steroids to that area.

### Differential Diagnosis

The differential diagnosis for SD includes anetoderma, scars, linear focal elastosis, lichen sclerosus (LS), polymorphic eruption of pregnancy (PEP), and Cushing syndrome.

- Anetoderma presents as macular depressions or outpouchings of skin on the trunk and extremities. They can also appear scarlike. Because they are typically smaller and rounder, they can be differentiated from the longer, more linear striations of SD. No effective therapy is available for this condition.
- Scars may clinically resemble striae because they are often linear and can become depressed over time. Scars, however, are not symmetrically distributed, and there is typically an accompanying history of trauma or surgical intervention in the area of scarring.
- Linear focal elastosis presents as atrophic linear plaques that are the result of elastic tissue abnormalities.

Although they may appear similar to SA, they are often raised with a yellow hue and tend to appear on the lower back and extremities. This condition is usually refractory to treatment.

- LS presents as white, cigarette paper–like atrophic plaques in the genitals, buttocks, thighs, and breasts. The affected areas tend to be larger and may have accompanying fissures and erosions. It is treated with high-potency topical steroids.
- PEP (also known as "pruritic urticarial papules" and "plaques of pregnancy") is an inflammatory disorder that presents at the end of the third trimester. The intensely pruritic and erythematous papules tend to involve SG but may spread to the back, buttocks, and proximal thighs with sparing of the umbilicus. There is no fetal risk associated with this condition and topical steroids can be used for symptomatic relief.
- Cushing syndrome is a disorder with a wide range of clinical manifestations that is characterized by excessive glucocorticoid exposure. The resulting progressive centripetal obesity may lead to the development of striae on the abdomen. These are often intensely pigmented, wider, and more depressed than SD. In addition, the patient may have other symptoms, such as buffalo hump, moon facies, and skin atrophy to indicate excess systemic glucocorticoid levels.

## Work-Up

SD is a clinical diagnosis based on its highly characteristic appearance and anatomic distribution. As such, it typically does not require a skin biopsy for confirmation.

- Physical examination and history of any conditions associated with rapid growth can be helpful when making the diagnosis.
- Patients who present with other systemic symptoms, such as weight gain, menstrual changes, ecchymoses, abnormal glucose tolerance, or new-onset hypertension, should be evaluated for Cushing syndrome.

## Initial Steps in Management

Because SD is asymptomatic and benign in nature, treatment is not medically necessary and typically not covered by insurance. The permanent cosmetic disfigurement, however, is often associated with psychological distress and frustration for the patient, so they may still opt for treatment. The goal of therapy should be to minimize the contrast from the surrounding normal skin. Given the treatment-resistant nature of this condition, patients should be counseled on realistic treatment expectations and the lack of likelihood of complete reversal even with different therapy modalities.

## Prevention

- Avoid rapid weight gain or excessive weight lifting, which can result in rapid muscular hypertrophy.
- For striae related to steroid use, the offending agent should be tapered down or discontinued. Patients should be counseled regarding the potential side effects of steroids (both systemic and topical) before starting these medications.

Treatment options and results can vary based on the type of SD.

## Striae Rubra

- Because SR represent earlier changes of SD, they are more likely to respond to treatment than SA.
- Recommend moisturizers containing vitamin C and fruit acids.
- Chemical peels containing glycolic acid or trichloroacetic acid can stimulate new collagen growth and decrease the width of striations.
- Topical tretinoin cream can be applied nightly to the affected areas. The therapy can be discontinued if no improvement is noted after 3 to 6 months.
  - Pregnant or breastfeeding women should not be treated with topical tretinoin because of the potential risk for teratogenicity.
- Superficial microdermabrasion mechanically ablates the affected skin and may improve the appearance of SR.
- Pulsed-dye laser therapy every 4 to 6 weeks can improve the appearance by reducing the erythema. Treatment should be continued for at least 3 months. If no improvement is noted, therapy may be discontinued.

## Striae Alba

- Ablative or nonablative fractional laser therapy (FLT) can stimulate skin pigmentation and improve the appearance of SA. Although ablative FLT may demonstrate faster improvements, the patients should be counseled that it is associated with a greater risk for side effects and longer recovery times.
- Microneedling stimulates the growth of new collagen through tissue remodeling. It can be performed alone or in combination with radiofrequency energy.

This may be a suitable option for darker-skinned individuals because of the decreased risk for postinflammatory hyperpigmentation.

- UVB phototherapy may result in increased pigmentation of the striations.

## Striae Gravidarum

- Treatment of SG in pregnant women should be delayed until after delivery because of the paucity of safety data for the different treatment modalities during pregnancy.
- Other therapies for SD may have some benefit based on anecdotal evidence; however, patients should be counseled on their varying efficacies.
- Moisturizing agents, such as cocoa butter and coconut oil, may improve the appearance of SD by increasing cutaneous hydration.
- Platelet-rich plasma can be injected intradermally to stimulate neocollagenesis.
- Intense pulsed-light therapy may decrease the width of striations and improve overall skin texture in both SR and SA.
- Infrared laser therapy can stimulate dermal collagen remodeling and new collagen growth.

## Warning Signs/Common Pitfalls

- Laser and microneedling therapies are the first-line treatments in SD, but the cost of these options may be a limiting factor.

- Pulsed-dye laser and FLT should be avoided in darker-skinned patients because of the risk for hyperpigmentation.
- SG associated with intense pruritus may be a sign of PEP, and a referral to a dermatologist should be considered to confirm the diagnosis.

## Counseling

The stretch marks on your body are called "striae distensae." The initial pinkness of these areas will ultimately resolve and leave lighter areas that are usually less noticeable with time. These are typically asymptomatic and benign, but they are a permanent condition that is difficult to treat. Keeping the affected areas moisturized may help. Other therapies may be offered; however, they are unlikely to completely reverse the process and would probably not be covered by insurance. If you have striae associated with pregnancy, it is recommended that you wait until after delivery to pursue treatment options. A dermatologist can review the different therapy modalities to help determine what the best option may be for you.

If you have other concerning symptoms, such as weight gain, menstrual changes, new onset hypertension, or difficulties controlling your blood sugar, then you should see a medical professional for evaluation of possible Cushing syndrome, which can present with striae.

# Skin Growths

# Acne and Acne-Related Conditions

# ACNE

**Payal Shah and Nikita Lakdawala**

## Clinical Features

- Acne is most commonly located on the face, neck, back, upper chest, and upper arms where pilosebaceous units are most densely concentrated.
- Acne most commonly affects adolescents.
- Adult women have a predisposition to a jawline distribution of papules.
- Acne in men commonly involves the trunk.
- Morphology ranges from comedones (i.e., clogged open and closed pores that create whiteheads/blackheads) to papules, pustules, cysts, and nodules. Inflammatory lesions can result in permanent scarring.
- Family history is often positive.
- All races are equally affected.
- Severe acne can result in disfiguring scarring (Fig. 9.1).
- The etiology of acne is complex and involves sebaceous gland hypersensitivity and the subsequent inflammatory response to circulating androgens, P acnes, and genetics. Some medications (such as lithium, steroids, and anticonvulsants) can precipitate acne, as can some endocrine disorders, such as polycystic ovarian disease. Finally, occlusive makeup and athletic gear can cause acne to worsen.

## Differential Diagnosis

The main differential includes perioral dermatitis and rosacea.
- A perioral predilection of inflammatory lesions is more consistent with perioral dermatitis.

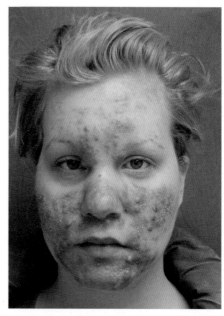

**Fig. 9.1 Cystic Acne (Acne Conglobata).** (From the University of Connecticut Department of Dermatology Grand Rounds Collection.)

- The presence of comedones helps differentiate acne from both rosacea and perioral dermatitis.

## Work-Up

- The patient's skincare routine should be reviewed because frequent rubbing, touching, and overcleansing of the face is known to exacerbate acne. Additionally, cosmetics and oil-based hair products can also exacerbate acne.

- Lifestyle contributions of grease/oils should be reviewed. Skin occlusion from occlusive make-up, sporting equipment, tight clothing, or backpacks may exacerbate acne.
- The patient's medication list should be reviewed for the possibility of drug-induced acneiform eruption. The sudden onset of monomorphic, inflammatory papules should raise suspicion of a drug-induced acneiform eruption. Triggering agents include, but are not limited to, systemic corticosteroids; topical corticosteroids; anabolic steroids; danazol; stanozolol; testosterone; lithium; isoniazid; phenytoin; cyclosporine; medroxyprogesterone; low-estrogen oral contraceptives; progesterone-only birth control; and vitamins B2, B6, and B12.
- Menstrual and medical history should be examined in females to consider hormonal acne, particularly in the setting of other signs of hirsutism. Endocrine disorders can cause hyperandrogenism that can predispose individuals to acne development. In these circumstances, checking the free and total testosterone, sex-hormone binding globulin, follicle-stimulating hormone, luteinizing hormone, and dehydroepiandrosterone is beneficial. Any hormonal imbalance is important to recognize because it guides treatment.
- Acne is usually a clinical diagnosis; routine histologic confirmation is not indicated.
- In the setting of small, itchy monomorphic follicular pustules on the upper back, shoulders, and scalp of an adolescents or young adult, scraping a pustule with potassium hydroxide (KOH) testing can assess for a diagnosis of *Pityrosporum folliculitis*.

## Initial Steps in Management
### General Management Comments

- A healthy skincare routine should be established that includes twice daily facial washing with a gentle cleanser. Cosmetic products that are used should be noncomedogenic and/or oil-free.
- An assessment of the severity of the acne guides the treatment.
  - Mild acne should be treated with benzoyl peroxide, a topical retinoid, or a topical combination therapy with benzoyl peroxide and either a topical antibiotic, a topical retinoid, or both.
  - Moderate acne should be treated with topical combination therapy or consideration of an oral antibiotic with adjunctive use of a topical retinoid, benzoyl peroxide, or both.
  - Severe acne should be treated with oral antibiotics and a combination topical therapy or oral isotretinoin; referral to dermatology to prevent progression of permanent scarring is recommended.
  - Patients with cystic acne and substantial pre-existing scarring should consider isotretinoin therapy.
- Topical antibiotic use is best used in combination with benzoyl peroxide to minimize antibiotic resistance.
- Topical retinoids should not be used at the exact time as benzoyl peroxide because the former may oxidize and be inactivated.
- Management strategies to consider if the desired response is not achieved include a change of topical retinoid, change to topical dapsone use, increase of the oral antibiotic dose, change to an oral antibiotic choice, use of oral contraceptives, use of spironolactone, and/or referral to a dermatologist.
- Noncompliance with therapies may lead to worsening of acne and the potential for scarring.
- In cases refractory to traditional antimicrobial therapy, skin and nasal swabs can be considered to exclude gram-negative folliculitis.

### Recommended Initial Regimen

For mild to moderate acne, the recommended initial regimen includes the use of 2.5% to 5% benzoyl peroxide, a daily face wash, and the gradually increased use of topical retinoids to daily at bedtime (tretinoin 0.025%–0.1%, tazarotene 0.05%–0.1% cream or gel, or adapalene gel 0.1%–0.3%).

- Retinoids are contraindicated in pregnancy.
  Topical antibiotics, such as clindamycin 1% lotion or solution, erythromycin 2% gel, dapsone 5% or 7.5% gel, or minocycline 4% foam, can also be used for mild to moderate cases.
- Topical antibiotics should be combined with a benzoyl peroxide wash or gel if possible to decrease antibiotic resistance.
- Adverse effects of topical therapies are common and expected. These include dryness, pruritis, peeling, burning, redness, and stinging. Daily oil-free moisturizer use can help handle these symptoms and maintain the skin barrier that is weakened by acne disease.

## Partial but Inadequate Response

If there is a partial but inadequate response after a 3-month trial of combination topical therapies, oral antibiotics can be tried for 3 to 4 months (doxycycline 100 mg daily or BID; minocycline 100 mg daily or BID; tetracycline 500 mg daily or BID).

- Tetracycline antibiotics are contraindicated in pregnancy.
- Known adverse effects of oral antibiotics include gastrointestinal (GI) upset, photosensitivity, and dizziness.

  Hormonal therapy can also be tried for female patients, particularly if the acne is in a perioral and jawline distribution (spironolactone 50–100 mg daily or BID).

## Continued Inadequate Response

If the response continues to be inadequate and you are confident that the patient has acne that is refractory to a combination of topical therapies and oral antibiotics, then the next step includes isotretinoin therapy.

- Registering isotretinoin use with the iPLEDGE program is required. Healthcare providers must be registered with iPLEDGE before they can prescribe isotretinoin and each individual patient must be registered.
- Isotretinoin initiation requires obtaining baseline and regular interval levels of the complete blood count (CBC), glucose test, liver function test, fasting lipids, and pregnancy tests for female patients (because isotretinoin is known to be teratogenic).
- Females should be on dual-contraception use during the course of treatment.
- Patients start typically with 0.5 mg/kg daily, which increases to 1 mg/kg daily after 1 month.
- Treatment duration of isotretinoin is typically 5 to 6 months, but the medication should be continued at least 2 months after total clearance of acne to increase the chance of a durable response.
  - Most healthcare providers use weight-based isotretinoin goals (150 mg/kg to 220 mg/kg).
- Known adverse effects include xerosis, cheilitis, elevated liver enzymes, and hypertriglyceridemia.

## Warning Signs/Common Pitfalls

Although acne is a benign skin condition, it can lead to permanent scarring or postinflammatory hyperpigmentation and significant psychological distress, making early treatment intervention critical for optimal patient outcomes.

Acne requires consistent treatment adherence for months to achieve the clinical response. Therefore lack of response before 6 to 8 weeks of treatment should not be assessed as refractory acne or a failure of treatment.

## Counseling

Your doctor has diagnosed you with acne, a very common chronic inflammatory condition of the pilosebaceous unit that presents because of a combination of factors, including increased sebum production, follicular hyperkeratinization, proliferation of bacteria (*Cutibacterium acnes*), and inflammation. It often is a self-limited disease that typically begins in adolescence because of androgen-stimulated sebum production and keratinization changes of the follicle.

Acne should be treated because it can cause permanent scarring of your skin. Acne treatment is targeted at preventing new lesions rather than treating existing lesions. The importance of treatment adherence cannot be overstressed because a clinical response is only expected after at least 8 weeks and ideally up to 2 to 3 months of strong adherence. Lack of adherence is the biggest reason for treatment failure. Treat the entire field of potential acne, rather than individual spots, with topical therapies.

The use of harsh cleansers and antibacterial soaps is discouraged because they may exacerbate acne. Additionally, pimples should not be squeezed because it may lead to scarring and infection.

Low glycemic diets that minimize the spike in blood sugar and insulin levels may improve acne, but more studies are needed to establish the relationship. Diets that are considered low glycemic can be found on the Internet.

# ROSACEA

**Payal Shah and Nikita Lakdawala**

## Clinical Features

- Facial distribution most often involves the nose, cheeks (Fig. 9.2), brow (Fig. 9.3), and chin (Fig. 9.4), usually with sparing of the nasolabial folds.
- Rosacea tends to predominate in individuals with lighter skin types.
- Episodic flushing with a sensation of stinging/burning is common.
- Episodes may be triggered by hot beverages, spicy foods, alcohol, chocolate, stress, extreme temperatures changes, and contact with *Demodex spp.*

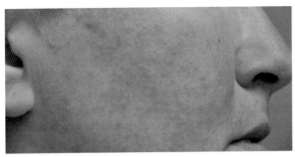

**Fig. 9.2** Rosacea, Cheek. (From the University of Connecticut Department of Dermatology Grand Rounds Collection.)

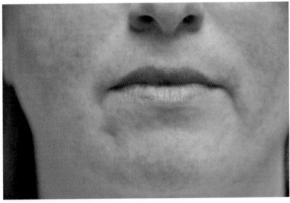

**Fig. 9.3** Rosacea, Brow. (From the University of Connecticut Department of Dermatology Grand Rounds Collection.)

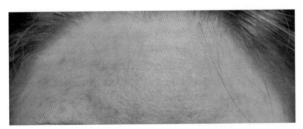

**Fig. 9.4** Rosacea, Chin. (From the University of Connecticut Department of Dermatology Grand Rounds Collection.)

- Facial edema is possible with sparing of the periocular areas.
- The morphology is a background erythema with telangiectasias, pustules, and papules.
  - By definition, rosacea lacks comedones.
- Severe disease may result in phymatous changes (i.e., a thickened, cobblestone appearance commonly on the nose) and enlarged pores in the skin.

- When ocular involvement occurs, patients may present with conjunctivitis and chalazia.
- The etiology of rosacea is complex and not completely understood. Nevertheless, it is multifactorial and likely involves vascular abnormalities, environmental triggers, microorganisms (such as *D. folliculorum* and *H. pylori*), and changes in the dermal matrix.

## Differential Diagnosis

The main differential includes acne and seborrheic dermatitis.
- The presence of comedones in acne helps differentiate it from rosacea.
- Additionally, unlike acne, rosacea is unrelated to hormones.
- Seborrheic dermatitis has scale, a greasy quality, and typically involves other areas like the retroauricular area and scalp that may help differentiate it from rosacea.

## Work-Up

- A review of the ocular symptoms, including dryness, itching, redness, and grittiness, should be performed to assess for ocular rosacea involvement.
- The patient should be asked about triggers and advised to avoid triggers to assess for improvement in symptoms.
- Because rosacea is a clinical diagnosis, routine histologic confirmation is not indicated.
- If the patient presents with flushing, rule out other serious conditions that can cause flushing (such as ordering urinary 5-hyroxyindoleacetic acid levels for possible carcinoid syndrome).
- Facial erythema in a malar distribution with other signs of lupus, such as photosensitivity, may warrant ordering the appropriate serologies.
- Monomorphic papules and pustules may suggest a drug-induced rosacea eruption and warrant a review of the medication history.

## Initial Steps in Management
### General Management Comments

An assessment of the predominant phenotype and severity guides treatment.
- Severe rosacea can be treated with oral and topical therapy with considered referral to an ophthalmologist if ocular involvement is suspected.

- Papulopustular rosacea is more effectively treated by topical therapies than the erythematotelangiectatic type.
- Topical therapies include 0.75% metronidazole, ivermectin 1% cream, 15% azelaic acid gel, and sodium sulfacetamide with 5% sulfur.
- Brimonidine 0.33% gel may improve rosacea erythema but may also cause rebound erythema.
- Alternative topicals include erythromycin or clindamycin lotion, calcineurin inhibitor, or permethrin 5% cream.
- Flushing may be treated with clonidine 0.05 mg BID, beta-blockers, or laser/light therapy.
- Rhinophymatous changes may require surgical or laser procedure for treatment.
- Do not treat rosacea with topical steroids. It will improve the rash initially but ultimately make it worse.

## Recommended Initial Regimen

The recommended initial regimen for rosacea includes 0.75% metronidazole gel BID for oily skin types and cream or lotion BID for normal/dry skin types. For all skin types, avoidance of triggers and the use of sun protection is recommended.

## Partial but Inadequate Response

If there is a partial but inadequate response after a 3-month trial of combination topical therapies, oral antibiotics can be tried for 12 weeks (doxycycline 40mg daily; minocycline 50mg BID).

- Tetracycline antibiotics are contraindicated in pregnancy.
- Known adverse effects of oral antibiotics include GI upset, photosensitivity, and dizziness.
- Alternative systemic therapies include oral metronidazole 200mg BID and azithromycin 250 to 500 mg TID.

## Continued Inadequate Response

If the response continues to be inadequate, severe papulopustular rosacea may be treated with systemic isotretinoin therapy, which requires obtaining a baseline and then regular interval levels of CBC, glucose test, liver function test, fasting lipids, and pregnancy tests for female patients (because isotretinoin is known to be teratogenic).

- Registration of isotretinoin use with the iPLEDGE program is required.

- Females should be on dual-contraception use during treatment course.
- Patients start typically with 0.5 mg/kg daily, which increases to 1 mg/kg daily after 1 month.
- The treatment duration of isotretinoin is 5 to 6 months.
- Known adverse effects include xerosis, cheilitis, elevated liver enzymes, and hypertriglyceridemia.

## Warning Signs/Common Pitfalls

Although rosacea is a benign skin condition, it can lead to significant psychological distress and possibly irreversible erythema and telangiectasias, making treatment intervention important for patients and their quality of life.

## Counseling

Your doctor has diagnosed you with rosacea, which is a common chronic inflammatory condition with a waxing and waning disease course that has no cure. The condition can be adequately controlled, however, with treatment adherence and lifestyle changes.

Your doctor will advise you to avoid hot beverages, spicy foods, alcohol, chocolate, topical steroids on this rash, stress, and extreme temperature changes because these may trigger your rash. Also, the use of broadspectrum sunscreens and sun avoidance to help control the condition are recommended. Gentle skincare products and cosmetic camouflage may also help.

Your doctor will prescribe some topical therapies and possibly some antibiotics. It will take several weeks to months for your condition to improve. Please know that this eruption can recur in the future but can be treated again if that occurs.

# PERIORAL DERMATITIS

**Nikita Lakdawala**

## Clinical History

- Perioral dermatitis is a benign, self-limited, inflammatory dermatosis.
- The condition can cause some pruritus or burning or be asymptomatic.
- Morphology of the lesions are acne like or rosacea-like and characterized by small, erythematous, papulopustular lesions. An eczema-like pattern with scale can also be seen.
- Distribution is most commonly around the mouth, including the upper cutaneous lip and chin. The

immediate vermilion border of the lip is spared. This can also affect periorificial sites, including the eyes and nose, which is termed "periorificial dermatitis."

- The demographic is variable, but the eruption commonly occurs in children. In the adult population, women between ages of 18 to 40 are mostly commonly affected

- The main differential includes acne vulgaris, rosacea, allergic or irritant contact dermatitis, fungal infection, and impetigo.
  - Acne vulgaris and rosacea typically have a broader distribution on the face.
  - In allergic or irritant contact dermatitis, a history of the inciting agent and pruritus are commonly present. Additionally, the rash is usually confined to the area of the contactant.
  - In impetigo, yellow-tinged or golden-crusted erosions and/or vesicles can be visualized.
  - Fungal infection may be difficult to distinguish clinically; KOH preparation can aid in diagnosis.

- The etiology of perioral dermatitis is unclear; the condition is frequently associated with topical or inhaled corticosteroid use.

- Perioral dermatitis can resolve without treatment in several weeks to months or persist for several years.

## Work-Up

- A diagnosis of perioral dermatitis can typically be made using the history and the physical examination.

- History should include timing, onset and duration of lesions, and symptomatology, including pain or pruritus secondary to eruption.

- An inquiry into the topical skincare regimen should be undertaken because it is thought to contribute to development of the condition; other associations include fluorinated toothpaste and topical skincare products.

- Reviewing the medication list is helpful because inhaled corticosteroids can be contributory.

- A physical examination should include an examination of the morphology and distribution of lesions.

- Skin swab culture may be beneficial to distinguish between perioral dermatitis and other infectious conditions.

- In select rare cases where clinical diagnosis cannot be made, histologic confirmation with skin biopsy can be helpful.

- Classification of severity of disease as mild, moderate, or severe can aid in management.

## Initial Steps in Management
### General Management Comments

- A gentle skincare regimen should be established in perioral dermatitis. This may include a gentle cleanser for the face.

- Topical products, particularly cosmetics, should be minimized. Should a patient chose to use cosmetic products, she or he should use products labeled non-comedogenic and/or oil-free. Once a patient's perioral dermatitis is under control, cosmetic products can be reintroduced, one at a time, to assess whether any individual cosmetic flares the perioral dermatitis.

- When possible, topical corticosteroids should be discontinued; inhaled corticosteroids may be necessary for the patient's other medical conditions.

- The therapeutic approach depends on the severity of the disease.

- Primary treatment options include topical antibiotics, topical calcineurin inhibitors, and oral antibiotics.

- Topical therapy is preferred, with oral antibiotics limited to cases refractory to topical agents and moderate to severe cases.

### Recommended Initial Regimen for Mild Perioral Dermatitis

- Treatment options include erythromycin 2% gel; metronidazole 0.75% or 1% (cream, gel); clindamycin 1% (solution, lotion, gel); and pimecrolimus 1% cream.

- Topical antibiotics, including erythromycin, metronidazole, and clindamycin, are typically less expensive and more readily available.

- Topical pimecrolimus has also shown benefit. The U.S. Food and Drug Administration (FDA) has approved a so-called "black box" on the association of the topical medication and malignancy risk; the significance of the risk is thought to be minimal.

- Twice-daily use of topical agents should be trialed for 4 weeks.

- Topical antibiotics and azelaic acid may be continued for another 4 weeks of treatment if partial clearance is noted.

- If no benefit is obtained from a topical regimen, it is preferred to trial an alternate agent before transitioning to oral therapy.

## Recommended Initial Regimen for Moderate to Severe Perioral Dermatitis

- Oral therapy may be necessary in cases with more severe disease presentation, symptomatology, or emotional distress related to the condition.
- Oral antibiotics options include erythromycin, tetracycline, doxycycline, and azithromycin.
- Tetracycline-class antibiotics carry a risk for gastrointestinal distress; additionally, doxycycline is associated with photosensitivity.
- In children 8 years of age and younger, erythromycin is a preferred approach because tetracycline antibiotics are contraindicated. Azithromycin may be also be considered as a second-line agent.
- In adults, a few different options may be trialed.
  - Tetracycline 250 mg or 500 mg can be tried twice daily for 4 weeks.
  - Doxycycline 100 mg can be used twice daily for 4 weeks.
  - Erythromycin base 333 mg three times daily or 500 mg twice daily can be tried for 4 weeks.
- If 4 weeks of therapy is insufficient, an additional 2 to 4 weeks of treatment may be of therapeutic benefit.

## Warning Signs/Common Pitfalls

Perioral dermatitis is a benign, self-limited, inflammatory dermatosis. It can present with significant symptomatology and be a source of emotional distress. Patients often are upset by this eruption and therefore it should not be ignored. History and physical examination are essential because clinical diagnosis can be made in a majority of cases. Counseling is important in management. Avoidance of topical corticosteroids and the limiting of topical skin products is essential to therapy. Consistent topical or oral treatment for at least 4 weeks is often necessary for therapeutic benefit. Expectations regarding the timeline of improvement can be helpful. Also, the eruption may recur and patients should be warned about this possibility. The condition carries a good prognosis and resolves spontaneously in weeks to months. Therapy can be undertaken to aid resolution and alleviate symptoms associated with the condition.

## Counseling

Your doctor has diagnosed you with perioral dermatitis, a benign rash on your face. Avoidance of topical steroids on your face is very important because use of topical steroids (e.g., hydrocortisone) is thought to keep this rash going. Your doctor may prescribe some creams or even oral antibiotics for this rash. It will take several weeks or even a few months for it to resolve. On occasion, the eruption may recur in the future, requiring a repeat course of treatment. The rash is not contagious and will resolve with time.

# FOLLICULITIS/FURUNCLES/CARBUNCLES

**Shivani Sinha, Gloria Lin, and Katalin Ferenczi**

## Clinical Features

Folliculitis refers to inflammation of the hair follicles, which can have infectious and noninfectious etiologies. It is most commonly caused by *Staphylococcus aureus,* which is also the causative agent for furuncles and carbuncles. Folliculitis typically affects the superficial portion of the hair follicle, whereas furuncles and carbuncles can also affect the surrounding skin and subcutaneous tissue. Untreated bacterial folliculitis may progress to furuncles, which, in turn, can transform into a carbuncle when multiple lesions coalesce together. This chapter will review bacterial and nonbacterial folliculitis, furuncles, and carbuncles.

- Folliculitis presents as multiple, erythematous, follicular-based papules or pustules. The associated hair shaft can sometimes be visualized in the center of each pustule/papule. There are several subtypes of folliculitis.
  - Pityrosporum folliculitis is characterized by intensely pruritic, monomorphic, erythematous papules, most commonly localized on the trunk. It is caused by the overgrowth of *Malassezia furfur,* a yeast present in the normal cutaneous flora.
  - Pseudomonas folliculitis, commonly referred to as "hot tub folliculitis," is caused by *Pseudomonas aeruginosa* and it is associated with recent hot tub or swimming pool exposure. Erythematous, follicular-based papules and pustules are typically found on the trunk and buttocks.
  - Gram-negative folliculitis is classically associated with chronic antibiotic therapy for acne and can be caused by *Klebsiella* or *Proteus* species.
- Furuncles, also commonly referred to as "boils," are tender, erythematous nodules, typically preceded by folliculitis. They can be firm or fluctuant with an overlying purulent crust, seen in areas constantly exposed to friction, heat, and maceration, such as the axillae,

buttocks, groin, and neck. Risk factors like obesity and immunosuppression may predispose individuals to furuncle formation. Rupture of a furuncle leads to discharge of caseous necrotic material and typically results in symptomatic improvement.

- Carbuncles are painful, erythematous, edematous multiheaded nodules that can have several purulent drainage sites. They are often localized on the skin of the back, nape of the neck, and thighs. Patients can present with systemic symptoms, such as fever and malaise.

## Differential Diagnosis

The differential diagnoses for folliculitis, furuncles, and carbuncles include acne, acne keloidalis nuchae (AKN), Grover disease (GD), ruptured epidermal inclusion cyst (EIC), and hidradenitis suppurativa (HS).

- Acne is characterized by inflammatory papules, pustules, and comedones on the face, trunk, and upper extremities. Acne most commonly affects adolescents. There can be resulting hyperpigmentation and long-term scarring after resolution of the inflammation. The presence of comedones, the anatomic distribution, and the absence of pruritus can differentiate it from folliculitis. Treatment of acne is often dependent on the patient and the severity but can include various topical agents (including antibiotics and retinoids), as well as systemic antibiotics, oral contraceptives, spironolactone, and isotretinoin.
- AKN typically presents on the posterior scalp and neck and predominantly affects darker-skinned individuals. Similar to folliculitis, AKN is associated with inflammation of the hair follicles; however, it presents as keloidal papules and plaques. There can be associated alopecia and so-called "tufted doll hairs," which manifest as multiple hairs arising from a single follicle. Topical or oral corticosteroids, retinoids, and antibacterial agents may be used, depending on the severity and need to minimize inflammation and improve the cosmetic appearance.
- GD is an acquired condition characterized by erythematous papules in middle-aged Caucasian men. This condition is most commonly localized to the trunk. Unlike in folliculitis, the lesions are not follicle based. Treatment of GD involves the avoidance of aggravating factors, such as heat and sun exposure, and symptomatic management using topical steroids and emollients.
- An EIC presents as a tender, erythematous nodule with a central punctum and malodorous caseous discharge, which can resemble a furuncle or carbuncle. Treatment of a ruptured EIC can include antibiotics, incision and drainage (I&D) for symptomatic relief, or surgical excision with removal of its capsule when the inflammation has resolved.
- HS is a chronic disease characterized by inflammatory nodules; persistent sinus tracts; double-ended comedones; and scarring in the axilla, inframammary, and inguinal areas. It is often misdiagnosed as recurrent furunculosis. Progression of HS can lead to debilitating sequelae and permanent disfigurement. Treatment depends on the severity of the condition and includes topical and oral antibiotics, biologics, and surgery.

## Work-Up

Folliculitis, furuncles, and carbuncles are clinical diagnoses based on a history and physical examination.

- Possible risk factors or exposures, such as recent hot tub use or chronic antibiotic therapy, may provide clues to the correct diagnosis and type of folliculitis.
- To identify the causative microorganism and determine appropriate therapeutic agents, a culture, Gram stain, and KOH preparation can be performed.
- If the diagnosis is uncertain, clinical findings are ambiguous, or there is no response to initial therapy, a skin biopsy may be done for further assessment.

## Initial Steps in Management

Superficial folliculitis often does not require treatment and resolves spontaneously with minimal or no scarring. Folliculitis that fails to improve within a few weeks, however, may require treatment.

### Staphylococcal Folliculitis

- Topical clindamycin with benzoyl peroxide can be used as first-line therapy.
- A 7- to 10-day course of oral antibiotics (cephalexin 500 mg four times daily) are indicated for deep, recurrent, or widespread recalcitrant folliculitis.
- A 7- to 10-day course of oral trimethoprim-sulfamethoxazole (TMP-SMX) two double-strength tablets twice daily, clindamycin 300 to 450 mg four times daily, or doxycycline 100 mg twice daily should be prescribed for patients with suspected or confirmed methicillin-resistant *S. aureus* (MRSA) infection.
- *Pseudomonas* folliculitis, also known as "hot tub folliculitis," is self-limited and will often spontaneously

resolve within 2 weeks. Severe cases may need treatment with a course of oral antibiotics, such as ciprofloxacin (500 or 750 mg twice daily).
- Treatment of gram-negative folliculitis is isotretinoin, a medication associated with multiple adverse effects including teratogenicity.

## Nonbacterial Folliculitis

- Pityrosporum folliculitis will improve with the use of topical azoles, such as ketoconazole 2% cream, because the causative agent is *M. furfur*. Recurrent fungal folliculitis can be treated with oral fluconazole (100–200 mg daily for up to 4 weeks or 300 mg weekly for 1–2 months) or itraconazole (100 mg daily).
- Viral folliculitis should be treated with a 5- to 10-day course of acyclovir 200 mg five times daily; valacyclovir 500 mg three times daily; or famciclovir 500 mg three times daily.

## Furuncles/Carbuncles

- Furuncles will often rupture and spontaneously resolve within 2 weeks of onset, whereas carbuncles are more likely to require intervention.
- A warm compress may be applied to the affected area for up to 10 minutes several times per day to encourage drainage of the lesion.
- I&D may be indicated to relieve pressure and hasten resolution. This is typically the first-line treatment for carbuncles. For carbuncles with multiple loculations, a hemostat can be used to break them up. Iodoform gauze may be packed into the incision site to facilitate drainage.
- Antibiotics may be indicated in severe cases with systemic symptoms. Patients should be closely followed up, with a low threshold for escalation of care if there is no improvement, especially if the patient is immunocompromised.
  - Oral cephalexin or dicloxacillin for 10- to 14-day courses can be used. If MRSA is suspected or isolated, consider doxycycline, TMP-SMX, or clindamycin.
  - Rarely, in severe cases, patients may need to be hospitalized and require intravenous antibiotics, such as vancomycin, linezolid, and clindamycin.

## Warning Signs/Common Pitfalls

- Untreated and unresolved furuncles or carbuncles may sometimes lead to bacteremia and sepsis.

Patients should be closely monitored for resolution or worsening of symptoms.
- Recurrent furunculosis may require evaluation for HS to prevent progression of misdiagnosed HS.
- In patients who have been on long-term antibiotics for chronic acne or folliculitis and fail treatment, a diagnosis of gram-negative folliculitis should be considered.

## Counseling

Your skin condition is called "folliculitis," "furuncle" (boil), or "carbuncle" (multiheaded boil), and it is caused by inflammation of the hair follicles. Folliculitis can sometimes spread to involve the surrounding skin, forming a furuncle. Multiple furuncles can coalesce to form a carbuncle. These lesions may be itchy or painful, but they are benign and treatable. Avoid scratching or picking at the involved areas and do not squeeze any boils because these behaviors may lead to spread and worsening of the infection.

Folliculitis is often self-limited and can resolve on its own within 2 weeks. Applying a warm compress to furuncles and carbuncles for up to 10 minutes several times per day can facilitate healing. When the boils rupture, you may notice a foul-smelling, cheese like drainage from the area. If the lesion persists for more than 2 weeks or continues to enlarge, your healthcare provider may need to make an incision to promote drainage.

Inform your physician if you notice a sudden increase in redness or tenderness and pain or if you develop fevers, chills, or malaise because these may be a sign of an underlying infection and you may need antibiotics.

# PITYROSPORUM FOLLICULITIS

## Clinical Features

Pityrosporum folliculitis is a common acneiform (acne-like) eruption caused by *Malassezia sp.*, the same yeast implicated in seborrheic dermatitis.
- It is clinically characterized by the development of 1- to 2-mm, monomorphic, acneiform papules and pustules in the absence of comedones, cysts, or nodules on the upper chest, shoulders, and/or forehead (Fig. 9.5).
  - Pityrosporum folliculitis is characteristically pruritic.
- Pityrosporum folliculitis most commonly occurs in adolescents and young adults (ages 10–30 years).

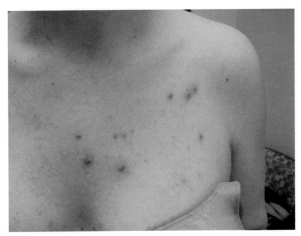

**Fig. 9.5 Pityrosporum Folliculitis.** Note the monomorphic nature of the papulopustules and the absence of comedones. (From the University of Connecticut Department of Dermatology Grand Rounds Collection.)

- Another population that disproportionately develops pityrosporum folliculitis is immunocompromised individuals, particularly organ transplant recipients.
- Almost all patients with pityrosporum folliculitis have a history of acne vulgaris and many of these patients have concomitant acne at the time of their diagnosis with pityrosporum folliculitis.
  - Both oral and topical antibiotic use are major risk factors for developing pityrosporum folliculitis
  - Some patients have concomitant seborrheic dermatitis, which would be expected because seborrheic dermatitis is also caused by *Malassezia sp.*

## Differential Diagnosis

The differential for pityrosporum folliculitis includes acne vulgaris, steroid acne, other drug-induced acneiform eruptions, and keratosis pilaris (KP).

- Acne vulgaris is the main differential for pityrosporum folliculitis. Differentiating between acne and pityrosporum folliculitis can be especially difficult because these two conditions almost always exist in some degree of overlap. Pityrosporum folliculitis can be distinguished from acne vulgaris by the monomorphic morphology of its papules and pustules, the lack of comedones in the affected areas, the lesional pruritis, and the failure to respond to antibiotics and other acne treatments. Unlike acne, pityrosporum folliculitis is also exquisitely responsive to azole antifungals.

- Clinically, steroid acne is almost indistinguishable from pityrosporum folliculitis because it also presents with monomorphic acneiform papules and pustules in the absence of comedones. Nevertheless, patients with steroid acne have a history of systemic or topical corticosteroid use, which suggests the diagnosis.
- Acneiform drug eruptions, like pityrosporum folliculitis, present with monomorphic acneiform papules and pustules without comedones. There are many agents that can cause this type of drug eruption, including, but not limited to, halogenated aromatic hydrocarbons, antibiotics like macrolides and penicillin, nystatin, isoniazid, naproxen, and hydroxychloroquine. A history of use of one of these medications is suggestive of a diagnosis of an acneiform drug eruption.
- KP is characterized by the presence of follicular-based keratotic papules most often on the upper arms. It can also occur on the cheeks and occasionally on the chest. KP can be distinguished from pityrosporum folliculitis because it lacks pustules, the lesions cannot be popped, it has a rough texture, and it is asymptomatic.

## Work-Up

Providers experienced with KOH preparations can confirm a diagnosis of pityrosporum folliculitis by examining pustular fluid under the microscope and identifying *Malassezia sp.*, which looks like spaghetti and meatballs.

Because many providers do not have the materials for KOH preparation readily available or are inexperienced in performing KOH preps, diagnosis can be made clinically and confirmed with a trial of treatment with topical azoles, which are effective in almost all cases.

There are no systemic associations with pityrosporum folliculitis and therefore no additional work-up is recommended.

## Initial Steps in Management

Pityrosporum folliculitis is impressively treatment responsive to azole antifungals. Topical azoles should be employed first, followed by oral azoles in refractory cases.

Start ketoconazole 2% shampoo applied topically every other day to affected areas and left in place for 3 to 5 minutes before rinsing.

- Patients should be counseled that the shampoo can be used as a body wash.

- Patients who initially clear with ketoconazole shampoo but who have recurrences can use the shampoo once weekly for maintenance of clearance.

Patients who inadequately respond to topicals can use oral fluconazole 200 mg daily for 7 days.

- Some patients require longer courses (up to 3 weeks).
- Fluconazole has many notable drug-drug interactions that may prohibit its use.
- Patients should not be started on oral ketoconazole in lieu of fluconazole because of the risk for hepatotoxicity with oral ketoconazole.

## Warning Signs/Common Pitfalls

The biggest pitfall when managing pityrosporum folliculitis is failure to manage patients' coexisting acne. Many patients have an overlap of the two conditions and become frustrated if they have remaining pimples despite treatment.

Patients with recurrent pityrosporum folliculitis often require maintenance therapy with weekly use of ketoconazole shampoo. Recurrence is not a sign of treatment failure and does not mean the patient is resistant to topical azole antifungals. It is also not an indication for oral antifungals. Using recurrent oral therapy in lieu of maintenance topicals is inappropriate.

Unlike gram-negative folliculitis, development of pityrosporum folliculitis does not require the affected individual to discontinue oral and/or topical antibiotic treatment for their associated routine acne vulgaris.

## Counseling

You have pityrosporum folliculitis. This is a condition that is similar to acne, except that it is caused by a yeast called *Malassezia*. This yeast lives on almost everyone's skin and is not infectious, which means you cannot spread this condition to other people. This yeast is also not dangerous and will not cause you internal harm.

Most people with pityrosporum folliculitis have regular acne as well and will need treatment for both conditions. For your pityrosporum folliculitis, your healthcare provider has prescribed you ketoconazole 2% shampoo, which you should use as a body wash in the shower every other day. Importantly, this product must be left on your skin for 3 to 5 minutes before rinsing for it to be effective. Most people have improvement or clearance of their pityrosporum folliculitis within 4 weeks of using this shampoo. If you stop using this shampoo, the pityrosporum folliculitis may come back.

It is safe to use this shampoo weekly to prevent recurrence of the rash.

# PSEUDOFOLLICULITIS BARBAE

## Clinical Features

Pseudofolliculitis barbae (PFB; so-called "razor bumps") is an acne like condition that occurs predominantly in the beard area of postpubertal men and on the chin of perimenopausal women.

- PFB is caused by a foreign-body reaction to curly hair shafts that repenetrate into the skin.
- It is characterized by the development of acne like papules and pustules occurring in areas with coarse hair that are shaved.
  - These acneiform inflammatory lesions frequently leave behind postinflammatory hyperpigmentation (dyschromia of the skin) that is cosmetically bothersome (Fig. 9.6).
  - In many cases, these lesions resolve with permanent scarring, including keloid scarring.
- It occurs most often in Blacks, then in Asians, and least frequently in white people.
- It is frequently painful and cosmetically bothersome.

## Differential Diagnosis

The differential for PFB includes acne vulgaris, tinea barbae, allergic contact dermatitis (ACD), irritant contact dermatitis (ICD), and seborrheic dermatitis.

- Acne vulgaris is in the differential for PFB because the primary lesions of both conditions look similar and the conditions can frequently coexist in the same individual. PFB can be distinguished from acne

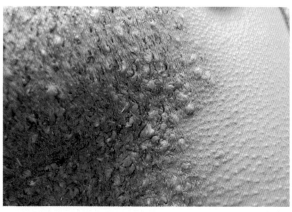

**Fig. 9.6** Pseudofolliculitis Barbae. (Courtesy Justin Finch, MD.)

vulgaris because it occurs predominantly in areas that are shaved and because hairs can be identified reentering the skin at the sites of inflammatory lesions in PFB.

- Tinea barbae is an infectious skin condition caused by dermatophytes that have infected hair shafts of beard hairs. Unlike PFB, tinea barbae presents with boggy, inflamed plaques and occurs focally within a beard rather than diffusely, like PFB does. Additionally, because of its genetic underpinnings, PFB is a typically chronic problem that affects afflicted individuals for the entirety of the time that they shave.
- ACD either from topically applied cosmetics or from an airborne contactant can cause ACD of the beard area. This typically does not present with the acneiform papules and pustules that PFB does; instead, it presents as an eczematous dermatitis.
- ICD frequently plagues individuals with PFB because individuals with PFB frequently use depilatories to try to eliminate beard hairs. Although effective, these depilatories frequently cause ICD, which can confound the clinical picture of PFB by creating a background of irritated, erythematous plaques.
- Seborrheic dermatitis of the beard area is common; however, it is characterized by pink plaques with greasy scale rather than acneiform lesions.

## Work-Up

Work-up for PFB involves obtaining a detailed history of an individual's shaving habits and ascertaining whether the patient is amenable to growing out a beard.

- History includes shaving frequency, type of razor, direction in which the patient shaves (with or against the grain), depilatory use, and before-shave and aftershave product use.

  In women, PFB is typically a sign of hyperandrogenism and should trigger a work-up for polycystic ovary syndrome (luteinizing hormone [LH], follicle-stimulating hormone [FSH], dehydroepiandrosterone sulfate [DHEAS], and free testosterone).

## Initial Steps in Management

In men, management of PFB is divided into men who are willing to grow a beard versus those who are not.

- If a man is amenable to growing a beard, he should be instructed to not shave for at least 4 weeks and to use an electric trimmer to trim his beard no closer than 1 mm to the skin.

- If a patient is interested in trying to grow a beard to treat their PFB but their job requires them to be clean shaven, a doctor's note can be helpful.
- Patients should be instructed that their disease will flare for 1 to 2 weeks while their beard is growing out.
  - This flare can be managed with topical corticosteroids, such as hydrocortisone 2.5% cream twice daily to the affected area for up to 2 weeks.
- This leads to disease resolution/control in almost all cases.
- For men who prefer to be clean shaven and who have beards that are not gray or white, the first-line therapy for PFB is laser hair removal with or without the use of topical eflornithine.
  - Insurance, as a rule, will not cover laser hair removal for PFB; however, in the long run, treatment with a laser is more effective and ends up being more cost effective for the patient.
  - If the patient is skin type V or VI, it is imperative to refer them to an experienced laser surgeon who is comfortable performing laser hair removal in individuals with this skin type.
- In cases where laser hair removal is not available, not financially feasible, or the patient does not want it, shaving modifications and prescription topical therapy is recommended.
  - Shaving modifications can include using more shaving cream or shaving gel if a patient uses a traditional razor.
    - Before shaving, the hair should be washed with warm water and brushed.
    - Some patients like a product called Magic Shave, which is a shaving cream or powder that contains a chemical depilatory.
    - Patients could also try different types of razors.
      - Use an electric razor with a guard to shave hair to a minimum length of 1 mm to keep hair beyond the length at which it readily repenetrates the skin.
      - Use a traditional razor twice daily, with the grain, to keep hair so short that it cannot repenetrate the skin.

### Recommended Prescription Therapy

In terms of prescription therapy, patients with PFB can use a topical antiinflammatory and topical retinoid.

They can also try hyperpigmentation therapy and using early laser hair removal for scar management.

- Topical hydrocortisone 2.5% cream or pimecrolimus 0.1% cream should be applied as an aftershave daily.
  - This helps with irritation and symptomatic control but does not prevent hairs from reentering the skin.
- Topical tretinoin 0.025% cream should be applied nightly to promote loosening of ingrown hairs and to prevent postinflammatory hyperpigmentation. Topical retinoids can be drying and irritating.
- Prescription hydroquinone-containing products (hydroquinone 4% daily) may help normalize pigmentation; however, their use should be limited to no longer than 6 months because prolonged use can cause permanent dyspigmentation; exogenous ochronosis is characterized by blue-black pigmentation in the skin secondary to long-term application of skin-lightening creams containing hydroquinone.
- The best way to manage scars in PFB is to prevent them by recommending early laser hair removal.
- Intralesional injection of corticosteroids or punch excision of scars can also be considered.
- We recommend avoiding antibiotics for the treatment of PFB because it is not an infectious condition and use of antibiotics may unintentionally propagate the false belief that it is infectious to patients.
- In women, hormonal therapies, such as oral contraceptives or spironolactone, can be considered to help control the hyperandrogenism that promotes the development of the condition's causative coarse hairs.

## Warning Signs/Common Pitfalls

The biggest pitfall when managing PFB is not offering a referral for laser hair removal at the first encounter to all patients who do not want to grow a beard. PFB can cause irreversible and cosmetically bothersome damage to the skin; therefore aggressive early management is indicated.

Historically, patients were counseled to shave less frequently (e.g., once weekly); however, this is now known to worsen the condition and should not be recommended.

Many providers place an emphasis on the number of blades that a razor has. This is likely less important than encouraging twice-daily shaving with the grain in those who choose to shave and promoting use of adequate amounts of shaving cream, gel, or foam.

This condition is drastically underdiagnosed in women. Strong suspicion for this diagnosis should be maintained in any perimenopausal female with hyperpigmentation on the chin.

## Counseling

You have pseudofolliculitis barbae. This is a genetic condition that is caused by your curly hairs curling back into the skin, which causes inflammation in these areas. Importantly, this condition is not an infection and is not because you are dirty. It is caused by the way your hair is made by your body. Because this condition is genetic, it is unlikely to ever go away without treatment.

The goal of treatment is to keep your hairs from reentering the skin. There are three approaches: 1) Grow a beard so that the hairs are so long that they do not reenter the skin. For this to be successful, your beard must be at least 1 mm (about half an inch) in length. If you do choose to grow out a beard, your skin will likely worsen for several weeks before it gets better because some of the hairs that you grow out will inevitably curl back into the skin. 2) Remove the hairs with a laser so that there are no hairs to reenter the skin. This is very effective, but it is not covered by insurance. 3) Keep the hairs so short with a razor that they are not given the chance to reenter the skin. To do this, you must shave twice daily with the grain. Before shaving, you should prepare the skin with warm water and use ample amounts of shaving cream. If you choose to do this, your doctor can prescribe you a topical antiinflammatory cream to use as an aftershave.

# HIDRADENITIS SUPPURATIVA

**Erisa Alia and Jun Lu**

## Clinical Features

HS, sometime referred to as "acne inversa," is a chronic, relapsing, inflammatory, debilitating skin disease, primarily affecting the apocrine gland-bearing areas. It is categorized as part of the follicular occlusion tetrad, which also includes acne conglobata, dissecting cellulitis, and pilonidal sinuses; these diseases most often present singly but can also present as a syndrome. HS is characterized by recurrent, deep-seated, painful nodules or abscesses; sinus tracts; fistulas; and prominent scarring (Fig. 9.7). Lesions involve intertriginous zones, favoring the axillae and inguinal folds (groins), but can also present in the inframammary folds, intermammary area, and perineal/perianal area. The scalp, face, neck, areolae, back, and thighs are considered atypical sites.

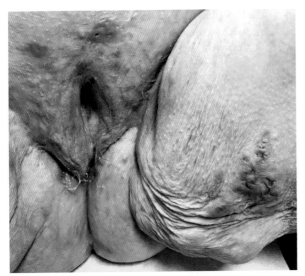

**Fig. 9.7 Hidradenitis Suppurativa, Hurley Stage IV.** (From the University of Connecticut Department of Dermatology Grand Rounds Collection.)

HS typically appears after puberty with a prevalence of 1% to 4%. People of African descent and women have a higher incidence of developing the disease; males have higher chances of developing severe disease. Smoking and obesity are widely accepted as major triggering factors of HS.

There is often a significant delay (7.2 years) between symptom onset and the confirmation of the diagnosis. Manifestations include a multitude of follicular lesions. Typical lesions for HS follow a specific path.

- Inflammatory, painful nodules and sterile abscesses (blind boils, furuncles, carbuncles) first develop in the axillae and groin, which are often the initial sites involved.
- Then, they spread to adjacent follicles and the coalescing of the nodules/abscesses forms sinus tracts.
- Sinus tracts eventually result in fistula formation, which drains purulent exudate, healing with fibrosis and scarring.
- Draining, scarring, the recurring nature of the abscess, and the lack of response to antibiotics are typical features of the sterile, noninfectious HS abscess.
- Double-ended pseudocomedones (DEP), which represent superficial sinus tracts, are also considered a typical clinical sign of this disorder.

The typical course of the disease involves acute exacerbations alternating with periods of quiescence. Classically, the lesions are accompanied by discomfort, pain, and pruritus. Because of its clinical course, features, and location, HS can be physically and emotionally debilitating, significantly impairing patients' quality of life.

## Classification

The most common classification system used to assess disease severity is the Hurley staging system. This 3-stage classification helps tailor the appropriate therapeutic approach for HS patients.

- Stage I involves single or multiple abscesses without sinus tract or scar formation.
- Stage II includes single or multiple widely separated recurrent abscesses with sinus tract and scar formation.
- Stage III has diffuse or near-diffuse involvement, or multiple interconnected sinus tracts and abscesses across an entirely affected area; more extensive scarring is present.

## Work-Up

HS remains a clinically defined disease, diagnosed based on the modified criteria of Dessau. In particular, three criteria must be met for the definitive diagnosis of HS.

1. The presence of typical lesions, as previously described.
2. Location in one or more of the predilection areas: the axillae, inguinal folds, inframammary and intermammary folds, or perineal/perianal area. If atypical sites are involved, one or more of the predilection areas must be involved as well to make the diagnosis.
3. Recurrence and chronicity are hallmarks of the HS clinical course. The occurrence of two or more episodes in a 6-month period is required for the diagnosis. It is crucial to follow patients who are in the midst of their first episode of typical lesions in predilected areas within 6 months to avoid delays in the diagnosis.
   - Complementary work-up, such as skin biopsy, is of limited use and indicated only in cases of diagnostic ambiguity. Bacterial culture of the lesions is necessary when there are signs of a superimposed infection.
   - A physical examination and a detailed review of the system is helpful to screen for obesity, metabolic syndrome, diabetes mellitus (DM), anxiety, depression, inflammatory bowel disease, PCOS, and smoking.

- Laboratory screening for DM in HS patients is recommended because the risk for DM is increased by 1.5-fold to threefold in this category.
- Because it is a chronic inflammatory pathology, HS increases the risk for developing anemia of chronic disease, which warrants a yearly evaluation with a CBC. It is recommended that a CBC be performed with differential to also assess a possible left shift in case of an acute flare and/or a superimposed infection.
- Serum inflammatory markers, C-reactive protein, and erythrocyte sedimentation rate are not required for diagnosis but are effective in assessing the disease severity and monitoring treatment success.
- Imaging studies, clinical photography, and high-frequency ultrasound can help characterize the surface lesion development and progression, as well as the extent of deeper dermal and subcutaneous changes.

## Initial Steps in Management

All HS patients should be informed about the importance of smoking cessation; weight reduction; the regular use of antibacterial soaps (i.e., benzoyl peroxide, chlorhexidine); the reduction of friction at the intertriginous areas; the use of absorbent powders and topical aluminum chloride in the axillae and groin areas; and the wearing of loose cotton clothing.

The initial management of axillae and groin HS is based on the severity of the disease as staged by the Hurley system.

### Hurley Stage I

In Hurley stage I, topical antibiotics, such as clindamycin 1% or erythromycin 2% with or without benzoyl peroxide, are applied to all affected area on a daily basis.
- Oral antibiotics can be taken as needed for a flare-up, such as doxycycline or minocycline 100 mg by mouth twice daily for 6 to 12 weeks. Clindamycin with or without rifampin are considered to be second-line treatment.
- Intralesional triamcinolone acetonide can be injected into inflammatory, painful lesions.

### Hurley Stages II and III

Topical and oral antibiotics should be used. Biologic therapies have also shown promising results, including the use of an adalimumab (Humira) 40 mg subcutaneous injection weekly; an infliximab (Remicade) 5 to 10 mg/kg intravenous infusion every 4 to 8 weeks; or other biologic therapies, such as secukinumab, ustekinumab, and anakinra (which have been shown to have various results).
- Oral retinoids, such as acitretin and isotretinoin, have also proven useful in some cases.
- Limited use of surgical excision may be indicated.
- $CO_2$ laser ablation can be used to achieve marsupialization.
- Systemic immunosuppressants, such as cyclosporine and methotrexate, are considered third-line options.

### Other Treatment Approaches

- The *Staphylococcal aureus* carriage can be eradicated using topical or oral antibiotics.
- Hormonal therapies in female subjects with PCOS have improved response rates.
- Antiandrogens therapy, such as finasteride and spironolactone, have shown to reduce HS severity.
- Metformin helps with weight reduction and has an antiandrogenic effect.
- Topical and oral analgesics (Tylenol, nonsteroidal antiinflammatory drugs, tramadol, and opioids) are recommended for appropriate pain control.

In general, HS management remains challenging and regular follow-up visits are encouraged. Referral to a dermatologist is recommended.

### Warning Signs/Common Pitfalls

- Patients with HS should be screened regularly for common associated comorbidities, such as metabolic syndrome, DM, anxiety, depression, inflammatory bowel disease (particularly Crohn disease), and PCOS.
- It is important to address smoking behavior.
- A new patient with typical lesions in typical areas should be re-evaluated within 6 months to avoid any diagnosis delays.
- Simple folliculitis must be differentiated from HS initial boil lesions because it typically resolves after topical antibiotics.
- Simple bacterial abscesses differ from HS abscesses in that they have a higher response rate to oral antibiotics and do not tend to result in sinus tract formation.
- Monitor and treat patients for superimposed infection.

## Counseling

Hidradenitis suppurativa (HS) is a chronic inflammatory disease that waxes and wanes over the years. Early diagnosis and management will improve your symptoms and quality of life.

There are several steps you can take (if applicable). First, stop smoking. Control your weight. Regularly use antibacterial soaps, such as benzoyl peroxide, chlorhexidine, and Dial soap. Avoid friction of the skin fold areas. Use absorbent powders and topical aluminum chloride in the axillae and groin areas. Lastly, wear loose-fitting cotton clothing.

Based on the severity of your HS, your healthcare provider may prescribe you topical and/or oral antibiotics, as well as other systemic medication to regulate your immune system. Medical therapy does not cure HS but may help control its severity.

You should work closely with your doctor to monitor and treat other comorbidities associated with HS, such as hypertension, diabetes, and heart disease. HS can cause scarring and pain. It can be very difficult to treat and may progress despite regular treatment. In some cases, you may consider surgery as a treatment option.

# ACNE KELOIDALIS NUCHAE

## Clinical Features

AKN is a scarring form of hair loss that presents with chronic folliculitis of the occipital scalp and nape of the neck. If left untreated, it causes keloid like scarring.

- It is diagnosed based on the clinical findings of folliculitis isolated to the nape of the neck and the occipital scalp with or without keloid like scarring (Fig. 9.8).
- AKN initially presents in the late teenage years and may continue until patients are in their 50s.

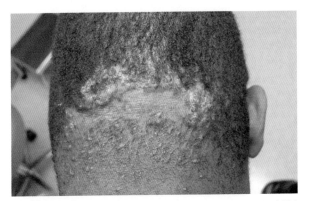

**Fig. 9.8** Acne Keloidalis Nuchae. (Courtesy Justin Finch, MD.)

- It most frequently occurs in Blacks, followed by Hispanics and then Asians, and is much more common in men than in women.
- It is frequently precipitated by irritation of the occipital scalp.
  - Common triggers include short haircuts, wearing a helmet, and wearing tight-collared shirts.
- It is not an infectious condition and there is no cure for it.

## Differential Diagnosis

The differential for AKN includes acne vulgaris, infectious folliculitis, and folliculitis decalvans.

- AKN can be distinguished from acne vulgaris because AKN exclusively affects the occipital scalp and the nape of the neck. It is also devoid of comedones and causes characteristic keloid like scarring that would not be seen in routine acne patients.
- AKN can be distinguished from folliculitis of the scalp because folliculitis more diffusely affects the scalp, is classically pruritic, and does not progress to keloid like scarring.
- AKN can be differentiated from folliculitis decalvans, another form of scarring alopecia, because AKN only affects the occipital scalp, whereas folliculitis decalvans scars the vertex as well. The scarring of folliculitis decalvans also is typically not keloidal.

## Work-Up

AKN does not require any systemic work-up or infectious work-up because it is not infectious.

A focused history to identify modifiable exacerbating factors should be performed to help identify interventions that may help prevent disease progression.

## Initial Steps in Management

Aggressive management of AKN should be undertaken at the time of diagnosis because this disease is frequently cosmetically bothersome to those who have it and difficult to treat once keloid like scars have formed.

Management of AKN is divided into prevention, medical strategies, and surgical approaches.

### Prevention

Modifiable exacerbating factors (e.g., avoidance of short haircuts or tight-collared shirts) should be discussed because lifestyle modifications can dramatically improve this condition.

## Medical Strategies

- Patients should be started on a combination of a high-potency topical corticosteroid (e.g., clobetasol propionate 0.05% solution) daily and a topical retinoid (e.g., tretinoin 0.025% gel) nightly. This combination is often helpful for inflammatory lesions of AKN; however, it does not improve scarring.
- Patients that are refractory to topical therapies can consider initiation of submicrobial dosing of tetracycline antibiotics for their antiinflammatory properties (e.g., doxycycline extended release 40 or 50 mg daily).
- Some patients benefit from benzoyl peroxide 5% wash; however, it may bleach the hair.
  - Combination products containing antibiotics typically do not provide added benefit because this condition is not infectious.

## Surgical Approaches

Surgical approaches may involve lasers, excision, and intralesional injections.

### Lasers

- Laser hair removal with long-pulse ND:YAG lasers and other modalities is effective for many patients with minimal morbidity and should be considered early in the disease course because of its potential disease-modifying abilities; however, there is a degree of cosmetic trade-off because this hair removal is permanent.
- An ablative $CO_2$ laser may be the most effective modality for inducing long-term remission of AKN; however, it is associated with significant postprocedural downtime.

*Excision.* Surgical excision of affected areas with subsequent cauterization and healing by secondary intention may be as effective as laser ablation and is widely available.

*Intralesional injections.* Keloid like lesions frequently benefit from intralesional injections of corticosteroids (e.g., triamcinolone 40 mg/cc); however, corticosteroids can lead to hypopigmentation and do not modify the course of the disease.

## Warning Signs/Common Pitfalls

The biggest pitfall when managing AKN is delaying management because this condition causes irreversible, progressive keloidal scarring.

- When prescribing topical therapies, it is important to consider the cosmesis of prescribed topicals because this condition affects hair-bearing areas, which frequently are poorly tolerant of creams and ointments.
- Do not perform repeated microbial testing to search for infection because this condition is non-infectious.

## Counseling

You have acne keloidalis nuchae (AKN). This is a very common condition. Although the exact cause of AKN is unknown, it is thought to be related to inflammation around your hair follicles. This inflammation is made worse by irritation of your scalp and neck, including by short haircuts, tight-collared shirts, and helmets (or other tight sporting gear). Importantly, AKN is not an infection and cannot be spread to others.

There is no cure for this condition, which means we cannot make it go away; however, the condition can often be improved. It is important that you treat your condition because the condition can cause irreversible scarring if not treated.

Your healthcare provider has prescribed you two medications to put on your skin. One is a topical steroid, which you can use in the morning. This helps decrease the inflammation in your hair follicles. The other is a topical retinoid, which helps prevent hair irritation. It may take weeks for these products to be helpful and your disease may worsen before it gets better.

# DISSECTING CELLULITIS OF THE SCALP

## Clinical Features

Dissecting cellulitis (also known as "perifolliculitis capitis abscedens et suffodiens") of the scalp is an autoinflammatory condition characterized by the development of many fluctuant, sterile abscesses and nodules, which ultimately ends in sinus tract formation on the scalp (Fig. 9.9).

- Patients frequently complain of having drainage from multiple areas on the scalp that is not cured by antibiotics despite having received multiple courses.
  - Drainage is typically expressed on examination during palpation of fluctuant nodules.
  - Pain and itching are other common symptoms.
- It occurs in men more often than in women and it occurs most frequently in Blacks.
- It frequently co-presents with acne conglobata, pilonidal cyst, and HS. These four conditions comprise the so-called "follicular occlusion tetrad."

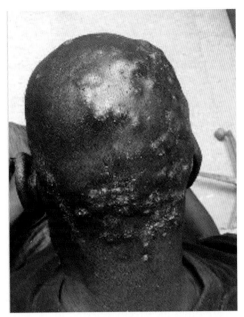

**Fig. 9.9** Dissecting Cellulitis Status Post Treatment with Radiotherapy. (Courtesy Reid Waldman, MD.)

- Over time, dissecting cellulitis can cause scarring hair loss.

## Differential Diagnosis

The differential for dissecting cellulitis of the scalp includes tinea capitis, folliculitis decalvans, pilar cysts, and AKN.

- Dissecting cellulitis can be differentiated from inflammatory tinea capitis (e.g., kerion) because dissecting cellulitis presents with multifocal involvement, it predominantly presents with nodules and abscesses rather than an actual rash on the skin, and it is a chronic process that patients have had for years.
- Dissecting cellulitis can be distinguished from folliculitis decalvans because it less frequently causes scarring hair loss, it presents with large abscesses and nodules rather than pustules and folliculitis-like lesions, and it often presents with hidradenitis elsewhere. Folliculitis decalvans presents with follicular pustules that evolve into patches of alopecia with pustules at the periphery of the patch, most commonly on the scalp.
- Dissecting cellulitis differs from pilar cysts because dissecting cellulitis presents with fluctuant abscesses and nodules rather than freely mobile, circumscribed

nodules. Both conditions are typically multifocal.
- Dissecting cellulitis is distinguished from AKN because it presents with large abscesses and nodules rather than pustules and folliculitis-like lesions, it is not typically associated with keloid like scarring, and it is not isolated to the neck and occipital scalp.

## Work-Up

Patients initially presenting with scalp abscesses suspected for a diagnosis of dissecting cellulitis should undergo a full-body skin examination. This examination should specifically look for signs of the other follicular tetrad conditions because this helps with diagnosis and management.

Unless suspicion for an acute infection is high, infectious work-up (e.g., cultures) is not recommended because it propagates the misconception among patients that their condition is infectious.

## Initial Steps in Management

Management of dissecting cellulitis is divided into acute management of individual painful lesions and chronic disease management.

### Acute Management

- Individual lesions can be treated with intralesional corticosteroids (e.g., triamcinolone 10 mg/kg).
- Surgical deroofing of abscesses with a #15 blade under local anesthesia can also provide symptomatic relief.

### Chronic Management

Chronic management is handled differently based on the disease severity and the presence of comorbid diseases.

- Patients with mild to moderate dissecting cellulitis can be initially started on oral antibiotics with or without the use of topical corticosteroids.
  - Suitable antibiotics that are antiinflammatory include doxycycline 100 mg by mouth BID, minocycline 100 mg BID, azithromycin 50 mg daily, clindamycin 300 mg BID, rifampin 350 mg BID, ciprofloxacin 250 mg BID, or Bactrim DS BID.
  - Antibiotics must be continued indefinitely to be effective. Disease almost always relapses after discontinuation.
  - Suitable high-potency topical corticosteroids include clobetasol propionate 0.05% solution or foam and betamethasone dipropionate 0.05% lotion.

- Patients with severe dissecting cellulitis and/or mild to moderate dissecting cellulitis and another follicular tetrad condition should be referred urgently to a dermatologist who is experienced in managing the condition.
  - Treatments used for patients with moderate to severe disease include isotretinoin and adalimumab.
- Patients with severe disease who have significant medical comorbidities or who cannot tolerate long-term medical management can consider laser ablation, laser hair removal, surgical excision, and radiotherapy to affected areas. These treatments can have curative potential but confer significant procedure-related morbidity and permanent alopecia.

## Warning Signs/Common Pitfalls

Dissecting cellulitis is a chronic, incurable condition. Chronic, uninterrupted therapy is required to maintain disease control. Short courses of antibiotics (e.g., doxycycline 100 mg BID for 14 days) are therefore unacceptable.

- Repeated testing for infection is not indicated and propagates the misconception that this condition is infectious.
- Failure to identify coexisting conditions in the follicular occlusion tetrad may cause patients to be undertreated.
- Patients with severe disease should receive early referrals for specialty care.

## Counseling

You have dissecting cellulitis of the scalp. This condition is a type of autoinflammatory condition, which means that it occurs because your immune system is attacking parts of your own skin. It is not known why your immune system is doing this; however, it is not caused by an infection or allergy. Furthermore, dissecting cellulitis is a chronic condition, which means there is no cure and you will need to be on medication for years to keep the condition under control.

Many people with dissecting cellulitis also develop severe acne, as well as boils in the armpits and the groin. If you develop these issues, it is important that you tell your healthcare provider because it may affect the way that your disease is treated.

Your healthcare provider has prescribed you an antibiotic and a topical steroid. You are receiving an antibiotic because it decreases skin inflammation, not because you have an infection. Antibiotics help the majority of individuals with your condition; however, if you stop them, it is likely that your rash will worsen. The topical steroid also helps decrease inflammation in the skin. It should be applied to the skin daily; however, it should be stopped if it is thinning your skin.

# EPIDERMOID CYST

Shivani Sinha, Gloria Lin, and Katalin Ferenczi

## Clinical Features

Epidermoid or epidermal inclusion cysts (EICs) are the most common skin cysts. They are most often found on the back, face, and neck but can occur anywhere on the body. EICs found in unusual locations, such as on the palms, soles, or buttocks, may be related to trauma. In most cases, these lesions occur sporadically; however, multiple lesions may be associated with Gardner syndrome, Gorlin syndrome, and pachyonychia congenita.

- EICs are often incorrectly referred to as "sebaceous cysts," which is a misnomer because they actually arise from the follicular infundibulum.
- They present as firm, flesh-colored nodules ranging in size from a few millimeters to several centimeters and often have a central punctum. They are asymptomatic and remain stable over time or demonstrate slowly progressive growth.
- Sudden onset of inflammatory symptoms, including erythema, pain, swelling, and foul-smelling caseous drainage, indicates rupture of the cyst and possible secondary infection. This rupture may lead to foreign-body granulomas, further enhancing the inflammatory response.

## Differential Diagnosis

The differential diagnosis includes pilar cysts, lipomas, abscesses, steatocystomas, and cutaneous metastases. Biopsy and histopathology may be required to distinguish these lesions from one another.

- Pilar or trichilemmal cysts are derived from the root sheath of hair follicles. They are most commonly seen on the scalp. Clinically, they may mimic EICs because they appear as flesh-colored nodules with a similar history of slow growth. Nevertheless, pilar cysts can be differentiated on the basis of being located predominantly on the scalp, lacking a central punctum, and other histopathologic findings. Treatment includes excision of the lesion.
- Lipomas are benign, soft-tissue neoplasms comprised of adipose tissue. They are typically larger,

softer, and lack a central punctum. They are diagnosed through physical examination, but rapid growth, functional limitation, pain, and firmer texture are indications for possible biopsy and surgical excision.

- Abscesses are localized infections with subsequent inflammatory response. They may appear similar to an infected or ruptured EIC because they are erythematous, painful nodules that can have malodorous discharge. Treatment includes incision with drainage and systemic antibiotics.
- Steatocystomas are cysts that most often present as part of steatocystoma multiplex as a sporadic or inherited condition. They can be single or multiple and associated with congenital diseases, such as pachyonychia congenita. Steatocystomas present as multiple, flesh-colored to yellow cysts. They are most commonly found on the chest but can be anywhere on the body. As opposed to EICs, they lack a central punctum and the wall of the cyst has a corrugated cuticle that resembles the lining of the sebaceous duct. The wall also may contain sebaceous lobules. Treatment includes excision with removal of the cyst wall.
- Cutaneous metastases may occur via lymphatic or hematogenous spread or through direct extension from the underlying soft tissue. They present as firm, erythematous nodules, usually on the head and trunk. If the patient has a history of malignancy, there should be a low threshold for referral to dermatology to rule out cutaneous metastases because this may be the first presenting sign of an underlying malignancy or recurrence. Cutaneous metastases often portend a poor prognosis.

## Work-Up

- This is usually a diagnosis based on the clinical presentation. If the diagnosis is unclear, biopsy of the lesion may be necessary.
- Patients with an unusually early onset of numerous EICs that are atypical in location, such as the extremities, or who have a family history of colon cancer should be evaluated for Gardner syndrome because this is associated with familial adenomatous polyposis and malignancies, such as colorectal and thyroid cancer.
- If erythema, pain, discharge, or other signs of inflammation develop, the lesion may be secondarily infected. The affected site should be cultured when

the lesion is incised and drained if there is no response to empiric topical and/or systemic antibiotic therapy.

## Initial Steps in Management

Although EICs are benign, treatment may be considered based on symptoms, size, and aesthetic concerns. If the cyst repeatedly becomes inflamed, painful, or infected, then definitive treatment should be considered. Patients should be counseled on the different treatment options and that recurrence is possible even with surgical excision.

- Nonsurgical therapies help with symptomatic management; however, because the cyst wall is not removed, the problem may persist.
  - Inflammation can be managed with intralesional injection of triamcinolone acetonide. To avoid rupture of the cyst, only a small volume should be injected. Given the variability in response and dosing schedules, intralesional steroids are best administered by a dermatologist.
  - Secondary infection should be considered if there is erythema, swelling, pain, and/or drainage because this should be treated with oral antibiotics, such as cephalexin or doxycycline. If indicated, the lesion should also be incised and drained.
- Surgical management may be considered for certain patients depending on the severity.
  - Incision and drainage can provide temporary symptomatic relief by alleviating the pressure caused by inflammation. Nevertheless, this procedure leaves the cyst wall intact, and the EIC is likely to recur.
  - Surgery is considered to be the most definitive treatment, but the patient should be counseled that the cyst can still recur, especially if the cyst wall is not entirely removed.
    - A punch biopsy can be performed to create a small skin opening to remove the cyst contents and wall. This method may not be suitable for ruptured cysts because the cyst wall is difficult to completely remove.
    - Elliptical excision may result in a larger surgical site but allows for visualization and removal of the entire cyst wall, thus minimizing the risk for recurrence. This is the preferred method for lesions that have ruptured, become infected, or have been surgically treated in the

past because the associated fibrosis may make the procedure more challenging.

- In the case of a ruptured or infected EIC, excision should be performed once these have resolved because it can be difficult to fully visualize the lesion in the presence of inflammation and/or infection. Delay in these cases will reduce the risk for infection, wound dehiscence, and cyst recurrence.
- Extruded contents and an excised cyst should be sent to be histopathologically evaluated for histologic confirmation and to exclude the presence of malignancy.

## Warning Signs/Common Pitfalls

- Secondary infection should be considered if there is erythema, swelling, pain, and/or drainage because this should be treated with oral antibiotics.
- Surgical removal of large cysts may result in sagging of the epidermis, which can be prevented by excising a small section of the overlying skin along with the cyst.
- Malignant transformation is rare but has been reported in about 1% of cases. If malignancy is suspected, the patient should be referred to dermatology for biopsy of the lesion. Although these growths are benign, there have been rare cases of malignancies developing within these cysts.

## Counseling

You have an epidermoid or epidermal inclusion cyst, which is a soft-tissue swelling filled with a cheese like material. They are usually asymptomatic and remain stable for years; however, they can rupture and become secondarily infected. Let your doctor know if you have multiple cysts or a family history of colon cancer because they may want to screen you for a condition called Gardner syndrome, which can predispose you to gastrointestinal or thyroid malignancy.

The cysts do not require any treatment, but if they become bothersome, multiple treatment options, including injectable steroids, antibiotics, and surgical excision, are available. These interventions are associated with different rates of recurrence, which should be considered when selecting a treatment option.

Inform your physician if you notice sudden symptoms of inflammation, such as redness, swelling, pain, or a foul-smelling, cheese like discharge because these signs may indicate that the cyst has ruptured or become infected.

# 10

# Benign Brown-Black and Pigmented Skin Growths

## CHAPTER OUTLINE

# SEBORRHEIC KERATOSES

**Layla Kazemi and Afton Chavez**

## Clinical Features

- Seborrheic keratoses (SKs) are common benign skin lesions found in nearly all older individuals.
- They typically begin to appear during the fourth decade of life and then continue to develop throughout one's lifetime.
- They can develop anywhere except the palms, soles, and mucosal surfaces.
- They are found most often on the head and neck, extremities, and trunk, especially the upper back and inframammary region (in women).
- SKs are macular, papular, or verrucous lesions and often have a keratotic plugging, a waxy stuck-on appearance, and/or overlying scale.
  - They typically evolve from a macule and may progress to become papular or verrucous.
- They are most commonly light brown but may appear white to waxy yellow to brown-black in color,

and within the same lesion, there may be a marked variation in color.

- SKs are occasionally solitary but more commonly present as multiple, pigmented, sharply demarcated lesions.
- Individual lesions may be of any size but usually measure about 1 cm in diameter, although they can become quite large (i.e., greater than 5 cm) in diameter.
- SKs may become inflamed or irritated because of friction or trauma or, rarely, from a secondary bacterial infection.
  - Irritated or inflamed lesions may become tender, pruritic, erythematous, crusted, and rarely, pustular.
- There are a few conditions associated with an abrupt appearance or increase in the number of SKs: pregnancy, coexisting inflammatory dermatoses, and malignancy. This would be followed by regression once the condition resolves.

## Differential Diagnosis

The differential for SKs includes solar lentigo, verruca vulgaris, condyloma acuminatum, Bowen disease, squamous cell carcinoma (SCC), melanocytic nevus, melanoma, acrochordon, and tumor of the follicular infundibulum.

- Solar lentigines are neither keratotic nor elevated, but over time, they can develop into SKs.
- Verrucae and condylomata acuminata are hyperplasias caused by human papillomavirus (HPV) that can clinically mimic SKs but differ in that they most frequently occur in younger individuals.
  - Verrucae present as rough papules with pinpoint red or black dots and favor acral locations, whereas condylomata acuminata occur in the anogenital region.
  - SKs can also have superimposed warts, which may present with overlying features as previously described or with filiform (finger like) projections.
- Differentiation between an irritated SK, an SCC *in situ* (known as Bowen disease), and SCC can be quite difficult and may require biopsy and histopathologic examination, but there should be no evidence of involvement of the dermis in irritated SKs.
- The keratotic plugging, stuck-on appearance, and/or overlying scale are helpful features in distinguishing SKs from melanocytic neoplasms, but they can still be extremely difficult to distinguish, so biopsy can be performed in any cases of uncertainty.
- Acrochordons have a pedunculated shape and are usually smoother and smaller in size than SKs.

- Tumor of the follicular infundibulum is a benign adnexal tumor that is distinguished from an SK by a biopsy.

## Work-Up

- SKs can usually be easily recognized clinically, but lesions that are difficult to diagnose by inspection alone can be biopsied.
  - Biopsy may be necessary if there is a history of recent change or inflammation or it is a larger dark lesion that causes concern for melanoma.
  - If biopsy is warranted, shave biopsy is recommended.
    - The specimen should be sent to a dermatopathologist experienced in interpreting keratinocytic lesions, given the difficulty of differentiating irritated/inflamed SK from SCC in situ.

## Initial Steps in Management

- Treatment of SKs is not necessary because they are harmless; however, they may be removed if they are symptomatic or cosmetically bothersome.
- Treatment options include cryosurgery, curettage, or shave removal.
- Because SKs are superficial lesions, their removal causes minimal scarring, but the skin may be lighter than the surrounding area; this may fade with time or stay permanently.

## Warning Signs/Common Pitfalls

- There are many entities that may have similar appearance to SKs, and therefore a malignancy can be misdiagnosed as an SK. Lesions should be biopsied if there is any concern for the possibility of malignancy.
- It is worth noting that there are instances where malignant neoplasms arise within or adjacent to SKs, but this is likely coincidental and because of the prevalence of both in the population at large.
- Sudden appearance of multiple SKs lesions may be associated with internal malignancy (the so-called "sign of Leser-Trélat"); however, the existence of this association is controversial.

## Counseling

You have seborrheic keratoses, which are very common benign skin lesions. They are seen in nearly all older individuals. You will likely continue to develop more throughout your lifetime and there is no way to prevent this, but they are not contagious or dangerous. The cause of seborrheic keratoses is unknown, but they seem to run in families and studies suggest that sun exposure may play a role.

Seborrheic keratoses are usually asymptomatic; however, they can become itchy and inflamed, and catch on clothing. If your lesions become symptomatic or you would like them removed for cosmetic reasons, there are options available. The most common option is cryosurgery, which involves freezing the lesion with liquid nitrogen. They can also be removed under local anesthesia by scraping the lesion from the skin or cutting it off with a small, flat blade. Their removal should cause minimal scarring, but the skin may be lighter than the surrounding area; this can either fade with time or stay permanently.

If you notice any changes in your lesions or a sudden increase in their number, you should make an appointment with a dermatologist so they can be reexamined.

# ACQUIRED DIGITAL FIBROKERATOMA

**Erisa Alia and Philip E. Kerr**

## Clinical Features

Acquired digital fibrokeratoma (ADFK) is a relatively rare, benign, fibroepithelial tumor with a predilection for the fingers and toes. Occasionally, it can be found on the dorsum of the hand, elbow, prepatellar area, nail bed, and heel. ADFK presents as small, firm, solitary, skin-colored to pink, exophytic papulonodules. Its surface is hyperkeratotic, and it is surrounded by a characteristic collarette of slightly raised skin at its base. ADFK is usually asymptomatic.

It has a tendency to gradually increase in size and occurs more often in middle-aged adults. The etiology remains unknown; however, trauma to the site may be contributory.

## Differential Diagnosis

ADFK is most commonly diagnosed based on history and physical examination. Nevertheless, to predict the response to treatment, it is important to differentiate ADFK from other cutaneous lesions in the differential diagnosis. These include verruca vulgaris (the common wart), supernumerary digits, periungual/subungual fibroma, and pyogenic granuloma (PG).

- ADFK's classic location on the lateral aspect of digits and its characteristic collarette of scale help distinguish ADFK from verruca vulgaris. Verrucae are also often tender or painful and demonstrate loss of surface dermatoglyphics. If magnified, multiple black or red dots can be easily appreciated. Biopsy of verruca is diagnostic and shows parakeratosis, papillomatosis, and koilocytes.
- A supernumerary digit is present at birth and usually located on the medial side of the fifth digit. Biopsy reveals nerve bundles in the dermis.
- With periungual/subungual fibroma, location is the distinguishing feature. Fibromas emanate near the proximal and lateral nail folds, whereas ADFK typically does not occur near the nail unit (although a periungual/subungual variant of ADFK exists, in which case histopathologic examination is required for diagnosis).
- Although location may be similar between PG and ADFK, they are unlikely to be confused with one another because PGs are vascular tumors that bleed profusely, whereas ADFKs are asymptomatic and do not appear vascular.

## Work-Up

Although clinical examination helps with the differential diagnosis, the gold standard for diagnosis remains excisional biopsy. Histopathologically, ADFK is characterized by epidermal thickening and hyperkeratosis, with abundant thick collagen bundles in the dermis admixed with dilated blood vessels.

## Initial Steps in Management

ADFK is a benign tumor that requires no further treatment; however, many patients prefer removal. Shave removal is the treatment of choice in cases where patients desire treatment because it is curative and allows for histopathologic confirmation.

Other therapeutic options include cryotherapy, curettage, and electrocautery.

## Warning Signs/Common Pitfalls

- ADFK is a benign tumor with no risk for malignant transformation.
- Spontaneous regression is unlikely.
- The periungual location may cause nail plate deformity and affect the function of the digit.
- Complete surgical excision is curative and recurrence is rare.

## Counseling

You have an acquired digital fibrokeratoma. It is benign but has no tendency to self-resolve. There is no risk for cancerous change, but a biopsy may be required to exclude other more concerning lesions. Treatment is not required, but if you elect to do so, the most effective treatment of choice is surgical removal.

# ACROCHORDON

**Erisa Alia and Philip E. Kerr**

## Clinical Features

Acrochordons, also called "skin tags" or "fibroepithelial polyps," are common benign neoplasms of the skin that share a few characteristics.

- They are sessile or pedunculated papules that are skin-colored to mildly pigmented.
- They are soft to palpation.
- The majority range in diameter from 1 to 6 mm, although occasionally they can be larger.
- They are typically located in the intertriginous areas of the neck, axilla, groin, and inframammary areas. Occasionally, they can be located on the chest.
- They are very common and affect men and women equally.
- They are more common in overweight individuals and develop increasingly with age.
- They are asymptomatic if not traumatized; they may become symptomatic because of rubbing or chafing against clothes or adjacent skin, which can lead to inflammation or even infarction.
- They often present as a solely cosmetic concern.

## Differential Diagnosis

The diagnosis of acrochordon is mainly clinical. Most mimickers of acrochordons are benign; however, rarely, malignancies can present in a tag like fashion.

- Benign lesions that may mimic acrochordons include melanocytic nevus, neurofibroma, seborrheic keratosis, and dermatosis papulosis nigra. Because all of these entities are benign, pathologic confirmation is not typically required.
- In instances where malignancy is expected, a skin biopsy is warranted. Rapidly growing papules or nodules, symptomatic lesions, and lesions with irregular texture and/or coloration should be biopsied.
- Fibroepithelioma of Pinkus is an uncommon variant of basal cell carcinoma. It classically presents as a

pink papule or plaque with a smooth surface. It can be differentiated from an acrochordon by its predilection for the lower back, more distinctly pink appearance, and generally larger size.

## Work-Up

Acrochordons are diagnosed clinically. As aforementioned, biopsy of probable acrochordons is only indicated in situations in which a malignancy is suspected. Acrochordons are often postulated as being associated with obesity and insulin resistance and have been reported as a skin marker for underlying diabetes mellitus (DM). Nevertheless, clinical studies undertaken to clarify this relationship have produced conflicting results and the relevant literature does not provide enough data to confirm the association. There is no indication that every patient with acrochordon should be evaluated for the presence of insulin resistance or DM.

## Initial Steps in Management

Patients should be reassured that skin tags are common benign skin growths. Unless irritated or infarcted, they represent more of a cosmetic issue.

The most common procedure used to remove skin tags is snip excision with scissors. Other destructive modalities include liquid nitrogen cryotherapy, shave removal, electrocautery, and ligation.

## Warning Signs/Common Pitfalls

The diagnosis of acrochordon is rarely clinically challenging.

Infarcted skin tags present as dark brown to black, involuting, pedunculated papules that will eventually fall off spontaneously, requiring no further intervention.

A recurrently bleeding skin lesion resembling an acrochordon but located in an atypical anatomic location may warrant further investigation to rule out more concerning lesions, such as basal cell carcinoma (especially the fibroepithelioma of Pinkus variant), SCC, dysplastic/atypical nevus, and malignant melanoma.

## Counseling

Skin tags are very common. They are benign, which means they are not a type of cancer. They are usually not concerning for your health and require no laboratory or radiologic work-up. If the skin tag bleeds recurrently; changes in size, shape, or color over a short period of time; or becomes inflamed, report this to a healthcare provider. If you have one or more skin tags and you are overweight, you may be at increased risk for developing diabetes. Because being overweight is a risk factor for developing acrochordons, practicing healthy eating habits and exercising is encouraged for weight loss. This will help reduce the risk for developing skin tags and will reduce your risk for developing diabetes.

# BLUE NEVUS

**Mohammed H. Malik and Philip E. Kerr**

## Clinical Features

Blue nevus refers to a type of benign nevus within the family of melanocytic nevi. Other names include "blue mole," "blue neuronevus," and "dermal melanocytoma." Clinical features include well-demarcated, bluish-black papules that are typically 2 to 5 mm; a predilection for the head, extremities, and buttocks; and single, acquired lesions in the vast majority of cases (rare congenital cases with multiple blue nevi exist). Blue nevi are more common in women and those of Asian descent.

The etiology of blue nevi is most likely failed melanocyte migration from the neural crest to the dermal-epidermal junction, resulting in melanocytes in the dermis. Many of these melanocytes (nevus cells) produce melanin. The placement of this brown pigment in the mid to deep dermis results in the blue-black color seen clinically. There are a variety of types of blue nevi. The two most frequent types are the common blue nevus and the cellular blue nevus. Common blue nevi occur as previously described. Cellular blue nevi are often somewhat larger and occur more commonly on the scalp and coccygeal region.

## Differential Diagnosis

By far, the most significant other diagnosis to consider is malignant melanoma. It is critical to distinguish melanoma from benign pigmented lesions, such as blue nevus. Using the well-known ABCDE screening tool can be of help.
- A: Melanoma is typically asymmetric, whereas blue nevus is usually highly symmetric.
- B: The border in melanoma is often indistinct and irregular, whereas the border in blue nevus is typically very sharp and distinct. Blue nevi are usually perfectly round or slightly oval.
- C: Melanoma often exhibits color variegation. Blue nevi are almost always uniformly blue-black.
- D: Melanoma can be quite large, with a diameter often less than 6 mm. Most blue nevi are 2 to 6 mm in diameter.
- E: A hallmark of melanoma is that it evolves or changes in appearance over 3 to 9 months, whereas blue nevi are typically stable for years.

## Work-Up

The diagnosis of a blue nevus is mostly clinical in nature. If the diagnosis is in question, a biopsy for histologic examination is recommended. Because blue-black pigment, regardless of whether it is the result of a melanoma or a benign nevus, indicates significant depth into the dermis, a deep shave or, preferably, excisional biopsy is recommended. An excisional biopsy can be performed with a scalpel or a punch instrument.

## Initial Steps in Management

All types of blue nevi should be monitored by the patient and clinician because of the possibility of misdiagnosis and potential for a blue nevus like melanoma. If the lesion remains stable, then continued clinical monitoring is appropriate.

## Warning Signs/Common Pitfalls

By far, the most significant potential pitfall is overconfidence in the diagnosis of blue nevus. Blue nevi are stable lesions that should change only slightly, if at all, over a 2- to 3-year time period. If a suspected blue nevus changes in size, shape, or color over a period of 3 to 9 months, then the clinical diagnosis should be reevaluated and a biopsy is likely indicated.

## Counseling

You have a blue nevus, which is a type of mole that appears bluish-black in color. Moles appear dark because melanocytes (the cells that produce pigment) are grouped together in that location. This mole is darker in color than typical brown moles because the pigment is deeper under the skin surface. This type of mole is benign, but these moles can look similar to more dangerous conditions like melanoma. Thus, if this mole changes in size, shape, or color over a few months, please let us know because we will likely recommend a procedure to remove the spot.

# CAFÉ-AU-LAIT MACULES

**Kathryn Bentivegna and Philip E. Kerr**

## Clinical Features

Café-au-lait macules (CALMs) are well-defined, evenly hyperpigmented macules or patches that develop in approximately 25% of the population. They range from light to dark brown in color and are named after their resemblance to "coffee with milk." They do not have any cancerous potential.

- CALMs may be present at birth but more typically appear in early childhood as one or two spots.
- The trunk and lower extremities are the sites of predilection.
  - They occur less commonly on the face and spare the mucous membranes.
- CALMs enlarge proportionately as the affected child grows older and larger.
  - They commonly become less clinically pronounced in adulthood.
- They can vary considerably in size (from 1 cm to over 20 cm).
- The presence of more than three CALMs may suggest that an individual has neurofibromatosis type 1 (NF1; Fig. 10.1).
  - Neurofibromatosis is an autosomal dominant genetic condition that is characterized by the development of CALMs, neurofibromas, and ocular tumors, among other findings.

CALMs are often the first sign of NF1 and therefore recognizing that a child has more than six CALMs may expedite diagnosis.
- Rarely, CALMs can have other syndromic associations.

## Differential Diagnosis

The differential for CALMS include congenital melanocytic nevus, linear nevoid hypermelanosis, nevus spilus, and lentigines.

- Congenital melanocytic nevi (Fig. 10.2) are a special type of mole that are present from birth. They can be distinguished from CALMs because they are almost invariably raised and lack the uniform pigmentation that is characteristic of a CALM. Additionally, they become hypertrichotic over time and if they are examined with magnification or a dermatoscope, they demonstrate a pigment network like other nevi.
- Linear nevoid hypermelanosis is a type of congenital hyperpigmentation that is distributed in a whorled pattern along Blaschko lines. It is distinguished from CALMs because it has a blaschkoid distribution and is not a solitary defined lesion like a CALM.
- Nevus spilus (also known as "speckled lentiginous nevus") is a type of birthmark that is likened in appearance to a chocolate chip cookie. They initially can present identically to a CALM; however, they subsequently develop a speckled appearance with multiple 1- to 2-mm, dark brown macules embedded

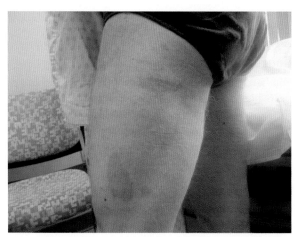

**Fig. 10.1 Multiple Café Au Lait Macules in an Individual with Legius Syndrome.** (From the UConn Grand Rounds Collection.)

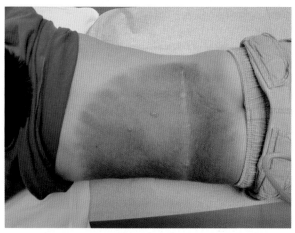

**Fig. 10.2 Giant Congenital Melanocytic Nevus.** (From the UConn Grand Rounds Collection.)

within a lighter brown hyperpigmented patch. The presence of this speckled appearance differentiates a nevus spilus from a CALM.

- Lentigines are acquired pigmented macules that are typically located in sun-exposed areas (especially the face, shoulders, and extensor arms) and that measure 1 to 5 mm in diameter. They can be distinguished from CALMs because they typically arise in adolescence or adulthood, are smaller than CALMs, and occur in multiples.

Patients with suspected NF1 are diagnosed based on clinical findings. The established criteria for diagnosis of NF1 include two of the seven following conditions.

1. Six or more CALM spots (equal to or greater than 0.5 cm diameter in the prepubertal or equal to or greater than 1.5 cm in the postpubertal child);
2. Freckling in skinfold areas, especially the axillary or inguinal regions;
3. Two or more neurofibromas or one plexiform neurofibroma;
4. Two or more Lisch nodules (raised tan hamartomas of the iris);
5. Optic pathway glioma;
6. Bony dysplasia (i.e., sphenoid wing dysplasia or cortical thinning of long bones);
7. A first-degree relative (parent, sibling, child) with NF1.

The differential for NF1 includes Legius syndrome, constitutional mismatch repair-deficiency (CMMR-D) syndrome, McCune-Albright syndrome, neurofibromatosis type 2 (NF2), and Noonan syndrome.

## Work-Up

A Wood lamp examination may be helpful for visualizing the spot on lighter-skinned individuals.

For solitary lesions in children younger than 6 years of age, no further workup is needed.

Greater than three CALMs in a Caucasian patient, more than five CALMs in a Black patient, and evidence of other signs of CALM-associated genetic condition (i.e., neurofibromas, Lisch nodules) warrant referral to a specialist.

## Initial Steps in Management

For solitary lesions, no treatment is needed. The patient should be reassured about the benignity of this finding.

- Cosmetically bothersome lesions can be treated with laser therapy.

For multiple lesions/concern for NF1, refer the patient to pediatric neurology, genetics, and ophthalmology.
- Patients meeting clinical criteria for NF1 do not need to undergo genetic testing for confirmation of the diagnosis; however, genetic testing is available for diagnostically challenging cases.

## Warning Signs/Common Pitfalls

Multiple CALMs, large segmental CALMs, CALMs appearing after 6 years old, and other associated skin findings or abnormal physical examination findings should increase suspicion of systemic disease.

## Counseling

Your child has a café-au-lait macule. One or two of these spots is common, occurring in about one out of every four children, and does not suggest that your child has any underlying illness. They are not dangerous and do not have the potential to become dangerous. They do not require any treatment. If this lesion is cosmetically bothersome, it can potentially be lightened with a laser.

If your child develops multiple café-au-lait macules (more than six), this may indicate that your child has an underlying systemic condition. If any new spots develop or you notice any change in size or shape of spots or other skin findings, your child should be reevaluated by your doctor.

## DERMATOFIBROMA

**Kathryn Bentivegna and Philip E. Kerr**

### Clinical Features

A dermatofibroma (DF) is a benign tumor that presents as a fibrotic dermal nodule and is generally less than or equal to 1 cm in diameter.
- It is typically smooth, firm, scar like, and nontender to palpation and may have overlying skin changes of tan-pink to red-brown discoloration.
  - A central white scar like area can almost always be appreciated within dermatofibromas and its presence can help distinguish DFs from mimickers.

[1]University of Connecticut School of Medicine
[2]Department of Dermatology, University of Connecticut School of Medicine, Farmington, CT

- In some cases, especially on the upper extremities, this central white area can develop blood vessels and/or milia like cysts within it, which can cause these lesions to look more haphazard to the untrained eye.
- The most common area of presentation is the legs, but DFs also frequently appear on the arms (the dorsal upper arm more often than the dorsal forearm) and neck.
- DFs most frequently develop in patients between the ages of 20 and 49 years and are more common in females.
  - Once acquired, they do not go away without surgical removal.
- Most DFs develop spontaneously; however, patients frequently endorse a history of trauma to the area, such as an insect bite.
- Most patients only present with a single DF; however, it is not uncommon to find multiple (two to three) DFs on the lower legs of predisposed women.
  - There is a rare DF-associated finding called multiple eruptive DFs (MEDF) in which a patient presents with at least five to fifteen nodules in fewer than 4 months.
    - MEDF occurs most frequently in immunocompromised patients with human immunodeficiency virus (HIV) infection or systemic lupus erythematosus (SLE).
- DFs are most often asymptomatic but may have associated pain and/or pruritus.
- Because they are benign, DFs do not need to be removed surgically unless they are bothersome to the patient or there is a need to confirm the diagnosis histologically because of atypical clinical presentation.

## Differential Diagnosis

The differential is broad because of its diverse clinical presentations; however, the most common mimickers are melanocytic nevi, hypertrophic scar, nonmelanoma skin cancer, dermatofibrosarcoma protuberans (DSFP), and juvenile xanthogranuloma (JXG).

- DFs are frequently misdiagnosed as acquired melanocytic nevi (moles) when they are tan-brown in color. They can be distinguished from melanocytic nevi based on the presence of a central white area, firmness on palpation, and a positive dimple sign.
- Based on texture and predilection for developing after trauma, many DFs get misdiagnosed as a scar. DFs

are well circumscribed, have a central white area, and a positive dimple sign, and do not respond to intralesional corticosteroids, distinguishing them from scars.

- DFs are most frequently biopsied to rule out nonmelanoma skin cancer (typically basal cell carcinoma) when they are pink. As aforementioned, the firmness, presence of a central white scar, and positive dimple sign are helpful for distinguishing these entities.
- DFSP is a locally aggressive malignant neoplasm that is important to distinguish from dermatofibroma. The borders of a DFSP are typically less well defined and by the time they are evaluated, they are frequently larger than 1 centimeter. A history of increasing size or presentation on an atypical location, such as the trunk, should increase suspicion for DFSP. If there is suspicion for DFSP, a biopsy is recommended because they can be distinguished by histopathology and immunohistochemical staining.
- JXG may also be mistaken for DF, but JXG is more likely to occur in infants and young children on the head, neck, and upper trunk. Again, skin biopsy can be performed to delineate these two entities.

## Work-Up

The diagnosis can typically be made by clinical examination alone, including visual inspection and palpation of a firm, nontender nodule centered in the dermis.

- The dimple sign is frequently positive in DF.
  - It is elicited by applying lateral pressure to the DF and is considered positive when the lesion dimples centrally.
  - Dermoscopy characteristically reveals a central white area with a peripheral pigment network.

## Initial Steps in Management

In cases where DFs can be diagnosed clinically, no intervention is necessary if the lesion is asymptomatic.

- Surgical excision can be performed if the patient desires removal.
- If the diagnosis is in doubt, performance of an excisional biopsy is recommended.

## Warning Signs/Common Pitfalls

DFs should be stable in size and appearance. In cases where patients endorse a history that the lesion is changing, a biopsy is recommended because the clinical features of DFSP can be very subtle.

If excision of a DF is being performed for cosmetic reasons, it is important to ensure that the lesion is excised with at least 2 mm clinical margins because they have a tendency to recur. For similar reasons, shave removal is not recommended.

## Counseling

You have a dermatofibroma. This is not a skin cancer and does not have the potential to turn into a skin cancer. Dermatofibromas are frequently described as being a "funny scar." They typically do not change or self-resolve over time; however, because they are not dangerous, we do not recommend treatment unless they are bothersome to you.

If the lesion is bothersome to you, it can be removed surgically; however, you will be trading it for a line scar that is longer than the lesion itself. Removing it is relatively safe; however, it can cause bleeding, infection, and scarring. There is also a chance that the dermatofibroma comes back after we remove it. If you notice any changes to the lesion, including increases in size, shape, or appearance, please notify your doctor and have the lesion reevaluated.

# 11

# Benign Flesh-Colored, Pink, and Red Skin Growths

## CHAPTER OUTLINE

# LICHEN SIMPLEX CHRONICUS

## Clinical Features

Lichen simplex chronicus (LSC; also known as "neuro-dermatitis") is a common secondary skin condition characterized by the development of thickened plaques with accentuated skin lines (i.e., lichenification).

- LSC is caused by chronic scratching or rubbing.
  - Patients do not always report frequent rubbing or scratching of the affected area.
- Plaques are typically well demarcated but can take on irregular, ovular, or angular morphologies and can vary in size.
  - Concomitant excoriations are frequently present.
  - Newly formed plaques are usually characterized by separate zones.
    - The peripheral zone (2–3 cm) is defined by marginal skin thickening, often with discrete papules.
    - The central zone has greater degrees of skin thickening and exaggerated skin lines.
    - Secondary pigmentation changes may be more dramatic in individuals with darker skin.
      - Plaques may be hyperpigmented or hypopigmented, depending on chronicity.
- LSC most commonly affects areas that are accessible to scratching, such as the scalp, legs, neck, genitals (Fig. 11.1), arms, and face.
  - It is more common on the patient's dominant side.

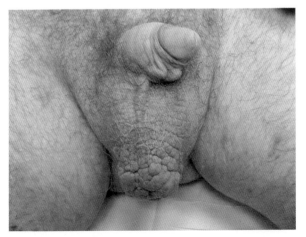

**Fig. 11.1** Lichen Simplex Chronicus, Scrotum. Note the accentuated skin lines. (From the UConn Grand Rounds Collection.)

- Unlike prurigo nodularis, LSC typically presents with one to five plaques, although in some cases many lesions are present.
- Although LSC can be seen in all age groups, it is distributed bimodally, peaking in childhood and then again in mid to late adulthood.
- LSC is more common in women than in men.

LSC can either arise in areas affected by a different primary dermatosis (e.g., atopic dermatitis [AD]) or de novo from idiopathic pruritus.

- In some cases of de novo LSC, it is thought to arise as a manifestation of an underlying psychiatric condition (e.g., generalized anxiety disorder, obsessive compulsive disorder [OCD]).

## Differential Diagnosis

The differential for LSC includes squamous cell carcinoma (SCC), lichen sclerosus, prurigo nodularis, lichen planus (LP), and psoriasis. Importantly, lichenification can arise secondary to a number of pruritic skin conditions. In all cases, it is important to recognize that patients may have a separate, underlying primary skin condition (including those in the differential diagnosis).

- SCC can also present as an isolated hyperkeratotic plaque. SCC is always in the differential for LSC. Cases of suspected LSC that demonstrate no response to occluded, super-potent topical corticosteroids or intralesional corticosteroids should be biopsied to rule out SCC. Importantly, this biopsy should be interpreted by a dermatopathologist because reaction changes seen in LSC can mimic SCC.
- Genital LSC can be confused with lichen sclerosus. Unlike LSC, which presents with thickened skin, lichen sclerosus presents with atrophic white plaques that burn in a perigenital distribution. The appearance of lichen sclerosus has been likened to that of cigarette paper. Untreated lichen sclerosus can cause genital disfigurement and can lead to development of SCC.
- Prurigo nodules are similar to LSC; however, they are nodular and frequently more widespread. Both conditions are caused by chronic scratching, rubbing, or picking.
- Hypertrophic LP can present with hyperkeratotic plaques, typically affecting the shins. It can be differentiated from LSC because hypertrophic LP typically presents with multiple lesions and typical LP lesions may be identifiable elsewhere.

- Other chronic inflammatory conditions (e.g., AD, psoriasis) can mimic LSC and can develop secondary lichenification from chronic scratching. In these cases, a primary dermatosis is also identified.

## Work-Up

LSC can typically be diagnosed clinically; however, histopathologic confirmation is occasionally necessary.

The presence of an isolated, lichenified plaque with accentuated skin lines and dyspigmentation is suggestive of a diagnosis of LSC.

- This is further supported by a patient history of repetitive scratching to the affected regions; however, many patients deny scratching.
- Visualization of broken hairs or excoriations may support a diagnosis of LSC because they are signs of chronic scratching.
- The presence of a primary dermatosis does not in and of itself rule out a diagnosis of LSC.

Patients who do not respond as expected to a 4-week course of occluded, super-potent topical corticosteroids or intralesional corticosteroids should undergo biopsy to rule out more significant pathology.

## Initial Steps in Management

### General Management Comments

Management of LSC differs based on whether or not the patient has an underlying primary dermatosis.

- If a primary dermatosis is present, treatment should initially be directed at managing the underlying condition.
- If there is no primary dermatosis, LSC-directed management should ensue.
  - Some providers screen for the presence of comorbid psychiatric illness in patients with LSC and refer appropriately based on the results of screening.

### Recommended Initial Treatment

Patients should be treated with either potent topical corticosteroids under occlusion or intralesional corticosteroids.

- For nonfacial, nongenital lesions, class I corticosteroids (e.g., clobetasol propionate 0.05%) can be occluded under saran wrap daily for 2 to 4 weeks.
- For facial or genital lesions, a 2-week trial of a non-occluded mid-potency corticosteroid (e.g., triamcinolone acetonide 0.1% cream) twice daily can be trialed.

- Intralesional corticosteroids (e.g., triamcinolone acetonide 10 mg/kg for nonfacial, nongenital skin; triamcinolone acetonide 5 mg/kg for facial or genital skin) can be performed and repeated at 4-week intervals as needed.
- Intralesional corticosteroids are highly effective for solitary lesions but should only be performed by an experienced healthcare provider because they can result in significant local AEs if injected inappropriately.
- Patients should also be advised to keep lesions covered with bandages and to apply a thick moisturizer (e.g., zinc oxide barrier cream) to the affected area every time that it itches. This is frequently helpful with breaking the itch-scratch cycle that drives this condition.

### Partial but Inadequate Response

If there is a partial but inadequate response after a trial of topical or intralesional corticosteroids, confirm the diagnosis, if it is in question, with a biopsy. Then add systemic anti-itch medications (e.g., gabapentin, pregabalin, n-acetylcysteine) or consider referral to a dermatologist.

- A punch biopsy is frequently required to obtain a sample of the entirety of the epidermis.
- You can also assess for patient willingness to seek cognitive behavioral therapy/psychiatrist evaluation to help break the itch-scratch cycle if an underlying psychiatric condition is suspected or known.

## Warning Signs/Common Pitfalls

SCC can mimic LSC and can develop concomitantly in patients with known LSC. If suspected LSC continues to grow despite treatment, a biopsy is always indicated.

Antihistamines and oral corticosteroids are frequently prescribed for the treatment of LSC but are unlikely to offer the patient any benefit.

A major pitfall in the treatment of LSC is failure to identify the primary driver of the patient's scratch–itch cycle.

- Failing to adequately address a mental health disorder that may be leading to LSC impedes treatment success.
  - In patients with OCD, significant depression, or anxiety, treatment success involves a multispecialty approach that may involve a psychiatrist, counselor, and primary care physician.
- Similarly, if the patient's pruritus is driven by a primary skin condition, such as psoriasis or AD, it is essential to adequately treat the primary condition.

LSC can become superinfected. Skin lesions demonstrating signs of warmth, erythema, or discharge should be cultured and treated with either a topical or oral antibiotic.

## Counseling

You have a condition called "lichen simplex chronicus." This type of rash is usually caused by excessive scratching or rubbing of the same area of skin over time. This condition is frequently difficult to treat.

There are several things you should do to treat your rash. First, you have been prescribed a topical corticosteroid. Apply this to the affected area and then wrap the area with saran wrap to help get the medicine into the skin. If this is not feasible, apply a bandage over the prescription cream. Second, keep the area covered with a bandage at all times, even when you sleep. Lastly, apply a thick moisturizing cream to the area every time that it itches as many times as is necessary throughout the day.

If your rash fails to improve despite this therapy, we will re-evaluate it.

# KELOIDS

**Shivani Sinha, Gloria Lin, and Katalin Ferenczi**

## Clinical Features

Keloids are characterized by an excessive growth of scar tissue in response to dermal injury; rarely, they have been reported to present spontaneously in patients prone to developing keloids. They are more commonly seen in younger, darker-skinned individuals, who may be genetically predisposed to developing these lesions. Their cosmetically disfiguring nature and lack of efficacious therapies can make this a challenging diagnosis because patients may be disappointed with the treatment outcomes.

- Given the prevalence of keloids, patients often self-diagnose this condition without the aid of a medical professional. They will complain of pruritus, tenderness, and enlargement of the lesions while relating a history of inciting cutaneous injury, including piercings, surgeries, vaccinations, burns, and acne.
- Keloids appear as smooth, shiny, flesh-colored to pink or red or hyperpigmented papules, plaques, or nodules, which are usually firm, rubbery, and can be pruritic or painful. They may present anywhere on the body but are often seen on the earlobes, chest, and back. The keloids may not appear until months after the cutaneous insult. Without intervention, progressive enlargement is possible because they are unlikely to regress on their own. Keloids may produce contractures, causing impaired function, which can be debilitating for the patient.

## Differential Diagnosis

The differential diagnosis for keloids include hypertrophic scars, dermatofibromas (DFs), dermatofibrosarcoma protuberans (DFSP), foreign body reaction, sarcoidosis, keloidal scleroderma, and lobomycosis.

- Hypertrophic scars are large, thickened scars that are confined to the wound borders, whereas keloids extend beyond it. They tend to appear quickly after the preceding trauma and can resolve. Keloids, on the other hand, may appear months later and are unlikely to improve without treatment.
- DFs are thought to arise in areas of trauma (i.e., shaving or arthropod bites) and are commonly seen in young females on the lower extremities, upper arms, and upper back. They present as firm, skin-colored or hyperpigmented papules or nodules, which can be pruritic or painful. On physical examination, DFs may have a positive dimple sign when squeezed because the skin will pucker inwards. Similar to keloids, these are unlikely to resolve on their own.
- DFSP is a locally aggressive soft-tissue sarcoma seen on the trunk or proximal extremities. DFSP appears as a firm, slow-growing plaque that becomes large and protuberant over time. Although this is a malignant condition, lymphatic or hematogenous metastasis is rare. Patients suspected of having a DFSP should be referred to a dermatologist for further evaluation and possible biopsy because it may require treatment with wide excision, Mohs micrographic surgery, radiation, and/or imatinib.
- A foreign body reaction may occur as a result of trauma and after implantation of foreign material in the skin and involves an inflammatory soft tissue response. It may appear as a painful, flesh-colored, erythematous, or hyperpigmented papule, nodule, or plaque at the site of injury. Referral to dermatology is recommended because the area may need to be biopsied or excised for diagnosis and therapy (to remove the foreign body).
- Sarcoidosis can mimic keloids because it can also occur at areas of trauma, injury, or pre-existent scars. Clinically, it can form hyperpigmented nodules that may be confused with keloids. On examination, compression

of the lesion with a glass slide (diascopy) can demonstrate an apple jelly like appearance that is often associated with granulomatous processes. A biopsy will demonstrate sarcoidal granulomas.

- Keloidal scleroderma is a rare variant of scleroderma that presents with multiple hyperpigmented nodules or plaques that are localized to the upper trunk. Although these lesions clinically resemble keloids, they are nontender and lack a history of an inciting injury and the systemic symptoms that may be seen with scleroderma.
- Lobomycosis, also known as "keloidal blastomycosis," is a fungal infection usually seen in more tropical areas, such as Central or South America. Chronic infection leads to the formation of nodules and plaques, whose growth and appearance resemble keloids. Treatment can be challenging, especially if there is widespread disease. A biopsy with special stains is often required to establish this diagnosis.

## Work-Up

This is usually a clinical diagnosis based on physical examination and history.
- The shape of the scar, growth progression, family history, and antecedent skin injury may support a diagnosis of keloid.
- If there is any uncertainty in the diagnosis, the patient should be referred to a dermatologist for further evaluation and treatment. A biopsy may be performed by a dermatologist to rule out serious skin conditions or malignancies that can mimic keloids.

## Initial Steps in Management

The initial management of keloids is complex and often requires a combination of therapies. The most important step in management is to educate the patient on avoiding cutaneous injury and to discuss realistic treatment expectations.
- Advise against any further insult to the skin, including piercings, elective surgeries, and burns. Caution should be taken when shaving to avoid any injury. If the patient has an active underlying condition, such as acne, this should be treated to prevent further keloid formation.
- Recommend counseling the patient that the management goal is symptomatic relief (decrease pain and/or pruritus). There may be some aesthetic improvement;

however, because there is scar tissue in the area, the skin cannot return to baseline. In addition, it is important to discuss that it will likely require multiple treatments to see maximum benefit. Many patients will often ask why the area cannot just be shaved down; thus it is important to discuss the high recurrence risk with this treatment method.

Management of keloids involves dividing cases by number, location, and size because this can affect the management plan. Based on the complexity and possible reactions to the treatments, a referral to dermatology is recommended.

### Small or Treatment-Naïve Keloids

- Intralesional triamcinolone acetonide (10–40 mg/mL) can be administered once or twice monthly to reduce inflammation and halt the proliferative process. This treatment may be beneficial for fast-acting symptomatic relief. Keloids treated with intralesional steroids may become softer in texture over time, making it easier to administer injections at a later time. Patients should be counseled on the risk for atrophy and dyspigmentation. Given the variability in the dosing and treatment schedule, the patient should be referred to a dermatologist.
- Occlusive silicone gel sheeting is used for both treatment and prophylaxis by providing hydration to the dermal layers.
- Pressure therapy involves applying dressing or bandages to the affected area to reduce the growth of scar tissue. For keloids on the ears, pressure earrings can be used and are highly recommended postoperatively to reduce the risk for recurrence.

### Larger or Treatment-Refractory Keloids

- Intralesional 5-fluorouracil (50 mg/mL) can be injected once weekly for up to 12 weeks to reduce inflammation. This option can be used in keloids that are unresponsive to steroid injections. Given the potential risk for side effects and need for biohazard precautions, the patient should be referred to a dermatologist.
- Cryotherapy (liquid nitrogen) can be performed to decrease the size of the keloid. Patients should be counseled on the risk for dyspigmentation in the treatment area.

- Laser therapy, including $CO_2$, Nd:YAG, or PDL, can be used on enlarging lesions to halt the progressive growth of scar tissue.
- Surgical excision of the keloid may be performed when the scar is large or linear, but the risks of the procedure should be clearly explained to the patient because the defect will likely be larger than the actual lesion, and the keloid can recur and worsen. For areas such as the ear, surgery may not be advisable because it can result in volume loss and asymmetry compared with the other side.
  - Many patients may not be ideal surgical candidates because it requires consistently following up with the healthcare provider. Further adjunctive therapy may be needed even after the procedure to decrease the risk for recurrence.
  - Intralesional steroids may be injected into the surgical site postoperatively on the same day and at subsequent follow-up visits.
  - Radiation therapy may also be used postoperatively to reduce the likelihood of recurrence after excision.
  - The patients may require multiple procedures to achieve the optimal outcome.
- Other emerging therapies, such as dupilumab, an IL-4 receptor inhibitor, have shown some promise in this condition.

## Warning Signs/Common Pitfalls

- Keloids are not malignant; however, there are nonbenign conditions that may visually resemble keloids. Patients should be referred to dermatology for possible biopsy and histologic examination to rule out malignancy if there is any doubt about the diagnosis.
- Keloids present with a high recurrence rate after treatment. Scars will often require multiple rounds of combination therapy. Even with treatment, there may not be significant improvement with the appearance of the lesions.
- Cosmetic disfigurement, functional limitation, and symptoms of pain and pruritus may cause decreased quality of life and should be addressed.

## Counseling

You have a keloid, which is an overgrown scar. It should be evaluated by a dermatologist, who may perform a biopsy to confirm the diagnosis. The primary goal is to minimize any associated symptoms, such as pain and itching. It is important to note that the area will not revert back to normal skin even with treatment, but there could potentially be some improvement with the size and texture of the lesions. Treatment could include steroid injections into the scar to halt its growth and decrease the size. This can be done in combination with other forms of therapy, such as occlusive or pressure dressings. Large scars may be surgically excised but are likely to recur and may appear worse than the original lesions. To decrease the risk for recurrence, postoperative steroid injections or radiation therapy may be recommended.

These lesions may have a genetic component because they tend to run in families. If you are predisposed to keloid formation, you should avoid ear and body piercings and elective cosmetic surgical procedures because these may result in keloid formation. If you are having a surgical procedure, inform the surgeon that you are prone to keloids because they may change the way they close the incision site. Try to reduce the incidence of minor cuts of the skin because these may also progress into keloids. Take care in shaving and treat acne without causing injury to the skin. If cuts do occur, keep them clean and moist while they heal. This can be done by applying gentle emollients, such as Vaseline or Aquaphor, and covering the affected area with gauze, Telfa, or a bandage.

# ERYTHEMA NODOSUM

**Campbell Stewart**

## Clinical Features

Erythema nodosum (EN) is a form of panniculitis (inflammation of the subcutaneous adipose tissue). It is a delayed hypersensitivity reaction associated with multiple infections, autoimmune/inflammatory disorders, and drugs. It can also be idiopathic.

## Classic Clinical Presentation

- The classic clinical presentation includes acute-onset, tender, painful nodules, which occur predominantly on the anterior aspects of the lower legs.
- The lesions are normally red in the acute setting; however, they usually resolve with associated pigmentary changes.
- Rarely, EN can present with lesions on the posterior lower legs, thighs, and upper extremities.
- Patients normally have associated symptoms of arthralgias and fever, with flu like complaints.

## Associations

The most common associations are *Streptococcal* infections (children and adults; Fig. 11.2, A–B) and sarcoidosis (adults).

Other infections with which EN may be associated include *Yersinia enterocolitica, Salmonella spp., Campylobacter spp., Mycoplasma pneumoniae,* tuberculosis, coccidioidomycosis, histoplasmosis, blastomycosis, viral hepatitis, herpes simplex virus (HSV), and human immunodeficiency virus (HIV).

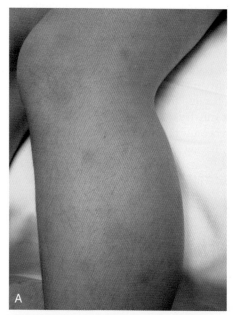

**Fig. 11.2AB** Poststreptococcal Erythema Nodosum in an Adolescent. Affected areas were firm to palpation. (From the UConn Grand Rounds Collection.)

Drugs can also be the cause, including oral contraceptives (pregnancy may also be associated), sulfa-based medications, antibiotics (including amoxicillin), nonsteroidal anti inflammatory drugs (NSAIDs; although this is uncommon), and gold.

Autoimmune and inflammatory conditions that can result in EN include sarcoidosis (Löfgren syndrome, involving uveitis, hilar adenopathy, fever, and arthritis), Crohn disease, ulcerative colitis, and Behçet disease.

EN tends to resolve over a period of 6 to 18 weeks, depending on the underlying cause. Idiopathic EN can last up to 6 months. Depending on the chronicity of EN, the lesions can leave behind postinflammatory pigment change. Residual focal atrophy or scarring is rare in EN.

EN can be chronic (i.e., lasting longer than 6 months) or recurrent, particularly if it is related to an underlying inflammatory disorder as opposed to an acute exposure (i.e., drug or infection).

## Differential Diagnosis

The clinical differential diagnosis includes other panniculitides, such as erythema induratum/nodular vasculitis, traumatic panniculitis, and skin-popping/foreign body panniculitis. These panniculitides tend to ulcerate and scar. Also included in the differential are arthropod bites (history and pruritis often establish this diagnosis) and cellulitis/erysipelas (in which lesions are generally warm and unilateral).

## Work-Up

Even if the diagnosis is immediately apparent, the underlying association should be determined to guide management. A careful history inquiring about oral medications and evaluating for recent illness, including gastrointestinal and genitourinary symptoms, should be performed. A full-body skin examination should be performed, particularly to look for cutaneous lesions of sarcoidosis. A biopsy is typically not needed except in clinically challenging/refractory cases.

- A deep-punch biopsy will reveal a mostly septal panniculitis with a variable inflammatory infiltrate. Telescoping punch biopsies (using a 4- to 6-mm punch followed by a 3- to 4-mm punch into the initial biopsy site to acquire deeper fat) can be used if adipose tissue is not acquired on the first attempt. Incisional biopsy into adipose can be performed if this technique fails.
- Sampling of the most acute or burned-out lesions may not reveal the classic findings, so it is important

to biopsy established but not resolving lesions. The sampled lesion should be indurated and tender to palpation, indicating disease activity. Depending on the quality of the sample, a biopsy may not be able to fully differentiate EN from other panniculitides.

- Blood work should also be completed, including a complete blood count (CBC)/differential to assess for leukocytosis; an antistreptolysin O (ASO) titer (if the value is low, it does not exclude the possibility of streptococcal infection); erythrocyte sedimentation rate/C-reactive protein (ESR/CRP) test; Quanti-FERON-gold test (or purified protein derivative [PPD] skin test); and viral serologies.

Other tests that can be used include a rapid strep and throat culture, stool examination and urine culture, and a chest x-ray to evaluate for tuberculosis and sarcoidosis.

## Initial Steps in Management
### General Management Comments

If a drug is suspected, then stopping the agent is essential. Remind patients that reexposure to the drug and similar compounds will likely trigger a flare of EN. Patients who react to oral contraceptive products may also flare during pregnancy.

- Infectious causes must be excluded and treatment rendered once an associated infectious cause is identified.
- Evaluating for sarcoidosis, with consultation of pulmonology or ophthalmology when necessary, is important.
- If no infectious cause is found and a patient has gastrointestinal complaints, referral to gastroenterology for evaluation of inflammatory bowel disease is recommended.

### Recommended Initial Regimen

- Most EN responds to rest, elevation of the lower extremities, and cooling/icing of the lesions.
- Scheduled NSAIDs (naproxen, indomethacin, and ibuprofen) are recommended.

### Partial but Inadequate Response

If there is a partial but inadequate response to the initial regimen after 4 to 6 weeks, a biopsy can be performed to confirm the diagnosis.

- Oral corticosteroids (prednisone 1mg/kg daily) tapered over a period of 3 to 4 weeks are usually adequate to provide relief.

### Continued Inadequate Response

If the response continues to be inadequate, colchicine (0.6 mg orally two to three times daily) can be tried.

If these therapies all fail, or if the disease progresses while on treatment, the diagnosis should be reconsidered. A repeat biopsy may be needed to investigate for other causes. Tissue culture of an active lesion should be done to evaluate for occult cutaneous infections, particularly if the lesions begin to ulcerate or drain.

### Other Treatment Options

Potassium iodide (SSKI) dosed as three to six drops three times daily (up to 1 g total per day) is effective.

## Warning Signs/Common Pitfalls

Warning signs for EN include a patient with fever, arthralgias, other flu like symptoms, and the classic tender lesions restricted to the anterior lower legs. Initial lesions may be small, and induration may be subtle at presentation, leading to a misdiagnosis of arthropod bites.

Larger, unilateral lesions may be mistaken for cellulitis/erysipelas. EN patients will progress and develop the classic bilateral presentation.

EN can present on the upper extremities as well.

One pitfall is missing an infectious cause when an easily identifiable trigger (such as oral contraceptives or sulfamethoxazole/trimethoprim) is present. Infections should always be considered and ruled out, ideally before systemic corticosteroids are initiated.

Another pitfall is missing an underlying cause, such as sarcoidosis or inflammatory bowel disease. Take a careful history and perform a comprehensive physical examination to avoid missing these conditions.

## Counseling

You have an inflammation of the fat layer of your skin called "erythema nodosum." There are many causes of this condition; however, in many cases, a cause is not determined.

We need to determine whether your EN is caused by any oral medications, infections, or autoimmune/inflammatory diseases. You will likely require cultures, blood work, possibly a chest x-ray or other imaging tests, and occasionally a biopsy of your lesions. The biopsy may leave a permanent scar.

The good news is that your lesions will likely resolve within a matter of weeks to months. Rarely, the disease can persist for over 6 months and can sometimes recur. The sites that are involved can be discolored for a long time.

Treatment for this condition hinges on resting your legs, elevating them as much as possible above the level of your heart, and cooling the area with compresses several times a day. Taking either prescription (indomethacin) or over-the-counter (ibuprofen, naproxen) nonsteroidal anti inflammatory medications regularly can help with the pain and shorten your course. If this does not work, we can trial oral steroids, such as prednisone. Other medications include a medication used for gout, called "colchicine," or a thyroid medication called "potassium iodide."

# DIGITAL MUCOUS CYST (DIGITAL MYXOID PSEUDOCYST)

**Erisa Alia and Philip E. Kerr**

## Clinical Features

Digital mucous cyst (DMC), also known as digital myxoid pseudocyst, is a benign pseudocystic lesion that more typically involves the dorsal or lateral surfaces of the distal phalanx of the hands than the feet.

- The cysts mainly occur between the distal interphalangeal joint (DIJ) and the proximal nail fold.
- Although there is a predominance for the index and middle finger of the dominant hand, toe lesions are less commonly observed.
- DMC usually presents as a solitary, rubbery, dome-shaped, rounded or oval, slow-growing papule/nodule of 3 to 10 mm in diameter. It may be translucent, skin-colored, or pink to bluish in color. It may drain a clear, gelatinous, viscous fluid after firm palpation or minor trauma.
- Multiple lesions can be found in the case of underlying osteoarthritis (OA) of the nearby DIJ.

  Etiologically, they may arise either de novo from fibroblastic overproduction of hyaluronic acid in the upper dermis or as an extension from the DIJ space after a small tear in the joint capsule or tendon sheath of an osteoarthritic joint, allowing synovial fluid extravasation.

- In the latter cases, a pedicle connecting the cyst to the adjacent joint space may be demonstrated.

  DMC is typically asymptomatic but may occasionally be associated with decreased range of motion, pain, nail dystrophy, and periodic discharge.

- Lesions that involve the proximal nail fold may affect the nail matrix, resulting in the characteristic groove sign, a longitudinal depression in the nail plate extending from the DMC proximally to the tip of the nail plate distally.
- The incidence is higher in middle-aged and older females, a population more likely to develop OA.
- For younger patients, trauma is a typical preceding factor.

## Differential Diagnosis

DMC is a relatively common periungual papule that is typically diagnosed by history and physical examination and rarely requires further work-up.

When encountering an atypical presentation of DMC, the differential diagnosis includes rheumatoid nodules, Heberden nodes, glomus tumors, pyogenic granuloma (PG), and periungual warts.

- Rheumatoid nodules occur deeper in the dermis and are firmer to palpation than DMCs. They occur in patients with a history of rheumatoid arthritis. Typically, they affect joints other than the DIP.
- Heberden nodes are not actually fluid-filled lesions. They are firm to palpation and noncompressible. They occur in individuals with a history of osteoarthritis.
- Glomus tumors typically develop in the nail unit. They present with the typical triad of pain, pinpoint tenderness, and cold sensitivity.
- PG involves vascular lesions that bleed easily. They also present with overlying scale.
- Periungual warts are an epidermal process and therefore have overlying skin change. They are hyperkeratotic and noncompressible. They do not have a cyst like appearance. They show multiple black or red dots on dermoscopy and hypertrophic epithelium.

## Work-Up

Noninvasive or minimally invasive modalities that can help confirm a diagnosis of DMC include transillumination; needle puncture and aspiration; plain radiographs, ultrasonography, and magnetic resonance imaging (MRI); and dermoscopy.

- With transillumination, cases of DMC are positive for fluid-filled lesions.
- In the case of needle puncture and aspiration, DMC shows an expression of clear, gelatinous fluid.
- Plain radiographs, ultrasonography and MRI can help identify deeper lesions, especially when located under the nail plate. MRI can detect lesions as small as 1 mm.

- On dermoscopy, the lesions appear mainly as vascular structures with different vessel patterns (arborizing, polymorphic, punctate, or linear vessels), oval or round red-purple lacunas, ulceration, and white-shiny structures.

Definitive diagnosis of particularly deep or unusual DMC may require skin biopsy. Histologically, there are two types of DMC, the myxomatous type and the ganglion type.

- The myxomatous type is superficial, well circumscribed, and has a dermal collection of mucin without an epithelial lining.
- The ganglion type is deeply seated, usually near the joint and consists of mucin-filled pseudocystic spaces surrounded by flattened fibrocollagenous tissue. A pedicle is noted in many cases.

## Initial Steps in Management

Patients must be reassured on the benignity of this condition. If asymptomatic, observation may be appropriate. If required, treatment generally involves repeated puncture and drainage, manual regular compression, cryotherapy, intralesional corticosteroid injections, electrosurgical destruction, and/or surgical excision.

Surgical intervention is reserved for cases that fail conservative treatment and/or larger lesions that are symptomatic. These are often deep-seated DMCs of the ganglion type that involve larger joints. Aggressive surgical therapy may cause scarring of the nail matrix, resulting in permanent nail deformity.

## Warning Signs/Common Pitfalls

- Despite their benign nature, DMCs rarely disappear spontaneously.
- There is no treatment consensus nor a generally agreed-upon treatment algorithm for its management.
- Recurrence rates are high after conservative treatments.
- In case the conservative therapy fails, a referral to a dermatologist subspecializing in nail pathology or a hand surgeon may be necessary.
- It is generally accepted that surgical excision has the highest cure rate (95%).

## Counseling

You have a digital mucous cyst. This is benign but has a low tendency to self-resolve. Observation is recommended if it is not painful or otherwise bothersome. If the lesion is located close to the nail bed, it may cause grooving of the nail. These cysts are highly associated with underlying osteoarthritis of the nearby joints. Individuals who are bothered by these lesions frequently require surgical excision because it has a very high cure rate.

## PEARLY PENILE PAPULES

**Erisa Alia and Philip E. Kerr**

### Clinical Features

Pearly penile papules (PPP) are common, benign, non-infectious, asymptomatic lesions that occur on the glans penis. The characteristic clinical appearance involves small (0.5–2 mm), uniform, dome-shaped or filiform, closely aggregated papules.

- Color varies from pearly-white to pink to skin-colored.
- In terms of distribution, they are arranged circumferentially in one or two rows around the corona or sulcus of the glans penis.
- Estimates of the prevalence of PPP in the male population vary widely, ranging from approximately 15% to 50%.
  - The condition most often presents during adolescence or young adulthood, then becomes less common with age.
  - They are more common in uncircumcised men.
  - Some studies have indicated they are more common in Black males.

PPP are benign, unrelated to any known infection, and unrelated to sexual activity. Despite this, PPP can cause significant distress to affected individuals and their partners because of the misconception that the lesions may be caused by a sexually transmitted infection (STI).

- PPP are technically a variant of angiofibroma akin to fibrous papules of the nose.

In rare instances, atypical presentations of PPP may resemble condyloma acuminata (genital warts) or molluscum contagiosum.

### Work-Up

The diagnosis of this condition is almost always made by history and physical examination and rarely requires further work-up.

When encountering an atypical presentation, examination with dermoscopy and/or biopsy is recommended.

- Dermascopically, PPP present as a whitish-pink cobblestone or grape like appearance in a few rows, with each papule containing central dotted or comma-shaped vessels. No irregular reflections are appreciated, which suggests a lack of desquamation, an important clue to distinguish PPP from genital warts.

- Histopathologically, PPP present as dilated vessels and increase collagen fibers in the superficial dermis.
  - If the location of the lesion is not specified in the pathology requisition form, then they are diagnosed as angiofibromas by the pathologist.

## Initial Steps in Management

Patients must be reassured on the benignity of the condition. The lesions have a tendency to regress with age. Treatment is not routinely recommended and generally is reserved for patients who suffer extensive embarrassment or request therapy for cosmetic reasons. All treatment options are painful and have the potential for scarring.

Treatment options include electrodessication, cryotherapy with liquid nitrogen, laser therapy ($CO_2$ laser, Er:YAG laser, Erbium laser, or PDL), and curettage.

## Warning Signs/Common Pitfalls

PPP must be distinguished from two STIs, condyloma acuminata (genital warts) and molluscum contagiosum.

- Genital warts are larger, clinically verrucous, and asymmetrically arranged on the affected area. They also frequently affect the shaft and pubic area in general.
- Molluscum contagiosum lesions typically exhibit a central umbilication and, like genital warts, are also larger and asymmetrically arranged.
  - In adults, molluscum are typically sexually transmitted, whereas in children they are common and spread by direct contact with other children.

## Counseling

You have pearly penile papules. This is a very common, harmless, noncontagious condition that tends to regress with age. The condition is unrelated to sexual activity and is not the result of an infection. You and your partner do not require any laboratory tests. No treatment is needed for PPP, unless you request to have them removed.

# CHERRY ANGIOMA

Mohammed H. Malik and Philip E. Kerr

## Clinical Features

Cherry angioma, also known as "cherry hemangioma" and "senile hemangioma," is a very common benign skin lesion. They are the result of a proliferation of vascular endothelial cells near the surface of the skin, forming firm red or purple papules.

- The majority are 1 to 5 mm in diameter, but they may occasionally grow to 1 cm.
- They often begin as small red macules before becoming papular.
- They are occasionally thrombose and appear black.
- Cherry angiomas affect all skin surfaces except the palms, soles and genitals; they have a predilection for the head, neck, trunk, and proximal extremities.
- Given the location in the very surface of the skin, they may bleed relatively easily with scratching or other minor surface trauma.
- They are common in males and females of any race beginning in their 20s; they often increase in number with age.

## Differential Diagnosis

Cherry angiomas are readily identifiable based on their characteristic appearance. They are well-circumscribed, red-purple, dome-shaped papules that are uniform in color. Importantly, not all red papules on the trunk are cherry angiomas. The differential diagnosis for cherry angioma includes amelanotic melanoma, nodular basal cell carcinoma (BCC), PGs, and angiokeratomas.

- Cherry angiomas can be differentiated from amelanotic melanomas because cherry angiomas are stable in size; they are evenly pigmented throughout; they are not nodular; and they demonstrate clear septation between vascular lobules if examined with magnification.
- Cherry angiomas can be differentiated from nodular BCCs because cherry angiomas have a near-homogenous appearance; cherry angiomas are not accentuated by vigorously rubbing an alcohol prep pad atop them like BCCs are; cherry angiomas are stable in size; and cherry angiomas are typically much smaller than BCCs.
- PGs are vascular tumors that are characterized by a propensity to spontaneously bleed profusely. Although they may appear clinically similar to

cherry angiomas, they are typically larger, have overlying scale, and bleed without provocation. These lesions, unlike cherry angiomas, require treatment for symptomatic reasons, even though they are benign.

- Angiokeratomas are another benign vascular tumor that can occur in isolation or as part of a diagnostic grouping (e.g., angiokeratomas of Fordyce). They typically are darker appearing than cherry angiomas and are usually distinguished from cherry angiomas based on their role as part of a diagnostic grouping as aforementioned. Distinguishing between cherry angiomas and angiokeratomas is usually not clinically relevant because they are both benign.

## Work-Up

Work-up is generally not necessary, but if the diagnosis is in question, a biopsy is recommended. Certain compounds have been noted to cause cherry angiomas. These include mustard gas, cyclosporine, bromides, and 2-butoxyethanol.

## Initial Steps in Management

Because cherry angiomas are benign, treatment is not required. If lesions are symptomatic, a biopsy is typically indicated to rule out malignancy. If the patient is cosmetically bothered by the cherry angiomas, however, the treatment of choice is pulsed dye laser (PDL). If PDL is not readily available, cherry angiomas can be treated with low-level electrodessication (3–6); however, electrodessication has a higher risk for scarring than PDL. As previously noted, if the diagnosis is in question, surgical removal for pathologic examination is recommended.

## Warning Signs/Common Pitfalls

Despite the name, cherry angiomas can rarely appear purple or black in color if thrombosis occurs.

## Counseling

You have a cherry angioma, which is a benign (noncancerous) skin lesion. These spots develop on almost all people and generally increase in frequency with age. They can be found on almost any part of the body. They most often are a bright red and range from flat dots to larger bumps.

Cherry angiomas do not usually require any treatment. Do not scratch or irritate the angioma because this can cause bleeding and may necessitate removal of the lesion. If the lesion is cosmetically unappealing, it can be removed through a few different methods, depending on how large and deep it is.

If the lesion changes in size, shape, or color over a short period of time (2–3 months), inform your doctor. Rapid change may indicate the spot needs to be surgically removed and examined for signs of skin cancer.

# CHONDRODERMATITIS NODULARIS HELICIS

**Tatiana Abrantes and Afton Chavez**

## Clinical Features

Chondrodermatitis nodularis helicis (CNH; also known as "chondrodermatitis nodularis chronica helicis et antihelicis"; "Winkler disease"; or, colloquially, "ear corn") is a benign inflammatory condition that affects the skin and cartilage of the outer ear.

- The precise etiology is unknown; however, most believe CNH is caused by local ischemia from chronic and excessive pressure.
  - It may be caused by same-side sleeping, prolonged use of hearing aids, or the wearing of headphones and other headgear.
- Other potential causes include actinic damage, cold exposure, trauma, and autoimmune and connective tissue disorders that lead to inflammation.
- CNH is not contagious.
- CNH can occur in all ethnicities; however, is usually seen in fair-skinned older adults with chronic sun exposure.
  - Men tend to develop lesions on the helix at an earlier age.
  - Women tend to develop antihelix lesions.
- CNH is typically unilateral and localized to the sleeping side, but it can be bilateral.
- Classically, on physical examination, CNH presents as a single, oval nodule with raised, rolled edges with central crusts or, occasionally, keratin-filled craters.
  - Papules can be skin colored to erythematous.
  - The most common site is at the apex of the helix.
  - The nodule is firm, tender, and usually fixed to the auricular cartilage on palpation.

- Some patients experience bleeding or discharge of a small amount of scaly material at the site of the lesion.
- Patients with CNH typically complain of pain or tenderness to the area surrounding the papule.
  - Nocturnal pain is the most frequent symptom.
  - Daytime pain occurs with touching the affected area.

## Differential Diagnosis

The differential diagnosis for CNH includes actinic keratosis (AK), SCC, BCC, cutaneous horn, verruca (warts), keratoacanthoma (KA), weathering nodule, calcinosis cutis, gouty tophi, and reactive perforating collagenosis.

- AKs are very common on sites repeatedly exposed to the sun, such as the back of the hands and face. AKs may be solitary, but they more frequently present as multiple keratoses with varying appearance (flat or thickened rough papule, white, yellow, or pigmented, tender or asymptomatic). Biopsy will help differentiate between the two.
- CNH may often be confused with malignant skin conditions like BCC because of its nodular appearance and central crusting, or SCC if the lesions are larger and inflamed. Keratoacanthoma is a subtype of SCC that erupts like a little volcano. KAs grow much faster than CNH, and some of them may resolve spontaneously after a few months.
  - A significant dermoscopic finding for CNH that differentiates it from BCC or SCC is a consistent global configuration (daisy pattern), consisting of radially arranged white thick lines surrounding a central rounded yellow/brown clod.
  - A biopsy would also help in differentiating BCC, SCC, and KA from CNH.
- Because cutaneous horns are more commonly found on sun-exposed areas, such as the head and ears, it may be confused with CNH. The appearance of the cutaneous horn will allow you to differentiate it from CNH.
  - A cutaneous horn presents as a straight or curved, hard, yellow-brown projection from the skin. The horn is typically taller than twice the width of the base, whereas CNH does not present as a projection but just as a raised area.

- Unlike CNH, verrucas (warts) are contagious, skin-colored papules caused by infection with human papillomavirus (HPV). Clinically, warts interrupt skin lines and may have tiny black dots (vessels) under the hard skin.
- Weathering nodules are often misdiagnosed as CNH because of their prevalence on the helices of ears. In contrast to CNH, weathering nodules typically show no inflammation and are asymptomatic.
- Calcinosis cutis is the accumulation of calcium salt crystals in the skin, presenting as hard, whitish/yellowish bumps that do not dissolve. Unlike CNH, calcinosis cutis typically does not present as solitary bumps.
- Gouty tophi typically present as multiple nodules that protrude from the skin in patients with gout. Although they may occur on the ear, they also may occur on fingers and toes.
- Reactive perforating collagenosis is a rare skin disorder commonly presenting with multiple lesions on the surface of hands, elbows, knees, or trunk, unlike CNH.
  - The inherited form of reactive perforating collagenosis typically presents in childhood, allowing for distinction from CNH's manifestation in later adulthood.

## Work-Up

Diagnosis of CNH can begin with a clinical examination; however, confirmatory testing may be necessary, especially in cases without history of pressure to the area.

- Histopathologic confirmation by skin biopsy is often warranted to rule out more serious skin malignancies like SCC or BCC.
  - A shave biopsy is the diagnostic test of choice. Many authorities recommend performing a shave removal of the entire lesion cartilage because this is frequently curative.
    - Too deep of a biopsy can result in permanent deformation of the helix, which can be very cosmetically bothersome.
- Other testing to rule out systemic illness, like scleroderma, thyroid disease or other collagen vascular diseases and autoimmune diseases, can be done, especially if the presenting patient is a young adult under the age of 40.

## Initial Steps in Management

The primary goal should be to relieve or eliminate pressure at the site of the lesion. There are several options for treatment of CNH, including both invasive and noninvasive procedures.

- Conservative treatment includes padding to relieve pressure on the lesion.
  - This is the most cost effective and inexpensive method.
  - This can be achieved by adhering a foam sponge, foam egg crate, or foam bandage to the affected area and providing doughnut pillows for sleeping or encouraging the patient not to sleep on the affected side.
- Surgical options include shave removal, primary wedge-shaped excision of skin and cartilage with minimal margin, and punch biopsy. Treatment with cartilage removal alone provides the most curative and best cosmetic results.
  - Excision makes histopathologic examination possible; therefore it allows for the secure differentiation of CNH from other differential diagnoses.
  - Recurrence rates after surgical excision are reported at 10% to 30%.
  - Possible complications of partial cartilage excision include postoperative asymmetry of the ears and infection.
- Cryotherapy, also known as "cold therapy," may also be used to destroy the lesion by freezing and thawing the cells.
- Corticosteroid injections and topical corticosteroids may reduce local inflammation, aiding in pain management.
- $CO_2$ laser ablation is another treatment for CNH, where the patient is treated with the laser and the wound is allowed to heal by secondary intention.
- Soft tissue fillers, like local collagen or hyaluronic acid injections, may provide relief by offering cushioning and insulation.
- Nitroglycerin gel and patches containing 1% to 2% glyceryl trinitrate have been shown to relieve both symptoms and appearance when applied twice daily to the affected area.
  - Side effects of nitroglycerin may include a transient headache and skin irritation; therefore it is generally not recommended for patients with low blood pressure or a history of headaches.

## Warning Signs/Common Pitfalls

Although CNH is benign and has a good prognosis, it is important to remind patients that long-term morbidity is common and that it can recur. Because spontaneous resolution is extremely rare, it is important for CNH to be treated properly.

- Establishing the correct diagnosis is crucial to ensuring the lesion is not a skin cancer.
- There is a lack of trials that study CNH; therefore there is no clear consensus on which treatment is the best. Educating the patient to avoid ear pressure should be of the utmost important to provide symptom relief.
- Testing for autoimmune diseases and connective tissue disorders can be done in rare cases, especially if the presenting patient is a young adult under the age of 40.

## Counseling

You have chondrodermatitis nodularis helicis (CNH), which is a benign, inflammatory condition that affects the skin and cartilage of the outer ear. Although it is not entirely well understood why CNH occurs, your condition was likely caused by chronic, excessive pressure on the outer ear, such as chronically sleeping on that side. CNH is not contagious.

Fortunately, there are treatments for CNH. The primary goal for treatment of CNH is to eliminate pressure at the site of the lesion. There are several options, including invasive and noninvasive remedies. The most conservative form of treatment involves using padding to relieve the area. This can be done by adhering a foam sponge or a foam bandage to the affected area. Using a doughnut pillow or avoiding sleeping on the affected side can also help. In addition to these methods of relieving pressure, we can also use corticosteroid injections or topical steroids to reduce local inflammation and aid in pain management and soft tissue fillers, like collagen injections, to offer more cushioning and insulation in that area.

Surgical options include a wedge-shaped excision of skin and cartilage. If the lesion is large, a punch biopsy followed by ear reconstruction may be necessary. Although surgical excision, primarily cartilage removal alone, provides the most curative and best cosmetic results, CNH can still recur after surgical excision at a 10% to 30% rate. As with all surgeries, there are some possible complications; these include postoperative asymmetry of the ears and infection. Cryotherapy, which involves freezing and thawing the cells in that area, is also a treatment option.

Depending on how aggressive you would like to be with your treatment and if your symptoms are manageable, it may be best to begin by following more conservative protocols of reducing pressure in the lesioned area. Unfortunately, long-term symptoms from CNH are common and it can recur, regardless of treatment type. CNH will rarely resolve on its own; therefore it is important for CNH to be treated for symptom relief. Additionally, if you are under the age of 40 and have other significant symptoms, it may be worth testing for other autoimmune and connective tissue disorders that lead to inflammation because those may be a cause of CNH.

# SECTION 5

# Hair Loss

# 12

# Common Skin Cancers

## CHAPTER OUTLINE

## BASAL CELL CARCINOMA

**Aziz Khan, Jonas Adalsteinsson, and Hao Feng**

### Clinical Features

- Basal cell carcinoma (BCC) of the skin is the most common type of skin cancer. It is most common in Caucasians and uncommon in individuals with darker skin types. When darker-skinned patients develop a BCC, it is often pigmented clinically.
- The major risk factor for BCC development is ultraviolet (UV) exposure in the setting of predisposing genetics.
- BCCs develop in areas of chronic actinic skin damage, especially the face (70%) followed by the trunk (15%) and lower limbs of women.
- BCC has many variants, with the most common being the nodular, superficial, and morpheaform subtypes.

### Nodular Basal Cell Carcinoma

- Nodular BCC is the most common subtype, accounting for 80% of cases of BCC.
- It most commonly occurs on the face, especially the nose, cheeks, forehead, nasolabial folds, and eyelids.
- It typically presents as a pearly pink or flesh-colored papule or nodule with surface telangiectasias and often has a rolled raised border.
- It may enlarge and ulcerate (the so-called "rodent ulcer" appearance).
- Recurrent crusting or bleeding is often reported by the patient.

### Superficial Basal Cell Carcinoma

- Superficial BCC is the second most common subtype, accounting for 15% of cases.
- It most commonly occurs on the trunk.

- It typically presents as a light red to pink, slightly scaly, macule, patch, or thin papule or plaque that may appear shiny when illuminated.
- It is often asymptomatic and may appear nonspecific and subtle on examination.

## Morpheaform Basal Cell Carcinoma

- Morpheaform BCC accounts for 5% to 10% of cases.
- It typically presents as a smooth, white or flesh-colored papule or plaque with a depressed area of induration and irregular borders.
- It may resemble a scar.
- It is more aggressive than superficial or nodular BCC with a greater propensity for local destruction.

## Other Variants

- Other rare variants of BCC include infundibulocystic, basosquamous, metatypical, or fibroepithelioma of Pinkus (a rare variant of BCC that may be benign-appearing and present as a pink pedunculated lesion that can resemble an acrochordon).
- Both nodular and superficial BCCs can produce a variable amount of melanin; when pigmentation is noted, the lesion is often termed "pigmented BCC" and can clinically be confused with melanoma.

## Work-Up

- A detailed history should be obtained, focusing on the personal and family history of skin cancer; the use of immunosuppressive medication; and the existence of other underlying medical conditions, such as transplant history.
- Careful examination of the skin should be performed.
- After a lesion is identified as clinically suspicious, it is recommended that the lesion be evaluated using a dermatoscope (a handheld magnifier with a light source that can be polarized or nonpolarized with a transparent plate) to help you see deeper into the skin unobstructed by skin surface reflections.
- Dermoscopy assists with establishing the diagnosis of a BCC and is especially useful for distinguishing BCCs from intradermal nevi and sebaceous gland hyperplasia. It often helps to rub the lesion gently with alcohol because this will make the vessels more visible on dermoscopy.
- Dermoscopic features of BCC are mainly arborizing vessels, blue-gray ovoid nests, shiny white structures,

leaf like structures, spoke-wheel areas, and the absence of findings typically associated with other skin conditions (such as the lack of a pigmented network, which is classically associated with melanocytic lesions).

- A full-body skin examination should be performed to identify concurrent BCCs or other types of skin cancers.
- Before removal, distant and close-up digital clinical photography should be undertaken to accurately portray the clinical location.
- In most cases, the suspected lesion should not be treated (using, for example, curettage or an electrodessication and curettage [ED&C]) before obtaining a skin biopsy. A skin biopsy is required to exclude less common mimickers (such as amelanotic melanoma) and establish the histologic subtype.
- Shave biopsies are, in most cases, sufficient to make an accurate diagnosis. Punch biopsies may be appropriate when the lesion is small and might have a deep extension. Incisional and excisional biopsies are rarely performed for diagnosing BCC.
- In areas where Mohs micrographic surgery (MMS) might be required, such as the face, only a small portion of the lesion is required to make the diagnosis. A biopsy with large margins might do the patient a disservice by removing an excessive amount of tissue.

## Initial Steps in Management

- Treatment options for BCC include both surgical and nonsurgical therapies.
- Treatment selection depends on patient age, gender, comorbid conditions, and tumor characteristics.
- BCCs can generally be classified into low and high likelihood of recurrence after treatment. Tumor size, site, and histopathologic subtype determine the risk for recurrence.
  - One risk feature is a tumor of any size on high-risk areas of the face (central face, nose, lips, eyelids, eyebrows, periorbital skin, chin, mandibles, ears, preauricular, postauricular areas, and temples), hands, or feet. The high-risk sites on the face include embryologic cleavage planes, which provide little resistance to tumor invasion.
  - Tumors that are larger than 10 mm in diameter on the head and neck and larger than 20 mm in diameter in all other anatomic areas are also risks for recurrence.

- Aggressive pathologic features, such as the morpheaform, micronodular, and basosquamous subtypes, may also suggest a risk for recurrence.
- Other high recurrence risk features include recurrent lesions, tumors in sites of prior radiation therapy, tumors in patients on immunosuppressive therapy or with immunocompromised conditions, and tumors with perineural invasion.
- Primary goals of therapy include complete removal of the tumor to prevent recurrence and the provision of an optimal cosmetic outcome.

## Surgical Treatment Options

Surgical treatment options include standard surgical excision, ED&C, and MMS.

- Standard surgical excision is the first-line therapy for tumors with a low risk for recurrence in suitable anatomic locations, such as the trunk and extremities.
  - Standard surgical excision may also be an alternative treatment option for select high-risk patients when MMS is not available or not preferred by the patient.
  - For low-risk patients, margins of 3 to 4 mm are considered to be appropriate. For high-risk patients, margins greater than 4 mm are more appropriate.
- ED&C is an option for small, low-risk BCCs on the trunk and extremities.
  - Its main advantages include that it is less invasive than wide excision and more convenient for many patients.
  - Disadvantages include a higher recurrence rates (inability to confirm clearance histologically) and a poor cosmetic outcome because a scar will result. Thus it is often used mainly for BCCs on the trunk and extremities.
- MMS provides the best long-term cure rates and a superior cosmetic outcome.
  - It is the first-line therapy for high-risk BCCs and recurrent BCCs on cosmetically and functionally sensitive areas.
  - Examination of all tissue margins during the procedure allows for the identification of inapparent subclinical tumor extension, resulting in excellent long-term cure rates.
  - It maximizes tissue sparing, thus allowing the preservation of vital structures and providing the best cosmetic outcome.

- Disadvantages include cost (although it is cost effective for appropriate lesions), lack of availability in many counties in America, and the lengthy procedure time (typically 2–4 hours).

## Nonsurgical Treatment Options

Nonsurgical treatment options include cryosurgery, topical therapies, and radiation therapy.

- Cryosurgery is a relatively quick, cost-effective procedure, which is in some cases indicated for smaller, superficial BCCs of the trunk for those wishing to avoid surgical procedures.
  - Liquid nitrogen is used to freeze the tumor and a small surrounding margin of normal-appearing skin.
  - Disadvantages of cryotherapy include a higher recurrence rate and poor cosmetic outcome (can cause hypertrophic scarring and permanent hypopigmentation).
- Topical therapies for BBC include 5-fluorouracil (5-FU) 5% cream and imiquimod 5% cream. Both are approved by the U.S. Food and Drug Administration (FDA) for the treatment of superficial BCCs.
  - Topical therapies are indicated for patients with multiple superficial BCCs, those who are poor surgical candidates, and those who do not wish to undergo surgery. It should not be done on tumors with high-risk features and cosmetically and functionally sensitive areas.
  - 5-FU 5% cream is generally applied twice daily for 4 to 6 weeks; however, some patients may achieve the desired inflammatory response (erythema, crusting, and scab formation) in as early as 2 weeks.
  - Imiquimod 5% cream is applied at bedtime 5 days per week for 6 weeks until the target inflammatory reaction is achieved. Imiquimod can be bothersome for patients to use because it comes in single-use packets. Each packet of cream, however, may be enough for multiple uses by the patient and therefore needs to be left open after each use. We recommend slicing a small opening in the packet from which the patient can squeeze a small amount of medicine daily.
  - Major disadvantages of topical therapy include application site reactions, hypopigmentation or hyperpigmentation, inability to confirm complete clearance of tumor histologically, and a higher recurrence rate. Some patients also complain of

flu like symptoms if the topical creams are applied to a larger area.

- Radiation therapy is an alternative option when surgery is contraindicated.
  - It can also be used as an adjuvant treatment of BCC when complete tumor removal is not achievable because of invasion of vital structures by tumor cells.
  - Disadvantages of radiation therapy include its high recurrence rate, high cost, prolonged course of therapy, poor cosmetic outcome, and increased risk for future skin cancers.
- Other nonsurgical treatment options for BCC include photodynamic therapy (which is a noninvasive, nonscarring treatment for superficial BCCs), systemic therapy with vismodegib or sonidegib (which are sonic hedgehog pathway blockers that are approved by the FDA for the treatment of advanced or metastatic BCC), and 500 mg of nicotinamide twice daily to decrease the incidence of nonmelanoma skin cancers.

## Warning Signs/Common Pitfalls

- After a first diagnosis of BCC, patients should be referred to a dermatologist because there is an increased risk for developing additional or recurrent BCCs as well as other cancerous or precancerous skin conditions.
- Pigmented BCCs should be distinguished from melanoma because therapy and prognosis differ significantly for both conditions.

**TABLE 12.1   Summary of Commonly Encountered Clinical Scenarios Involving Basal Cell Carcinomas**

| Clinical Scenario | Treatment Recommendations |
| --- | --- |
| **BCC of the trunk or extremities, with positive margins after biopsy** | • A standard excision with 4-mm clinical margins provides the highest chance of a cure.<br>• ED&C if patient would prefer to avoid surgery and stitches. There is a higher risk for recurrence and the patient must be counseled on the scar that will result.<br>• Topical imiquimod or 5-FU for small/superficial lesions if the patient wants to avoid surgical intervention. Close clinical follow-up is recommended. |
| **BCC of the trunk or extremities with negative margins after biopsy**<br>**Note: negative margins on biopsy may not reflect true clinical negative margin** | • Do nothing and clinically follow the patient.<br>• A standard excision or ED&C.<br>• Imiquimod or 5-FU for 3–6 weeks; chance of recurrence is still 10%–20%. |
| **BCC of the trunk or extremities, less than 20 mm diameter: positive margins after standard excision** | • Standard re-excision.<br>• Consider an MMS referral. |
| **BCC of a cosmetically or functionally critical area on the face/neck/hands/feet with positive margins** | • MMS |
| **BCC of a cosmetically critical area on the face/neck with negative margins**<br>**Note: negative margins on biopsy may not reflect true clinical negative margin** | • Strongly consider MMS referral to minimize chance of recurrence and optimize cosmetic outcome.<br>• Watch with a close clinical follow-up.<br>• Imiquimod or 5-FU for 3–6 weeks; chance of recurrence is still 10%–20%. |
| **Multiple BCCs** | • Topical therapy using 5-FU or Imiquimod.<br>• Photodynamic therapy.<br>• Sonic hedgehog pathway inhibitors for extreme cases, such as Gorlin syndrome. Often not tolerated because of side effects. |

*BCC*, Basal cell carcinoma; *ED&C*, electrodessication and curettage; *MMS*, Mohs micrographic surgery; *5FU*, 5-fluorouracil.

- The differential for BCCs includes Merkel cell carcinoma and amelanotic melanoma, tumors which both have high metastatic potential. Therefore biopsy is strongly recommended in most cases to confirm the diagnosis. A Merkel cell carcinoma or amelanotic melanoma treated with ED&C without a biopsy could have disastrous consequences. BCCs, especially superficial BCCs, can also be confused with inflammatory skin conditions, like nummular dermatitis or psoriasis. The possibility of a superficial BCC should be considered if a presumed inflammatory lesion does not respond to topical steroids.
- If a biopsy is undertaken and margins are clear, there is still a 20% to 30% risk for tumor recurrence as negative margins on biopsy may not reflect true clinical negative margin. Topical therapy with imiquimod or 5-FU can be used to reduce recurrence risk, or standard surgical treatment can be performed to ensure full clearance. For areas of high cosmetic importance, MMS should be strongly considered despite biopsy margins being negative.

## Counseling

Skin cancers occur when healthy skin cells transform into abnormal cells. Basal cell carcinoma is a common type of skin cancer and the least dangerous type of skin cancer. Basal cell carcinoma can be, in most cases, entirely removed when caught early. Very rarely, it spreads to other parts of the body; however, it can spread locally if left untreated.

Skin cancer can present as a nonspecific abnormal area of skin. It can present as a pink, crusty, bleeding bump or as a wound that will not heal. You should always show your doctor any skin changes you think might be abnormal. Your doctor will examine the spots and check the skin all over your body. Further tests, including a skin biopsy, will be suggested if your doctor suspects a skin cancer.

Skin cancer is often caused by chronic sun exposure. Sun exposure is the most important and most preventable risk factor for all skin cancers, including basal cell carcinoma. Damaging effects of sun are cumulative and therefore sun protection is urged, no matter what your age is.

You can prevent skin cancers by helping protect your skin from sun damage. Apply sunscreen to all exposed areas, preferably a water-resistant sunscreen with a Sun Protection Factor (SPF) of at least 30 that provides broad-spectrum protection from both ultraviolet A (UVA) and ultraviolet B (UVB) rays. Reapply every 2 hours, even on cloudy days, and after sweating or swimming. Sunscreens are not perfect because some ultraviolet light may still get through; do not use them to allow you to prolong your sun exposure. You should seek shade when possible and be aware that the sun's rays are the strongest between 10 AM and 4 PM. Wear sun-protective clothing, such as pants, a wide-brimmed hat, a long-sleeved shirt, and sunglasses, when possible. Some sunlight will still get across your clothing. You can wear sunscreen underneath, or you can buy clothing that has been treated to give additional sun protection.

Protect children from sun exposure by dressing them in protective clothing, applying sunscreen after they are older than 6 months, and having them play in the shade. Use extra precaution when near water, snow, and sand. These surfaces reflect the damaging rays of the sun and can increase your chance of getting sunburnt. Get vitamin D safely through a healthy diet rather than seeking the sun for vitamin D.

Avoid tanning beds. UV rays from tanning beds can also lead to wrinkling and skin cancer. Perform a regular self-skin examination. If you notice anything changing, growing, or bleeding on your skin, see a dermatologist. Skin cancer is very treatable when caught early.

# SQUAMOUS CELL CARCINOMA

**Aziz Khan, Jonas Adalsteinsson, and Hao Feng**

## Clinical Features

Cutaneous squamous cell carcinoma (SCC) is the second most common type of skin cancer in the United States.

- Incidence increases with age; it is uncommon in those under 45 years of age and it is more common in Caucasians.
- The major risk factor for SCC development is UV exposure in the setting of predisposing genetics, immunosuppression and/or HPV (human papilloma virus)
- SCCs can develop on any cutaneous surface. SCCs most commonly arise on sun-exposed areas in Caucasians and non–sun-exposed areas in individuals with darker skin types.
- They can clinically present with so-called "horns" with thick, vertically oriented hyperkeratotic scale.

This type of lesion should always be biopsied to sample the base of the lesion.

## Squamous Cell Carcinoma in Situ (Bowen Disease)

- SCC in situ typically presents as a well-demarcated, erythematous, scaly patch or plaque on sun-exposed areas. The lesion can also be pigmented, particularly in people with darker skin types.
- The lesions are usually asymptomatic and tend to grow slowly over many years.
- SCC in situ of the penis, termed "erythroplasia of Queyrat," may present with pruritus, pain, or bleeding. The lesion is usually a well-demarcated red plaque.
- SCC is on a spectrum with its premalignant counterpart, actinic keratosis (AK).
- SCC in situ or early invasive SCC can sometimes be clinically difficult to distinguish from some AKs, especially bowenoid AK and hyperkeratotic AK.

## Invasive Squamous Cell Carcinoma

- The clinical appearance of invasive SCC varies with the degree of tumor differentiation.
- Well-differentiated tumors present as indurated, firm hyperkeratotic papules, plaques, or nodules. Ulceration is infrequent.
- Poorly differentiated tumors present as fleshy papules or nodules that lack hyperkeratosis. The lesions usually ulcerate and bleed.
- The lesions are typically asymptomatic; however, patients might present with pain, itching, or bleeding. Tumors with perineural invasion present with local neurologic symptoms, such as numbness, burning, paresthesia, and paralysis.

## Clinical Variants of SCC

Clinical variants of SCC include keratoacanthoma, cutaneous SCC of the lip, oral SCC, verrucous carcinoma, and Marjolin ulcer.
- Keratoacanthoma is believed to be a subtype of a well-differentiated SCC.
  - These tumors are predominantly found on sun-damaged skin, and present as rapidly growing dome-shaped or crateriform nodules with a central keratotic core.
- Cutaneous SCC of the lip mostly occurs on the lower lip.
  - Lesions may present as indurated nonhealing ulcers, nodules, or white plaques.

- Oral SCC primarily occurs on the floor of the mouth and the lateral or ventral tongue.
  - Lesions may present as indurated, nonhealing ulcers, nodules or white plaques.
  - Lesions may present clinically as erythroplakia or leukoplakia and are often associated with tobacco and/or alcohol use. It should be noted that erythroplakia is in most cases associated with malignancy, whereas leukoplakia is more likely to be premalignant or because of chronic trauma.
- Verrucous carcinoma is an uncommon variant of SCC, which manifests as well-defined, exophytic, cauliflower-like growths resembling large warts.
- Marjolin ulcer is a rare type of SCC arising in sites of long-standing chronic wounds or scars.
  - The malignant transformation is often very slow, with an average latency period of around 30 years.
  - It presents as a nonhealing ulceration. Other features include rolled wound margins, excessive granulation tissue, brisk growth, and easy bleeding.

## Work-Up

- A detailed history should be obtained, focusing on the patient's personal and family history of skin cancer, as well as the use of immunosuppressive medication and other underlying medical conditions, such as transplant history.
- A careful examination of the skin should be performed.
- After a lesion is identified as clinically suspicious, it is recommended that the lesion be evaluated using a dermatoscope (handheld magnifier with a light source that can be polarized or nonpolarized with a transparent plate) that helps you see deeper into the skin unobstructed by skin surface reflections.
- Dermoscopy assists with establishing the diagnosis of a SCC and is especially useful for distinguishing SCCs from intradermal nevi and sebaceous gland hyperplasia.
- SCCs are often covered with thick scale, making dermoscopic evaluation difficult. It often helps to rub the lesion gently with alcohol to remove the scale.
- Dermoscopic features of SCC in situ and SCC are dotted and/or glomerular vessels (hairpin vessels can be more commonly seen in the KA type of SCC); white to yellowish surface scales; blood spots; white, shiny structures; and the absence of findings typically associated with other skin conditions (such

as the lack of a pigmented network, which is classically associated with melanocytic lesions).

- A full-body skin examination should be performed to identify concurrent SCCs, precancerous lesions, or other type of skin cancers.
- Before surgical biopsy or removal, digital clinical images should be obtained at a distance as well as close up to accurately document the anatomic location.
- The suspected lesion should be biopsied before treatment. A skin biopsy is required to exclude less common mimickers, confirm the diagnosis, and establish the histologic subtype.
- Shave biopsies are, in most cases, sufficient to make an accurate diagnosis. Punch biopsies can be suitable when the lesion is small and/or might have a deep extension.
- In cosmetically and functionally sensitive areas where Mohs surgery might be required, such as the face, only a small portion of the lesion is required to make the diagnosis. A biopsy with large margins might do the patient a disservice by removing an excessive amount of tissue.
- A portion of the dermis (at least up to the upper or midreticular dermis) should be included in the biopsy specimen to evaluate possible tumor invasion and to best guide appropriate therapy.

## Initial Steps in Management

- In contrast to BCC, SCC has a considerably higher potential to metastasize to regional lymph nodes and more distant sites.
- Early recognition and treatment provide the best opportunity to cure SCC.
- Treatment options for SCC include both surgical and nonsurgical therapies.
- Treatment selection depends on patient age, gender, comorbid conditions, and tumor characteristics.
- SCC can generally be classified into low-risk and high-risk SCCs. Tumor size, site, depth of invasion, and histopathologic differentiation determine the risk for recurrence and metastasis.
  - A tumor of any size on the lip or ear increases the risk for recurrence.
  - Tumors greater than or equal to 20 mm in diameter on the trunk and extremities also increase the risk for recurrence.
  - Tumors equal to or greater than 10 mm in diameter on the cheeks, forehead, scalp, neck, or pretibial area increase the risk as well, as do tumors

equal to or greater than 6 mm in diameter on high-risk areas of the face, hands, or feet.
  - Other features that increase the risk for recurrence include recurrent tumors; tumors in patients on immunosuppressive therapy, with immunocompromised conditions, or with history of transplantation; tumor location in sites of chronic wounds, scars, or the site of previous ionizing radiation; and certain histologic features, such as perineural invasion, poor differentiation, and deep microinvasion beyond subcutis.
- Primary goals of therapy include complete removal of the tumor to prevent recurrence and the provision of an optimal cosmetic outcome.

## Surgical Treatment Options

Surgical treatment options include standard surgical excision, MMS, and CCPDMA.

- Standard surgical excision is the first-line therapy for tumors with a low risk for recurrence in suitable anatomic locations, such as the trunk and extremities.
  - A clinical margin of 3 to 4 mm of uninvolved skin is recommended for low-risk SCCs.
  - Standard surgical excision is not the preferred method for high-risk SCCs. If performed, however, a margin of 5 to 10 mm is recommended.
- MMS is performed under local anesthesia and provides the best long-term cure rates and a superior cosmetic outcome.
  - It is the first-line therapy for high-risk, localized SCCs.
  - It should be considered in low-risk patients for sites where function is at risk (such as the hands, feet, or genitalia) or cosmetics and tissue sparing is important (like the face).
  - Examination of all tissue margins during the procedure allows for the identification of inapparent subclinical tumor extensions, resulting in excellent long-term cure rates.
  - It maximizes tissue sparing, thus allowing preservation of vital structures and providing the best cosmetic outcome.
  - Disadvantages include cost (although it can be cost effective for appropriate lesions) and the lengthy procedure time (typically 2–4 hours).
- CCPDMA is an alternative to MMS.
  - It is typically performed for larger tumors that require excision under general anesthesia.

## Nonsurgical Treatment Options

Nonsurgical treatment options include cryosurgery, ED&C, radiation therapy, topical therapies, and chemo-prevention.

- Cryosurgery is a relatively quick, cost-effective procedure for those wishing to avoid invasive procedures.
  - It may be used for small, low-risk in situ SCCs.
  - Liquid nitrogen is used to freeze the tumor and a small surrounding margin of normal-appearing skin.
  - Disadvantages of cryotherapy include a higher recurrence rate, poor cosmetic outcome (can cause hypertrophic scarring and permanent hypopigmentation), and inability to confirm complete clearance of tumor histologically.
- ED&C may be used for small, well-defined, superficial, low-risk SCCs on noncritical sites.
  - It is inexpensive, convenient, and associated with a low complication rate.
  - It is contraindicated for large, poorly defined, or high-risk SCCs.
  - Disadvantages include higher recurrence rates (inability to confirm clearance histologically) and a bad cosmetic outcome because a scar will result. Thus it is mostly used for BCCs on the trunk and extremities.
- Radiation therapy is not routinely used as mono-therapy because of the high risk for recurrence.
  - It can be used an alternative therapy for patients who are not surgical candidates.
  - It can also be used as an adjuvant treatment for high-risk SCC to decrease the risk for local recurrence.
  - It may also be used to control symptoms or salvage therapy when complete tumor removal is not achievable because of perineural invasion or invasion of vital structures by tumor cells.
  - Disadvantages of radiation therapy include the high cost, prolonged course of therapy, poor cosmetic outcome, and increased risk for future skin cancers.
- Topical therapies, including 5-FU 5% cream and imiquimod 5% cream, are not approved by the FDA for the treatment of SCCs; however, they have been used off-label to treat SCC in situ.
  - They are often preferred by patients who have had multiple surgical treatments in the past and prefer noninvasive therapy. They may be used for patients who refuse surgery and other therapies for SCC in situ.
  - 5-FU 5% cream is generally applied twice daily for 4 to 8 weeks; however, some patients may achieve the desired inflammatory response (erythema, crusting, and scab formation) in as early as 2 weeks.
  - Imiquimod 5% cream is applied at bedtime 5 days per week for 6 to 16 weeks until the target inflammatory reaction is achieved. Imiquimod can be bothersome for patients to use because it comes in single-use packets. Nevertheless, each packet of cream may be enough for multiple uses by the patient and therefore needs to be left open after each use. We recommend slicing a small opening in the packet from which the patient can squeeze a small amount of medicine daily.
  - Major disadvantages of topical therapy include application site reactions, hypopigmentation or hyperpigmentation, and an inability to confirm complete clearance of tumor histologically. Some patients also complain of flu like symptoms if the topical creams are applied to a larger area.
- Chemoprevention, through the use of oral retinoids (such as acitretin or isotretinoin) may reduce the development of new primary SCCs but has not been shown to decrease the risk for recurrence in high-risk SCCs.
  - Oral retinoids may be considered in patients who develop SCCs frequently (three to five SCCs per year) to reduce the development of subsequent SCCs, especially in transplant patients.
  - 500 mg of nicotinamide twice daily may decrease the incidence of nonmelanoma skin cancers.
- Other nonsurgical treatment options for SCC include systemic chemotherapy and chemoradiotherapy, which are primarily used in advanced locoregional and metastatic disease.

## Warning Signs/Common Pitfalls

- After a first diagnosis of SCC, patients should be referred to a dermatologist because there is an increased risk for developing additional or recurrent SCCs and other cancerous or precancerous skin conditions.
- A full-body skin examination should be performed by a dermatologist to identify coexisting skin cancers or precancerous conditions.

**TABLE 12.2    Summary of Commonly Encountered Clinical Scenarios Involving Squamous Cell Carcinomas**

| Clinical Scenario | Treatment Recommendations |
|---|---|
| SCC of the trunk or extremities with positive margins on biopsy. | • Standard excision with a 4 mm clinical margins.<br>• ED&C if patient would prefer to avoid surgery; there is a higher chance of recurrence and the patient must be counseled on the scar that will result. |
| SCC of the trunk or extremities with negative margins after biopsy.<br>Note: negative margins on biopsy may not reflect true clinical negative margin. | • Do nothing, and clinically follow the patient.<br>• Standard excision or ED&C. |
| SCC of the trunk or extremities, less than 20 mm: positive margin with standard excision. | • Strongly consider MMS referral.<br>• Resection with complete circumferential margin assessment. |
| SCC of a cosmetically critical area on the face/neck with positive margins. | • MMS. |
| • SCC of a cosmetically critical area on the face/neck with negative margins.<br>• Note: negative margins on biopsy may not reflect true clinical negative margin. | • Strongly consider MMS referral to minimize chance of recurrence and optimize cosmetic outcome.<br>• Watch with close clinical follow-up. |
| • Bowen disease (SSC in situ). | • Standard excision with a 4-mm clinical margin.<br>• Topical therapy (not FDA approved).<br>• ED&C if patient would prefer to avoid surgery.<br>• Photodynamic therapy. |
| • SCC, locally advanced, nonresectable. | • Radiation therapy.<br>• Chemoradiotherapy. |
| • SCC, metastatic. | • Chemotherapy.<br>• Anti-PD-1 and PD-L1 inhibitors. |

*ED&C*, Electrodessication and curettage; *FDA*, Food and Drug Administration; *MMS*, Mohs micrographic surgery; *PD-1*, programmed cell death-1; *PD-L1*, programmed cell death-1 ligand; *SCC*, squamous cell carcinoma; *5FU*, 5-fluorouracil.

- AKs can resemble early SCC. Although the malignant transformation of AKs to SCC is very low, approximately 60% of SCC arise from prior AKs. Tenderness, induration, and bleeding suggest the possibility of underlying SCC and such lesions should be biopsied.
- SCC in situ can be confused with inflammatory skin conditions like nummular dermatitis or psoriasis. Possibility of SCC in situ should be considered if a presumed inflammatory lesion does not respond to topical therapies.

## Counseling

Skin cancers occur when healthy skin cells transform into abnormal cells. Squamous cell carcinoma is a common type of skin cancer. Squamous cell carcinoma can be easily treated when diagnosed early; however, it can spread to other parts of the body if the diagnosis is delayed or if it is left untreated.

Skin cancer can present as a nonspecific abnormal area of skin. It can present as a pink, crusty, bleeding bump, or a wound that will not heal. You should always show your doctor any skin changes you think might be abnormal. Your doctor will examine the spots and check the skin all over your body. Further tests, including a skin biopsy, will be suggested if your doctor suspects a skin cancer.

Skin cancer is often caused by chronic sun exposure. Sun exposure is the most important and most preventable risk factor for all skin cancers, including squamous cell carcinoma. Damaging effects of the sun are cumulative and therefore sun protection is urged, no matter what your age.

You can prevent skin cancers by helping protect your skin from sun damage. Apply sunscreen to all exposed areas, preferably a water-resistant sunscreen with an SPF of at least 30 that provides broad-spectrum protection from both UVA and UVB rays. Reapply every 2 hours, even on cloudy days, and after sweating or swimming. Sunscreens are not perfect because some ultraviolet light may still get through; do not use them to allow you to prolong your sun exposure. You should seek shade when possible and be aware that the sun's rays are the strongest between 10 AM and 4 PM. Wear sun-protective clothing, such as pants, a wide-brimmed hat, a long-sleeved shirt, and sunglasses, when possible. Some sunlight will still get across your clothing. You can wear sunscreen underneath, or you can buy clothing that has been treated to give additional sun protection.

Protect children from sun exposure by dressing them in protective clothing, applying sunscreen, and having them play in the shade. Use extra precaution when near water, snow, and sand. These surfaces reflect the damaging rays of the sun and can increase your chance of sunburn. Get vitamin D safely through a healthy diet rather than seeking the sun for vitamin D.

Avoid tanning beds. UV rays from tanning beds can also lead to wrinkling and skin cancer. Perform a regular self-skin examination. If you notice anything changing, growing, or bleeding on your skin, see a dermatologist. Skin cancer is very treatable when caught early.

## MALIGNANT MELANOMA

### Clinical Features

Malignant melanoma (MM) (Fig 12.1) is a malignant tumor made up of melanocytes that is responsible for around 75% of skin cancer–related deaths. Early detection of MM is imperative because survival is very good for melanoma that remains localized in the skin.

- MM is more common in men than women; however, the incidence has been noted to be reversed during women's childbearing years.
- It most frequently presents in individuals aged 55 to 74 years; however, it occurs in all ages and is actually the second most common malignancy in women between the ages of 20 and 29 years.
- Most common location for MM is the upper back in men and calves in women, although MM can develop anywhere on the body.
  - It is especially common on heavily sun-damaged skin.

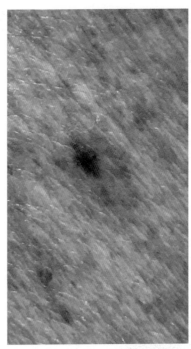

**Fig. 12.1 Malignant Melanoma.** Note the variegated pigmentation. (Courtesy Jonas Adalsteinsson, MD.)

- Major risk factors include fair skin, light eyes, a history of extensive sun exposure or tanning bed use, a history of sunburns, more than 50 melanocytic nevi, more than five clinically atypical nevi, a personal history of melanoma, a family history of melanoma in a first-degree relative, and personal history of organ transplantation.
- The vast majority of melanomas are asymptomatic; however, ulceration is an important clue for cutaneous malignancy and has prognostic implications

For clinical diagnosis of flat pigmented lesions based on visual inspection alone, the ABCDE criteria are recommended.

- Asymmetry asks, "Can the lesion be folded on itself in a way that the internal appearance of both halves of the lesion appear near-identical?"
  - Symmetry involves not only lesion shape but also an evaluation of the internal appearance or pattern of the lesion.
- An irregular border is defined as a border that is either difficult to define and not well circumscribed or

appears as though it is reaching out asymmetrically in a specific direction suggesting active growth.

- Importantly, nevi do not have to be perfectly circular or oval to be benign.
- In terms of color, more than three colors within a pigmented lesion are highly suspicious for melanoma.
  - Although many providers are concerned about "dark" nevi, these are not necessarily malignant especially if the patient has multiple nevi that are equally dark .
- In terms of diameter (or different, see the so-called "ugly duckling" sign), most melanomas are greater than 6 mm at the time of diagnosis; however, this finding is neither sensitive or specific for melanoma; therefore this feature would be better viewed as "changing diameter" because malignancies tend to change and enlarge over time.
- With evolution, patient reports of change or presence of objective change on serial digital photography are suggestive of a melanoma; this could involve change in symmetry, border, color, diameter or surface features of the lesion.
  - A major caveat to evolution is in children and adolescents. Children and adolescents have changing nevi. This is particularly noticeable around puberty.

## The Ugly Duckling Sign

- When examining a patient, there is presence of a pigmented lesion that is obviously different than the patients other pigmented lesions, which is a sign concerning for malignancy.
- Similarly, pigmented lesions that are in isolation (e.g., the only pigmented lesion on a patient's thigh) can be suspicious for malignancy, especially if these lesions are newly noted.

## Primary Types of Cutaneous Melanoma

There are four primary types of cutaneous melanoma. They are superficial spreading, nodular melanoma, lentigo maligna (LM), and acral lentiginous.

- With the exception of some variants of desmoplastic melanoma, all types of cutaneous melanoma are prognostically equal based on AJCC staging.
- Superficial spreading is the most common type of melanoma.
  - It has a prolonged radial growth phase and is the prototypical melanoma that the ABCDEs of melanoma were created to identify.

- Nodular melanoma is the second most common type of melanoma and presents as an indurated nodule that frequently ulcerates.
- LM is sometimes called "melanoma on sun-damaged skin" and involves broad, frequently bland-appearing pigmented lesions on heavily sun-damaged locations (e.g., the nose, cheeks) that have a prolonged radial growth phase.
  - Although only 3% to 10% of LM become invasive (becoming lentigo maligna melanoma), all are capable of becoming invasive over time if neglected.
- Acral lentiginous is the most common type of melanoma in Blacks and Asians.
  - It can involve either acral skin or the nail unit (see ch 15, longitudinal melanonychia).
  - Diagnosis is frequently delayed, especially in patients of color.
- Additional types include amelanotic and desmoplastic.
  - Amelanotic is a clinical subtype of melanoma comprising around 8% of melanomas, in which the malignant melanocytes are either making no pigment or so little pigment that the pigment is not clinically appreciable.
    - This subtype frequently presents as pink to flesh-colored nodules.
    - It is often misdiagnosed as BCC or vascular neoplasm.
  - Desmoplastic is a rare histologic subtype with prognostic and management implications. The melanoma cells in this variant are often spindled and the stroma is desmoplastic or fibrotic.
- Several other rare subtypes, including malignant blue nevus and spitzoid melanoma, also exist. Discussion of these entities is beyond the scope of this chapter given their rarity.
  Dermoscopy (also called "epilumenesce microscopy and dermatoscopy") detects up to two-thirds of melanomas that would not be identified based on visual inspection alone by a dermatologist (around 20% of all melanomas).
- Dermoscopy is as indispensable to the evaluation of pigmented lesions as a stethoscope is to the evaluation of heart murmurs.
- A review of the dermoscopic features of MM is beyond the scope of this chapter.
  - Primary care providers who are interested in learning dermoscopy are advised to refer to Cliff

Rosendahl's "Chaos and Clues" algorithm for primary care providers and to review dermoscopy terminology on dermoscopedia.org

## Differential Diagnosis

Differentiating melanoma from other cutaneous neoplasms is one of the most difficult facets of dermatology. As such, the differential diagnosis for MM is incredibly broad and includes acquired melanocytic nevus, congenital melanocytic nevus (CMN), dysplastic nevus, SK, solar lentigo, lichen planus-like keratosis, dermatofibroma, angiokeratoma, BCC, and many others. When there is clinical concern for MM, a biopsy can differentiate it from all mimickers.

- Distinguishing banal nevi and dysplastic nevi from MM can be difficult. Use of the aforementioned ABCDE rule, "ugly duckling" sign, and dermoscopy (if trained) can be helpful. Equivocal pigmented lesions that are flat can be photographed and reevaluated for change at 3-month intervals. Changing suspicious lesions should be referred to a dermatologist or biopsied.
- CMNs are a type of benign melanocytic neoplasm that is present at birth. CMNs are classified based on their size and the risk of malignant transformation of a CMN is directly related to the size of the lesion. CMNs are frequently identifiable as they are present at birth and have many terminal hairs emanating from the lesion. Patients with CMN should be referred to a dermatologist for close monitoring.
- Aside for banal nevi, SK (Chapter 10) is the most common skin lesion to be misdiagnosed as melanoma. SKs are often concerning to patients because they develop during adulthood, change, and can get irritated and inflamed. SKs are often concerning to healthcare providers because they are raised, may have variegated colors, and are frequently noted to be new and often changing by patients. SKs can be identified based on their characteristic stuck-on and/or waxy appearance, and because they often readily crumble after rubbing with gauze.
  - Importantly, SK and melanoma do occasionally collide and therefore identification of features of SK does not necessarily rule out an underlying melanoma.
- Solar lentigines are sun-induced, flat pigmented lesions that are present in almost all fair-skinned individuals over the age of 50 and can develop as early as adolescence in heavily sun-damaged individuals. They are typically uniform in color and appearance and often are present in crops. They are most frequently misdiagnosed as melanoma on the face where they may be broad, growing, and changing like a lentigo maligna.
- Lichen planus-like keratoses (LPLK) are a subtype of inflamed solar lentigines or seborrheic keratoses that is regressing because of the inflammation. LPLKs can be exceptionally difficult to distinguish from MM clinically and as a result they are frequently biopsied.
- Dermatofibromas (DF; Chapter 11) [NE(5)are scar-like neoplasms that most frequently occur on the legs and shoulders. They can be distinguished from melanoma based on identification of a positive dimple sign and stability of lesion. Although nodular melanoma are firm, they do not typically dimple.
- Angiokeratoma (ch 11) are benign vascular neoplasms that can appear dark black when thrombosed. When magnified or examined with a dermatoscope, obvious lacunae can frequently be appreciated, distinguishing them from MM.
- BCC, in the case of amelanotic melanoma, and pigmented BCC, in the case of melanoma in general, are common mimickers. Because both BCC and MM are malignant, they both must be biopsied. BCC is typically dome-shaped, pearly, and translucent, with notable telangiectasia.

## Work-Up

MM are typically identified either because they are brought to the attention of a healthcare provider by a patient or because they are identified by a provider during a full-body skin examination.

- Although the USPSTF does not routinely recommend regular full-body skin examinations, all patients with suspicious skin lesions, a personal or family history of melanoma, a personal history of nonmelanoma skin cancer, greater than 50 nevi, severe sun damage, history of sunburns, and/or with multiple risk factors for skin cancer should be referred for skin cancer screening by a dermatologist, if one is available.
  - Some authorities recommend that all adults over the age of 35 should be referred for skin cancer screening.

When a lesion that is concerning for melanoma is identified, a full-body skin examination, which includes an examination of the nails, scalp, and mucosa, should also be performed.

- The potential presence of additional suspicious lesions, in-transit metastases, and distant cutaneous metastases should be evaluated for on examination.
- Lymph node examination and palpation of the liver and spleen should also be undertaken.

All suspicious lesions should be biopsied. Determining whether or not an individual pigmented lesion requires a biopsy is exceptionally difficult, as noted previously. In cases where equivocal lesions are identified, several options are widely available.

- If the lesion is flat, it can be photographed and measured and then reevaluated at 3-month intervals for 6 months. All changing lesions should be biopsied.
  - Serial digital photography is not recommended for raised lesions.
- Refer the patient to a dermatologist.
- Consider a teledermatology consult. Several companies now provide dermoscopic evaluation of lesions by using mail-order kits. In areas where a dermatologist is not available, this may be a reasonable option.

All concerning lesions should be biopsied. Biopsy of pigmented lesions concerning for melanoma requires a very specific approach to ensure adequacy of sampling.

- The entirety of the lesion should be sampled.
- The biopsy should extend at least 2 mm deep to avoid transection of the lesion because melanoma is primarily staged based on depth of tumor invasion.
  - Small lesions (less than 6 mm) can often be excised in toto with a punch biopsy.
- All specimens concerning for melanoma should be referred to a dermatopathologist for evaluation, if possible, because melanocytic neoplasms are very difficult to interpret for individuals who do not evaluate them with some degree of regularity.

## Initial Steps in Management

Management of MM is based on AJCC staging. Initial staging is dependent on tumor depth and the presence or absence of ulceration.

- All melanomas should be referred to a dermatologist for longitudinal skin cancer monitoring, if possible.
- Stage 0 melanoma (malignant melanoma in situ [MMIS]) resides entirely in the epidermis.
- Surgical excision is definitive management for MMIS.
- MMIS occurring in cosmetically sensitive areas where tissue sparing is desired (e.g., the face) should be referred to a provider who performs staged excision (also known as "slow Mohs").
- MMIS occurring in areas where tissue sparing is not required can be excised with 5 to 10 mm clear margins depending on the location and degree of background sun damage.
  - All individuals with invasive melanoma need active monitoring by a dermatologist for recurrence and development of second primary melanomas every 6 months for 2 years and then at least annually thereafter.
- Stage I melanoma is melanoma that has a Breslow depth (measured from the top of the granular layer of the epidermis to the deepest extension of the melanoma into the skin) of less than 1 mm.
  - Stage I melanoma is further stratified into stage Ia and Stage Ib melanoma.
    - Ia has a Breslow depth smaller than 0.8 mm and is not ulcerated.
    - Ib either has a Breslow depth ranging from 0.8 to 1 mm or less than 0.8 mm but is ulcerated.
  - Stage Ia MM can be excised by an experienced practitioner down to fascia with 1 cm clear margins.
  - Stage Ib MM should be referred to a surgical oncologist for discussion of sentinel lymph node biopsy and surgical management.
- All melanomas with a Breslow depth of greater than 1 mm with clinically palpable lymph nodes or with known distant metastases should be referred to both a medical oncologist and a surgical oncologist for further management.
- All individuals with invasive melanoma need active monitoring by a dermatologist for recurrence and development of second primary melanomas every 3 months for 2 years and then at least annually thereafter.

## Common Pitfalls

The biggest pitfall when managing melanoma is delaying diagnosis and definitive management. Patients with lesions highly suspicious for melanoma should have the lesions biopsied as soon as possible. Once a diagnosis is confirmed, surgical excision should ideally be performed within 2 weeks.

Transecting a melanoma (i.e., not reaching the base of the lesion on biopsy) is a critical error because it robs the patient of critical prognostic information that will directly dictate their subsequent management. Of note is that transecting a melanoma does not induce metastasis or activation of the melanoma. If you are not comfortable biopsying a highly suspicious pigmented lesion and a dermatologist is not readily available, an excisional biopsy can often be performed by a general surgeon or plastic surgeon. If a patient is going to be referred to a surgeon for biopsy, photos of the concerning lesion should be faxed to the surgeon's office so that the correct lesion is biopsied.

Similarly, tangential (i.e., partial) sampling of a pigmented lesion is inappropriate because it can result in sampling errors. If a pathologist is not provided with the entire lesion, then the diagnosis may be missed.

All patients who have had a melanoma require indefinite active monitoring by a dermatologist for recurrence of the melanoma, development of a second primary melanoma, and development of other skin cancers. Failure to provide patient with adequate follow-up can lead to a delay in diagnosis of additional neoplasms.

## Counseling

Given the gravity of this diagnosis, we recommend that patients receive the patient information leaflet that is freely available from the National Cancer Institute. Patients should be provided with the leaflet that is specific to the stage of melanoma that they have.

# Diffuse Hair Loss

## ANDROGENETIC ALOPECIA

### Clinical Features

Androgenetic alopecia (AGA; also known as "female-pattern hair loss" and "male-pattern baldness") is the most common type of hair loss in both men and women. It is caused by androgen-mediated effects on hair follicles, which result in miniaturization of hairs, decreased hair count, and observable hair thinning in a male-patterned scalp distribution.

- AGA presents differently in men and women and treatment differs, too.
  - In men, AGA presents with frontotemporal hairline recession and diffuse thinning of the crown of the scalp. Importantly, hair on the occipital and temporal scalp is never lost in AGA because the hairs in these areas are androgen insensitive.
  - The first sign of AGA in men may be kinking of hairs in the frontotemporal scalp (Fig. 13.1), which causes these hairs to become increasingly difficult to style.
- In women, AGA presents with thinning of the crown and frontal aspects of the scalp despite preservation of the frontotemporal hairline.
  - AGA is less common in black women in whom central centrifugal cicatricial alopecia, a scarring hair loss affecting the crown of the scalp, is the most common form of hair loss.

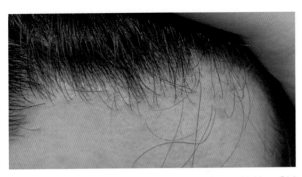

**Fig. 13.1 Early Androgenetic Alopecia in a 26-Year-Old Male.** Note the decreased hair density and variability in hair shaft diameter.

- For men and women, AGA is characteristically asymptomatic, nonpatchy, lacking in overlying skin changes, and nonscarring, which helps to distinguish it from other causes of hair loss.
- Close examination, especially with a magnifying glass and bright light (trichoscopy or dermoscopy of the hair and scalp) of affected areas reveals hairs with varying widths, which is diagnostic for AGA.

## Differential Diagnosis

The differential for AGA is broad and includes telogen effluvium (TE), lichen planopilaris (LPP), traction alopecia, central centrifugal cicatricial alopecia (CCCA), and alopecia areata. Importantly, multiple types of hair loss can coexist in the same individual, making accurate diagnosis difficult in some cases.

- TE is a nonscarring alopecia characterized by diffuse shedding and thinning of the scalp. It is caused by hairs entering the telogen phase of the hair cycle prematurely. This typically presents 3 to 4 months after a significant illness, major stressor, or the initiation of a new medication. TE can be distinguished from AGA because it is characterized by diffuse, nonpatterned thinning of the scalp rather than the thinning characteristic of AGA. Furthermore, patients with TE report a significant increase in the amount of daily shedding that they experience. This shedding can be objectified by performing a pull test on unwashed hair; it is positive if more than 10 telogen hairs are removed by a gentle pull. TE is also typically more transient than AGA; however, chronic TE can occur.
- LPP is a scarring alopecia that is characterized by the presence of perifollicular erythema and scaling that

progresses to scarring hair loss on the scalp vertex. A clinical variant of LPP, frontal fibrosing alopecia (FFA) presents with identical clinical findings to LPP; however, it affects the frontal scalp and causes marked recession of the hairline. LPP is distinguished from AGA because it is symptomatic (burning and itching), it presents with perifollicular erythema, and it scars. FFA should be considered in any woman with significant hairline recession because hairline recession is not frequently seen in AGA in women.
- Traction alopecia is a common type of nonscarring alopecia that can progress to scarring alopecia overtime. It is caused by tight hairstyling that chronically puts significant traction on the hair follicles. It is characterized by frontotemporal hair loss, almost exclusively in women, that demonstrates a positive fringe sign where the hairline appears grossly normal despite significant thinning of the hair directly behind it. Traction is distinguished from AGA by its characteristic distribution, history of tight hairstyling (especially braiding), and the absence of hair loss elsewhere on the scalp.
- CCCA is a common form of scarring alopecia that predominantly occurs in black women. It should be considered in all black women who present with AGA-like hair loss. It is characterized by progressive scarring of the vertex scalp in the absence of clear primary lesions. It can be differentiated from AGA because it scars.
- Alopecia areata is an autoimmune hair loss that frequently presents with discrete patches of hair loss. Typically, it is not misdiagnosed as AGA because it is very patchy, comes and goes, and occurs in areas that are not characteristic of AGA. Less common variants of AGA that affect the entirety of the scalp (e.g., alopecia totalis, alopecia universalis) can occasionally be mistaken for AGA. These variants can be distinguished from AGA based on their quick development, their distribution (which is beyond that which is typical for AGA), and their responsiveness to steroids.

## Work-Up

AGA is typically a clinical diagnosis; however, in some cases, additional work-up is required to distinguish it from mimickers.

- Examining distribution of hair loss is helpful in narrowing down the differential.

- In all patients, examination of hairs on an affected area with magnification can be helpful because AGA presents with easily appreciable variation in the diameter of hairs, which is not seen in other forms of hair loss.
- In cases where diagnosis is uncertain, punch biopsy can be helpful for securing a diagnosis. This should only be performed by an experienced healthcare provider because performing biopsies on the scalp is technically difficult.
  - The specimen must be sent to a dermatopathology lab that is experienced in processing scalp specimens because they are prepared differently than regular skin biopsies.
- Women with early-onset and/or severe AGA with other masculinizing features benefit from a hormonal work-up to evaluate for polycystic ovarian syndrome (luteinizing hormone [LH], follicle-stimulating hormone [FSH], dehydroepiandrosterone [DHEA], and free testosterone).

## Initial Steps in Management

Management of AGA is different in men than it is in women. Regardless, early, aggressive management is recommended because maintenance of hair is much easier to achieve than hair regrowth.

### In Men

- First-line treatment is topical minoxidil 5% once daily. Minoxidil is available both as a foam and a solution. Men frequently prefer the foam; however, neither vehicle is particularly cosmetically appealing.
  - Patients should be reassessed 6 months after minoxidil initiation.
  - Patients should be instructed that transient, early shedding is an expected side effect of minoxidil use.
  - Some patients experience significant burning with preparations containing polyethylene glycol.
  - Discontinuation of minoxidil results in loss of benefit and shedding within months.
- Men who are not amenable to a topical medication, who do not respond to minoxidil, or who receive inadequate benefit from minoxidil alone can try finasteride 1 mg orally (PO) daily.
  - Routine counseling of patients about potential sexual side effects is controversial because these side effects are rare and counseling is associated

with an increase in the rate of finasteride-related sexual adverse events.
- Patients should be counseled that oral finasteride will lower their prostate specific antigen.
- Topical finasteride 1% is available from compounding pharmacies and has been shown to be as efficacious as PO finasteride in small studies.
  - Many healthcare providers compound it with minoxidil 5% to improve compliance; however, the cost of these compounded products is typically prohibitive for most patients.
- Low-level laser therapy (LLLT, also known as "laser comb") has also been cleared by the U.S. Food and Drug Administration (FDA) for treatment of androgenetic alopecia; however, its clinical utility is debatable and it is very expensive.
- Other therapies include platelet-rich plasma (PRP) injections and hair transplants, which should only be performed by experienced healthcare providers.
  - Patients with advanced disease often require hair transplantation to achieve satisfactory results.

### In Women

- Topical minoxidil 5% is the first-line treatment in women as well. Many women prefer topical minoxidil solution over foam for cosmetic reasons.
  - Low-dose oral minoxidil is effective and typically well tolerated in women; however, it almost invariably causes hirsutism.
    - Oral minoxidil (0.5–2.5 mg daily) requires blood pressure monitoring and some experts recommend electrolyte monitoring as well.
- Oral finasteride is less well established in women. Studies suggest that women require higher doses of finasteride (5 mg daily) to receive benefit.
  - Finasteride can feminize a male fetus and should not be used by pregnant women or women who may become pregnant during their treatment.
  - Topical finasteride may also be effective in women; however, the data supporting its use is less robust than the data for men.
- Oral spironolactone is occasionally used for management of AGA in women; however, dosing recommendations are currently unclear.
- LLLT, hair transplant, and PRP are also available to women.
  - PRP may be less effective in women than it is in men.

## Warning Signs/Common Pitfalls

The biggest pitfall when managing AGA (or any hair loss) is downplaying the patient's concern. Different patients experience hair loss differently and for some patients, hair loss can be deeply emotional. Early initiation of aggressive therapy is always recommended in concerned patients because hair maintenance is easier to achieve than hair regrowth.

If there is any concern for a scarring alopecia, the patient should be urgently referred to a dermatologist for a biopsy because these scarring alopecias are progressive and irreversible.

Patients should be thoroughly counseled that no treatment for AGA modifies disease course and that lifelong treatment is necessary for hair maintenance.

Patients with advanced AGA are unlikely to achieve satisfactory results with medical management alone. These patients frequently require hair transplantation to achieve the results that they want.

## Counseling

You have a type of hair loss called "androgenetic alopecia" (AGA). It is the most common type of hair loss in both men and women and it is caused by the effect of hormones on hairs in certain locations on the scalp. Unfortunately, AGA tends to worsen over time.

To help you regrow hair and to keep you from losing additional hair, your healthcare provider has recommended that you obtain minoxidil 5% solution or foam, which is available over the counter. It is marketed under the brand name Rogaine. You should massage this product into the scalp once daily. It works by increasing blood flow to your hair, which helps your hair continue to grow. You are unlikely to notice significant benefit for around 3 to 6 months. In fact, sometimes minoxidil actually makes hair loss more apparent before it is helpful. Additionally, if you discontinue the minoxidil, the benefit that you gained from it will be lost over a period of several months, so it is important that you stick with it.

The main side effect from minoxidil is that it may cause unwanted hair growth. This occurs if you allow the minoxidil to come into contact with areas where you do not want hair. For example, if you allow the minoxidil solution to drip down your forehead, you may grow excess hair there. For that reason, do not apply the medication to the scalp right before bed because you do not want it getting on your pillow and then transferring to your face.

We would like to see you in 6 months to see how your hair loss is doing. Additional treatment options are available if you are not seeing the results that you would like.

# LICHEN PLANOPILARIS

## Clinical Features

- LPP occurs more commonly in women than in men, in white people than in other groups, and in people in their 50s and 60s than in other age groups.
- Clinically, LPP is divided into three subtypes based on distribution of involvement that may demonstrate overlap.
  - Classic LPP involves the frontal and parietal scalp.
  - FFA is considered by some to be a variant of LPP that exclusively involves the frontal scalp (often presenting as hairline regression) and the eyebrows.
  - Graham-Little-Piccardi-Lasseuer Syndrome is the rare triad of scalp LPP, nonscarring alopecia of the axillae and pubic hair, and an eruption of follicular papules all over the body.
- In a minority of cases, LPP coexists with lichen planus on non–hair-bearing skin or on the mucosa.
- Although there are specific clinical findings that are more common in different subtypes of LPP, all types of LPP can present with eyebrow loss, other nonscalp hair loss (including the beard area and the extremities), and flesh-colored facial papules (which likely represent involvement of vellus hairs on the face).

## Differential Diagnosis

- Early LPP is often misdiagnosed as AGA occurring in combination with seborrheic dermatitis.
  - Early LPP can be differentiated from androgenetic alopecia because it presents with discrete patches of alopecia, has perifollicular erythema and scaling (although it may be subtle), and causes scarring (and therefore follicular ostia will not be identifiable in areas of scarring).
- Other common mimickers of LPP include the other primary cicatricial alopecias (e.g., central centrifugal cicatricial alopecia, chronic cutaneous lupus erythematosus).

## Work-Up

- In all cases of LPP, a full-body skin and mucosal examination should be performed and a targeted history should be obtained to evaluate for disease activity elsewhere (e.g., extremities, groin, axillae).

- In cases where a diagnosis of LPP cannot be rendered on clinical grounds alone, a punch biopsy is required to confirm the diagnosis. A biopsy should be obtained from an active area of inflammation, not from a scarred area.
- Thyroid function tests should be ordered in all patients with LPP because around 10% of patients with LPP have hypothyroidism.

## Initial Steps in Management

All patients with presumed primary cicatricial alopecia, including LPP, should be referred urgently to a dermatologist who is comfortable treating scarring alopecia because the scarring that results from these conditions is permanent but can be curtailed with appropriate management.

There is no cure for LPP and the scarring that it causes is irreversible. The goal of therapy is to stop active inflammation and prevent disease progression. A secondary goal of therapy is to hasten hair regrowth in nonscarred areas; however, this should not be emphasized until the inflammatory component of the disease is under control. It is important to convey this to patients.

Most patients with LPP require the combination of an ultrapotent topical corticosteroid with an oral immunosuppressive agent (e.g., mycophenolate mofetil, cyclosporine, methotrexate) or an antimalarial (e.g., hydroxychloroquine) to obtain complete remission of their disease. These medications should be started and monitored by a dermatologist.

### Recommended Initial Regimen

- Clobetasol propionate 0.05% scalp solution, spray, or foam (depending on patient preference and the insurance formulary) is recommended daily or twice daily. Patients should be counseled that daily use is mandatory and that this can safely be continued for months. On average, it takes almost a year of continuous therapy to obtain complete remission of LPP and it may take months of continuous use to notice any clinically significant benefit. Before obtaining complete remission, no topical steroid drug holiday should be employed.
  - Patients should be counseled that topical steroids do not hasten hair regrowth and that their hair

will grow, if scarring has yet to take place, at its normal growth rate once the inflammation is stopped.

- A nonexhaustive list of alternatives to clobetasol propionate include in decreasing order of potency: halobetasol propionate 0.05% lotion or foam, betamethasone dipropionate 0.05% lotion or spray, fluocinonide 0.05% topical solution, betamethasone valerate 0.12% foam, and fluocinolone 0.025% oil or solution.

## Extensive Inflammation or a Delay in Access

If there is extensive inflammation or if there is going to be a delay in access to a dermatology appointment, oral corticosteroids can be used.

- As previously mentioned, the majority of patients require either an oral immunosuppressant or an antimalarial to obtain control of their LPP; however, in cases where there is going to be a delay until the initiation of one of these agents, oral corticosteroids can be used. Nevertheless, initiation of oral corticosteroids is not a replacement for requesting an urgent dermatology referral so that a steroid-sparing oral medication can be initiated.
- If you are going to start oral corticosteroids, they should be started in most cases with prednisone 1 mg/kg PO every morning with a plan to down-titrate the dose by 10% per week to the lowest dose possible that still maintains satisfactory disease control.
  - It is important to consider the significant systemic toxicities of long-term, high-dose corticosteroids before starting treatment.
    - Most patients need a baseline dual-energy x-ray absorption (DEXA) scan and qualify for osteoporosis prophylaxis.
    - Some patients qualify for pneumocystis pneumonia prophylaxis.
  - Patients who are titrated off oral corticosteroids without substitution of an appropriate steroid-sparing agent are at a high risk for disease relapse.
  - Short-course steroids (e.g. a 5-day dose pack) are not helpful and may trigger severe disease rebound.

## Warning Signs/Common Pitfalls

This disease causes irreversible scarring hair loss and therefore requires aggressive management to prevent progression. Once scarring has occurred, there is nothing that can be done to reverse it. If you are suspicious that a patient may have LPP or another primary cicatricial alopecia, refer them urgently to an experienced dermatologist.

Patients with LPP often have coexistent AGA. The presence of AGA does not rule out LPP or any other primary cicatricial alopecia, nor does it make these diagnoses less likely.

Do not stop place a stop date on the use of ultrapotent topical corticosteroids out of fear of local corticosteroid-induced adverse effects because these adverse effects are unlikely to develop on the scalp and long-term therapy is necessary to achieve clinical benefit.

## Counseling

You have an uncommon type of hair loss called "lichen planopilaris," or "LPP" for short. This type of hair loss is caused by inflammation in your hair follicles. It is unknown why people develop LPP; however, it is a chronic condition, which means that it lasts for a long time and it is currently incurable (Fig. 13.2).

If left untreated, LPP can cause permanent scarring and hair loss. Permanently scarred areas will never regrow hair. This is why it is important to treat LPP early and to continue treatment until the condition has burned out, which may take years. The goal of treating your condition is to reduce the inflammation, prevent additional scarring from occurring, and allow hair regrowth to occur in nonscarred, areas.

You have been prescribed an ultrapotent topical corticosteroid. It is important that you use this medication every day. It is important that you do not stop this medication without consulting your healthcare provider first. It may take months of daily use for you to notice improvement. If you stop your medication, your disease may come back. You should not put this medication on your face or on other areas of your body that your healthcare provider has not specifically instructed you to use this medication on. It can cause thinning of the skin and visible blood vessel formation.

Many patients will also need an oral medication in addition to this topical medication to get satisfactory control of their disease. It is important that you see a dermatologist to determine whether you are a patient who might benefit from a pill for this condition.

# FRONTAL FIBROSING ALOPECIA (FFA)

**Lynne J. Goldberg**

## Clinical Features

FFA was first described in postmenopausal women by Kossard in 1994. It is a type of cicatricial or scarring alopecia where the hair follicle is destroyed permanently. Its incidence has increased dramatically over time, and both premenopausal women and men have been affected. FFA is now a common cause, if not the most common cause, of scarring alopecia seen by dermatologists. Although many hypotheses exist, the etiology remains unknown.

Patients with FFA often present with either recession of the frontal hairline or symmetric thinning of the eyebrows, findings that are the two major criteria for the disease. Other findings include loss of hair on the face (particularly the preauricular areas) and extremities, and subtle, fine, skin-colored facial papules. When severe, the disease can extend onto the crown of the scalp and/or posteriorly behind the ears to involve the occipital hairline.

Examination reveals a smooth scalp surface in the area of the hair loss, with isolated remaining terminal hairs. When the disease is active, close inspection with a dermatoscope will reveal a cuff of white scale around affected hair shafts, especially on the frontal scalp and preauricular areas.

## Differential Diagnosis

Other causes of hair loss of the peripheral scalp include alopecia areata and traction alopecia.
- Alopecia areata can also involve the eyebrows, body hair, and scalp and can therefore mimic FFA. Nevertheless, it is a nonscarring alopecia, and close inspection with a dermatoscope will reveal retained follicular orifices on

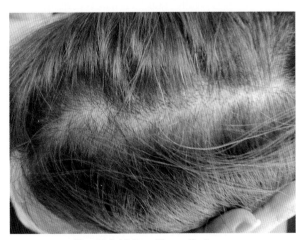

**Fig. 13.2** Lichen Planopilaris.

the scalp surface and sometimes exclamation point hairs (truncated hairs that are thicker distally and thin toward the scalp surface). It also lacks perifollicular scale.

- Traction alopecia should be suspected in patients whose hairstyling results in repeated or constant pull on the hair shaft. It can closely mimic FFA. Loss of eyebrows is a clue to the presence of FFA.
- Many patients with FFA are misdiagnosed with pattern hair loss or AGA. This is the most common nonscarring alopecia, and although it can affect the frontal hairline, close inspection will reveal a decrease in hair shaft diameter not present in FFA. The two diseases can occur together.

## Work-Up

Patients with suspected FFA should be referred to dermatology. Patients with classic FFA can be readily diagnosed clinically by healthcare providers experienced in the evaluation of hair loss. When the diagnosis is in doubt, a scalp biopsy can be very helpful.

FFA is a lymphocytic scarring alopecia. In active disease, a scalp biopsy will reveal a cuff of lymphocytes and/or fibrosis (scar tissue) surrounding the upper hair follicle. Loss of the sebaceous glands that are normally associated with the hair follicle is an early finding. This is in contrast to traction alopecia, where sebaceous glands are spared.

There are no characteristic laboratory abnormalities in FFA. Although an increase in autoimmune thyroid disease has been reported, routine screening is not recommended.

## Treatment

Treatment of FFA is mostly based on case studies because there have not been controlled clinical trials. Most dermatology providers adopt a tiered approach based on healthcare provider experience/comfort and patient preference. Treatment is all off label and includes topical steroids, injectable steroids, and oral agents, such as hydroxychloroquine, doxycycline, and 5-alpha reductase inhibitors. These are frequently used in combination. Although the disease can stabilize on its own, it does not always respond to treatment.

## Warning Signs/Common Pitfalls

- FFA can coexist with pattern hair loss, so the finding of the latter does not exclude the former.
- Eyebrow loss can precede scalp hair loss, so patients presenting with brow loss should be examined carefully for early FFA.

- FFA can coexist with traction alopecia, so a biopsy can be especially useful in this differential diagnosis.
- Providers need to keep in mind that all forms of alopecia, especially scarring alopecia, have a significant effect on patients' quality of life and well-being.

## Counseling

You have been diagnosed with a type of permanent hair loss, which we are aware is distressing. The aim of treatment is to stop any symptoms and halt further hair loss. Hair follicles that have been partially affected can recover, but completely destroyed hair follicles can no longer produce a hair shaft. We will refer you to a dermatologist who will likely prescribe topical and possibly systemic medications to help you.

There are patient resources available, including an excellent organization called the "Cicatricial Alopecia Research Foundation" (CARF). Their website, CARFintl.org, contains information on FFA and other types of scarring alopecia, as well as dates and locations of local support group meetings.

# TELOGEN EFFLUVIUM

## Clinical Features

TE is a common cause of diffuse hair loss that can affect both men and women, although women more commonly complain of this disorder than men.

- Unlike other types of hair loss, TE presents with a chief complaint of hair shedding.
  - Patients typically state their hair is coming out in clumps in the shower.
- Patients can also complain of trichodynia (so-called "painful hair"), which is typically described as scalp prickling in areas of hair loss.
- TE is a diffuse hair loss and by definition does not present with patches of alopecia.
- TE is caused by premature, inappropriate transition of hairs from the anagen (growth phase) to telogen (resting phase), which results in premature expulsion of hair from the hair bulb.
  - There are many causes of TE; however, stress, postpartum, surgery, and major medical illness are the most common causes of TE.
    - Hair loss is typically observed 3 to 4 months after these events.

- Patients with TE are often anxious out of proportion to their healthcare provider–perceived hair loss (healthcare providers frequently tell these patients, "Don't worry; you look like you have a full head of hair"), which often can increase the distress that these patients experience.
- Patients with AGA can also develop TE, which can make diagnosis of TE more difficult.
- TE typically slowly self-resolves after withdrawal of the causative stressor; however, a small subset of patients develops chronic TE, which persists for years.
  - Even in self-limited cases of TE, cosmetically apparent hair regrowth is typically not appreciable for 12 to 18 months.

## Differential Diagnosis

The differential for TE includes AGA, anagen effluvium, alopecia areata, and psychogenic pseudoeffluvium.

- AGA frequently coexists in patients with TE; however, pure AGA is distinguishable from TE because AGA presents with a frontotemporal to occipital hair density ratio of less than 1; there is visible variability in the width of hairs in the frontotemporal scalp when magnified; it does not present with hair shedding but rather with rarefaction of hair; and it favors the crown of the scalp in women and can cause true thinned or bald spots.
- Anagen effluvium is similar to TE; however, AE occurs almost exclusively from chemotherapeutic agents, which lead to apoptosis of hair follicles, triggering immediate release of hairs. In contradistinction, TE develops 3 to 4 month after exposure to new medications.
- Alopecia areata, particularly a variant of alopecia areata called "alopecia areata incognito," can mimic TE by causing diffuse hair loss without patchy bald spots. This variant is very difficult to distinguish from TE and typically can only be distinguished by biopsy or by the presence of typical AA lesions elsewhere.
- Psychogenic pseudoeffluvium is a rare psychological condition where patients complain of hair loss that is not actually occurring for secondary gain. This is a diagnosis of exclusion in patients in whom examination, biopsy, and a hair washing test do not reveal a cause and when there is strong suspicion of a psychiatric origin for a patient's complaint.

## Work-Up

Work-up for TE is divided into history taking, clinical examination, and laboratory work-up.

### History Taking

- Patients should specifically be queried about recent changes in their health, including history of acute febrile illnesses, surgery, pregnancy, psychosocial stressors, and new medications.
  - Specific medications that are frequently implicated in the development of TE include oral retinoids, oral contraceptives, beta blockers, angiotensin-converting enzyme (ACE) inhibitors, anticoagulants, anticonvulsants, amphetamines, lipid-lowering agents, and antithyroid drugs.

### Clinical Examination

- In the office, a hair pull test should be performed if the patient has not washed their hair in more than 24 hours.
  - A hair pull test is performed by putting gentle traction with the thumb and middle finger on 40 to 60 hairs on the patient's vertex scalp.
    - Testing is positive if more than 10% of the hairs on which traction is placed are easily removed.
- At home, patients should perform the modified hair washing test (MHWT) and should repeat this monthly to track their progress. It cannot be overstated how much patients appreciate being asked to perform this test because it validates their concerns.
  - An MHWT is performed by having the patient go without washing their hair for 5 days. The hair should then be washed and shampooed in the sink with gauze over the drain so that all of the hairs that are removed by washing are collected. The patient should then count their hairs and divide them into those that are less than 3 cm in length and those that are greater than 3 cm.
    - Shedding of more than 100 hairs is diagnostic of TE. Most patients will shed more than 300.
    - This testing can be used to monitor the activity of hair loss because cosmetically appreciable regrowth lags behind the reduction and ultimate termination of TE.

## Laboratory Work-Up

- This should be undertaken in all patients regardless of symptoms because it not infrequently identifies a treatable cause of TE and makes the patients feel that their concerns have been taken seriously.
  - Laboratory work-up should include complete blood count (CBC), urine analysis, thyroid-stimulating hormone (TSH), T3, T4, ferritin, zinc, vitamin D, and antinuclear antibody (ANA).

## Initial Steps in Management

Management of TE is divided into management in patients in whom a treatable cause has been identified and management of patients in whom no underlying cause is identified.

- If a treatable cause is present (e.g., hypothyroidism), treat the underlying cause.
- If no treatable cause is identified, proceed as follows.
  - Start clobetasol 0.05% scalp solution daily to entire scalp.
    - Topical steroids may be helpful because they allow patients to actively participate in their recovery and there is some evidence that some cases of TE arise from stress-mediated inflammation in the hair follicle, which is combatted by the steroids.
  - Although off-label topical minoxidil has historically been recommended as a treatment for TE, we generally do not recommend its use because minoxidil can cause TE upon initial use and after discontinuation, which can be very distressing to patients.
    - The exception to this recommendation is for patients with coexisting TE and AGA in whom minoxidil will be beneficial for treating the AGA component of their hair loss.
- All patients should monitor their hair loss at home with monthly MHWTs.

## Warning Signs/Common Pitfalls

The biggest pitfall when managing TE is downplaying a patient's concern. There is nothing more distressing to these patients than being told to not worry "because no one else will notice their hair loss." By virtue of the patient scheduling an appointment with a healthcare provider to discuss their hair loss, the hair loss is of significance to them and should be treated that way by the healthcare provider.

As aforementioned, use of topical minoxidil is not recommended for management of TE because it triggers TE acutely and after discontinuation, which can contribute to patient stress.

## Counseling

You have a type of hair loss called "telogen effluvium." This is very common and fortunately it goes away on its own in most cases. It occurs because some of your hairs have stopped growing prematurely, which has caused them to fall out. There are many reasons why your hair may have done this, including hospitalization, surgery, stress, pregnancy, and new medications. These stressors typically precede hair loss by 3 to 4 months.

To confirm your diagnosis, your healthcare provider recommends that you perform a hair washing test at home. This test will help you and your healthcare provider know exactly how much hair you are losing and will help track your progress as your hair recovers. To do this test, you must not wash your hair for 5 days. Then, you must wash and shampoo your hair in the sink with the drain covered by gauze so that all the hair you shed is collected. Then count the number of hairs you collect and write this number down so you can share it with your healthcare provider. Repeat this test every month to track your hair loss. Importantly, showering is not causing your hairs to fall out. The hairs that come out when your hair is washed will come out regardless of what you do.

To better understand why you might be having hair loss, your healthcare provider has ordered some blood work. Please complete this to help with your assessment.

Additionally, to help promote hair regrowth, your healthcare provider has prescribed you a steroid solution for your scalp. This steroid is meant to decrease the inflammation that may be playing a role in causing your hair to fall out. You should use this once per day.

# ALOPECIA TOTALIS/UNIVERSALIS (SEE CHAPTER 14, ALOPECIA AREATA)

# 14

# Focal Hair Loss

## CHAPTER OUTLINE

## ALOPECIA AREATA

**Rana Abdat**

### Clinical Features

Alopecia areata (AA) is a common cause of hair loss that affects men and women equally and can affect patients of all ages.

- AA is the second most common cause of nonscarring hair loss after androgenetic alopecia (AGA; also known as "male/female pattern hair loss").
  - It is of unclear etiology but is thought to be immune mediated via loss of tolerance and has a link to other autoimmune diseases.
- This disease happens in all age groups but is more common in younger individuals.

- AA can affect any hair-bearing area, but the scalp is most commonly affected (Fig. 14.1).
  - Other affected areas include the eyebrows, facial hair (Fig. 14.2), and body hair.
- There are multiple different clinical subtypes. These include patchy, pattern, totalis, and universalis.
  - Patchy is the most common subtype and involves one or more (typically annular) patches, which can present on any hair-bearing area.
  - Pattern is less common but comes in many patterns, ranging from diffuse to ophiasis, sisiapho, and reticular.
  - In totalis AA, all of the hair on the scalp is affected.

**259**

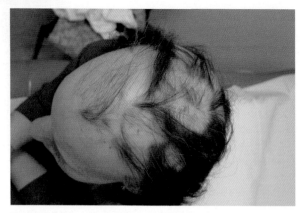

**Fig. 14.1 Alopecia Areata.** Scalp, patchy variant. (From the UConn Grand Rounds Collection.)

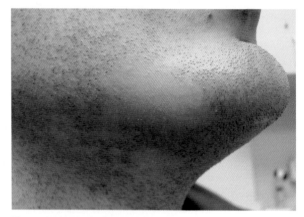

**Fig. 14.2 Alopecia Areata.** Alopecia areata on the beard. (Courtesy Justin Finch, MD.)

- In universalis AA, all of the hair on the body is affected.
- There may also be nail findings of AA, typically involving pitting.
- AA involves one or more painless patchy areas of hair loss, although white hairs may be spared and when new hair growth (short hair) is visible, it may also be white.
- The area of hair loss does not appear to be red or inflamed on a physical examination.
- AA typically presents as a sudden patch of hair loss on the scalp. The process is painless and noninflammatory.
  - Patients often state, "I lost this patch of hair overnight." The patient does not report clumps of hair coming out as is reported in telogen effluvium (TE).
- AA is an autoimmune disease, which is associated with other autoimmune diseases, including rheumatoid arthritis, vitiligo, and autoimmune thyroid disease.
  - AA is also strongly associated with atopic dermatitis (AD).
- Because AA has a strong genetic component, it is important to ask about family history.
- As with all conditions, AA may exist within the context of other hair pathologies (i.e., a patient with AGA may have coexisting AA).
- Prognosis depends on age of first presentation (younger is worse) and extent of disease (more extensive is worse).
- About 50% of patients have hair regrowth without treatment within 1 year.

## Differential Diagnosis

The differential for AA includes tinea capitis, AGA, trichotillomania, TE, anagen effluvium, and psychogenic pseudoeffluvium.

- Tinea capitis, especially in children, can present as one or more patches of hair loss. It is distinguished from AA because tinea capitis has inflammation and scale. If the diagnosis is unclear, a fungal culture can differentiate between the two. Tinea capitis also resolves with antifungal treatment and has classic potassium hydroxide (KOH) of hair scraping, showing a hyphae (long) and yeast (round) with spaghetti (long) and meatball (round) appearance.
- AGA can coexists in middle-aged to older patients with AA where the patient will present with a new patch of hair loss in the background setting of AGA. Other subtypes of AA, including the diffuse subtype, can present with diffuse hair thinning and can be easily mistaken for AGA. Timing is very important here. AGA is a much slower process (years) compared with AA (days or weeks) and thus completing a patient history is critical before providing additional work-up. The pattern of hair loss (location on the head) is also important because AGA favors the frontotemporal and occipital areas.
- Trichotillomania, which commonly presents in children, is caused by obsessive hair pulling/twisting and can cause patchy hair loss, which resembles AA.

Patients can be observed for hair-pulling behavior and there are various physical examination findings, including hairs of various different lengths and an abundance of split ends, which should raise suspicion. Trichotillomania often coexists with other psychiatric conditions, including obsessive-compulsive disorder (OCD).

- TE patients typically present with complaints of hair shedding in clumps. This type of hair loss is diffuse; therefore it should be easily distinguished from the classic patchy AA. Distinguishing between diffuse AA and TE can be very difficult and relies on biopsy findings or results of a modified hair wash test.
- Anagen effluvium is a form of diffuse hair loss that is triggered by chemotherapeutic-based destruction of hair follicles, leading to rapid, diffuse hair loss. Patient history is critical for establishing this diagnosis.
- Psychogenic pseudoeffluvium is another psychiatric-associated hair condition, and it occurs when patients are intentionally causing hair loss for secondary gain. This is usually discovered when work-up, including biopsy, is not revealing.

## Work-Up

Work-up for AA is divided into history taking, clinical examination, and laboratory work-up.

### History Taking

- Patients should specifically be queried about the duration of hair loss. When did it start? How long has it been happening?
- AA is a recurrent disease that can involve any area of hair, so asking about prior episodes or other affected areas is important. AA is an autoimmune disease, so asking if the patient has a history of another autoimmune disease, such as thyroid disease, systemic lupus erythematosus, or vitiligo, is important.
- Ask about any treatments and their effects and inquire about a family history of AA.

## Clinical Examination

- History and visual examination are all that are required to diagnose the common variants of patchy AA. Document the pattern of hair loss, including whether there is a single patch or multiple patches and what the specific patterns are (diffuse, ophiasis, sisiapho, reticular).

- Evaluation with a dermatoscope or other form of magnification (such as a jeweler's loupe, which is very inexpensive and readily available online) can be helpful. The classic findings on magnification are yellow dots (keratin in the follicles) and exclamation mark hairs (thinner proximally), although these findings are nonspecific. A positive hair pull test (during active disease) can be helpful in differentiating AA from trichotillomania and psychogenic pseudoeffluvium, but this is not typically done. Biopsy can also be done in cases of diffuse AA that are more difficult to diagnose.
- White hairs can be spared, and new hair growth may be white.
- Pictures should be taken (with a ruler) to document changes in future visits.

## Laboratory Work-Up

Laboratory work-up is not necessary unless there is suspicion for thyroid disease, which is a common coexisting disease (both are autoimmune). In that case, thyroid-stimulating hormone (TSH), T3, and T4 should be tested.

## Initial Steps in Management

There are no U.S. Food and Drug Administration (FDA)–approved treatments for AA, and the literature lacks high-quality randomized trials for this disease. Nevertheless, there are multiple treatment options. Patients should be counseled on this and on the fact that hair regrowth, even with treatment, will take a minimum of 3 months.

- The most common treatment modality for patchy disease on the scalp is local injection of corticosteroids. Triamcinolone acetonide is the most commonly used option and treatment involves multiple injections approximately 1 cm apart and 0.1 mL in volume. These injections are painful, require multiple treatments at 1-month intervals, and can result in skin atrophy, among other complications. It should be noted that these treatments do not prevent AA from developing in other areas. If there is no response after 6 months, local injections should be stopped.
- Topical corticosteroids can be trialed for isolated AA patches on the scalp. Options include clobetasol foam and lotion. This treatment is less likely to work than local corticosteroid injection. Moreover, clobetasol is a very potent steroid and can cause local

atrophy. Patients should be counseled to only use this on areas on the scalp. Similar to injections, the treatment should only last for 6 months. Patients should take 2 days off treatment per week and should have regular follow-up visits to assess progress and check for side effects.

- Systemic corticosteroids (either pulsed-dose oral steroids or intramuscular steroids) have also been used for treatment, but the side effects can be significant and rebound after discontinuation is common. This treatment is only reasonable in cases of debilitating hair loss where patients are accepting of the inherent risks of long-term corticosteroids.
- About 50% of patients have regrowth within 1 year with no treatment. Some male patients prefer to shave their heads to cover up the areas of disease.
- Trichopigmentation is a form of nonpermanent hair tattooing that has been helpful for concealing areas in some patients, especially eyebrow loss in severe cases.
- Laser treatments (by excimer lasers) are another nonmedical option, but the evidence for these treatments is not robust.
- In terms of upcoming treatments, Janus kinase (JAK) inhibitors offer promising hope for severe and treatment-resistant diseases. Multiple biologic antibodies are also currently being tested and the next 10 years are sure to bring exciting developments for therapy.
- Hair prosthesis (i.e., medical-grade wigs) should be considered in all cases of diffuse hair loss, especially in children, where current therapies are poorly tolerated,
- Although it will not affect the AA, treat a thyroid disease if it is identified.
- Topical minoxidil has not been shown to have any benefit for patients with AA.
- All patients should monitor their hair loss at home with serial pictures.

## Warning Signs/Common Pitfalls

Do not downplay the patient's concern regarding the alopecia, no matter how limited the disease may be. Patients should be counseled regarding the risks and benefits of treatment. Scheduling regular follow-up visits and assessing the need for psychological support, especially for severe AA cases, are also important steps. Children with this disease are often bullied extensively and special precautions warning teachers and counselors may be necessary.

## Counseling

You have a type of hair loss called "alopecia areata." It is caused by an autoimmune reaction against the hair follicles. The trigger for this is not clear, but there is a strong genetic component. There is a large spectrum of disease. Most commonly, one or a few patches of hair are lost, and this can happen anywhere on the body. The disease fortunately goes away on its own in about a year in half of all cases. The most common treatment for this disease involves steroid injections into the affected region on the scalp. There are also multiple cosmetic options we can explore. This type of hair loss can be very distressing, and we are here to help should you need any type of emotional support.

# TRICHOTILLOMANIA

Sonal Muzumdar and Andrew Kelsey

## Clinical Features

- Patients with trichotillomania (also known as "hair-pulling disorder") compulsively remove their own body hair. Methods of removal often include pulling, plucking, and twirling.
- This condition should be considered a variant of OCD.
- Although any part of the body may be involved in trichotillomania, hair loss is most frequently found on the scalp. Eyebrows, eyelashes, and genital hair may be involved.
- Characteristic physical examination findings include irregular, patchy areas of alopecia. Hair within a patch of alopecia may be of different lengths and in different stages of regrowth (Fig. 14.3). Underlying skin is typically normal in appearance, without scarring or inflammation.
- Trichotillomania is often associated with trichophagia, which is the eating of the pulled hair. This can lead to intestinal obstruction with trichobezoars.
- Trichotillomania is found in females more often than males (in a 5:1 ratio).

## Differential Diagnosis

The differential diagnosis for trichotillomania of the scalp includes AA and tinea capitis.

- Trichotillomania may be differentiated from alopecia areata in that AA typically presents with circular patches of nonscarring alopecia. In contrast, the

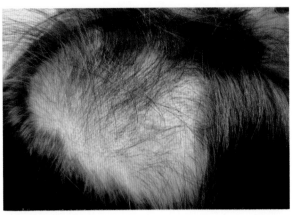

**Fig. 14.3 Trichotillomania.** Notice the different lengths of hairs within the alopecic patch. (Courtesy Justin Finch, MD.)

patches of alopecia in trichotillomania are typically irregular in shape and may contain hair of different lengths.

- In AA, the hair pull test may be positive at the edges of the patches of alopecia. The hair pull test is typically negative in trichotillomania.
  - The hair pull test involves grasping about 40 hairs and gently tugging on them. If at least 6 hairs (or more than 10% of the hairs tugged on) are removed, the test is considered positive.
- Trichotillomania may be differentiated from tinea capitis in that tinea capitis may present with scaling. Scaling is not found in trichotillomania.
  - Tinea capitis may also cause occipital lymphadenopathy, which is not found in trichotillomania.
  - A KOH preparation of a skin scraping may also be used to distinguish between tinea capitis and trichotillomania because it will show hyphae in tinea capitis.

## Work-Up

- Trichotillomania is diagnosed with a careful history and physical examination.
- According to the fifth edition of the American Psychiatric Association's Diagnostic and Statistical Manual (DSM-5) the following five criteria must be present for the diagnosis of trichotillomania:
  - The patient must be removing their own body hair.
  - The patient must have tried to stop removing their body hair.
  - Removal of body hair must cause significant emotional distress or impairment in functioning.

- Hair loss must not be caused by another medical condition.
  - Hair pulling cannot be explained by another mental disorder.
- Although a biopsy is not necessary for the diagnosis of trichotillomania, it may show traumatized or empty hair follicles in a dermis without inflammation.
- The confirmatory test is the hair growth window. This test involves repeated shaving of a specific area of hair. As the hair grows in, it will grow with a normal density because these hairs are too small for the patient to remove.

## Warning Signs/Common Pitfalls

- Given the stigma associated with hair loss, patients may be reluctant to divulge a history of pulling out their own hair. It is important to consider this diagnosis in all patients with alopecia.
- Some patients may eat their hair after removing it. Patients with trichotillomania who present with abdominal pain should be evaluated for a trichobezoar, a mass of hair found in the intestines.
- Hair loss in trichotillomania is typically temporary. Nevertheless, long-standing disease may lead to scarring of the involved hair bulbs and permanent hair loss.

## Management

- In children, trichotillomania may be self-limited. The prognosis is generally better in children than in adults.
- In adults, trichotillomania is difficult to treat. It is important to explore the psychosocial factors causing this condition. Patients should be referred to a psychologist or psychiatrist. Therapies such as behavioral therapy, clomipramine, or selective serotonin reuptake inhibitors (SSRIs) may be considered.
- In both children and adults, there is increasing evidence for the efficacy of taking N-acetylcysteine 600 mg orally daily.

## Counseling

Your hair loss is caused by a condition called "trichotillomania." Trichotillomania is a medical condition related to obsessive-compulsive disorder where patients feel compelled to remove their own hair. Some patients may not even be aware that they are doing it. Many factors can cause trichotillomania, including emotional stress. We recommend that all patients with trichotillomania see both a dermatologist and a psychologist or psychiatrist who will try to help you understand the underlying causes behind your condition. Although trichotillomania is hard to treat in adults, behavioral therapy and certain antidepressant medications have been shown to help patients.

# CENTRAL CENTRIFUGAL CICATRICIAL ALOPECIA

**Sonal Muzumdar and Andrew Kelsey**

## Clinical Features

- Central centrifugal cicatricial alopecia (CCCA) classically presents with alopecia on the vertex scalp that slowly expands in a centrifugal, spiraling pattern (Fig. 14.4).
- In late-stage disease, alopecia may involve the whole scalp. Affected areas of the scalp are smooth, without visible follicles. Patients may complain that the scalp is tender or pruritic.
- The etiology of CCCA is complex. It was originally thought to be secondary to the use of hot combs; hot oils on the scalp; chemical relaxers; and excessive tension from braids, hair rollers, or extensions. Heredity (family history) also appeared to play a role. Because the biopsy of the involved scalp demonstrates a lichenoid inflammatory process, however, CCCA is now thought to possibly be a variant of frontal lichen planopilaris (LPP).

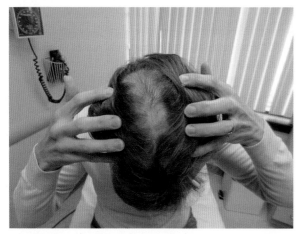

**Fig. 14.4 Central Centrifugal Alopecia.** Notice the scarring and total obliteration of hair follicles in the alopecic patch. (From the UConn Grand Rounds Collection.)

- A recent study identified a gene mutation that is possibly causative of CCCA in a subset of women.
- CCCA most commonly occurs in Black women in their 20s and 30s. As previously noted, it is often associated with the use of pomades, hot combs, chemical relaxers, and tight hairstyles.

## Differential Diagnosis

The differential diagnosis for CCCA includes AGA. CCCA may be differentiated from androgenetic alopecia in a few ways.

- Although CCCA typically begins on the vertex of the scalp and expands radially, AGA classically involves both the frontal scalp (in women this is usually seen with frontal thinning behind a retained frontal hairline) and the vertex and presents with a widened medial part.
- The scalp in CCCA may be tender. In AGA, the scalp is typically asymptomatic.

## Work-Up

CCCA is diagnosed by clinical examination, dermoscopy, and histopathologic corroboration.

### Clinical Examination

Patients typically present with hair loss at the vertex of the scalp, which then extends radially to the periphery.

### Dermoscopy

Gray or white peripilar halos under dermoscopy are sensitive and specific for CCCA. There may be several hairs growing from one apparent follicle. This is known as "tufted hair" or "doll's hair."

### Histopathology

Biopsy should be performed at the site of a peripilar halo. The specimen should be sent to a dermatopathologist because it requires sectioning horizontally for more complete follicular evaluation. Histopathology will show decreased follicular density and absent or greatly diminished sebaceous glands. Early in the course of the disease, there may be follicular lichenoid inflammation. Later on, this may progress to follicular fibrosis. The dermatopathologist may see polytrichia, which correlates to fusion of several follicles, giving the clinical appearance of tufted hairs.

## Management

The management of CCCA focuses on preventing further hair loss.

- Patients should avoid chemical relaxants, thermal treatments, and traction on the hair.
- Topical or intralesional steroids or topical calcineurin inhibitors may be used on affected areas. Topical minoxidil 2% or 5% is another therapeutic option. Oral minocycline or tetracycline may also be considered for their antiinflammatory effects.
- In severe cases, hair transplantation may be considered.
- All patients should be counseled on the nature of the disease and emotional support should be provided, given the distress that may result from alopecia.

## Counseling

Your hair loss is caused by a condition called "central centrifugal cicatricial alopecia" (CCCA). In this disease, patients initially lose hair on the top of their scalp. This hair loss may progress outwards to involve most of your scalp. Your healthcare provider can diagnose this condition with a careful physical examination, dermoscopy, and a biopsy of your scalp.

Once you have lost hair, regaining it may not be possible. Treatment for CCCA is focused on preventing further hair loss. Your healthcare provider may prescribe you topical steroids or perform steroid injections in the affected area. Topical calcineurin inhibitors, topical minoxidil (such as Rogaine) and oral antibiotics may also halt further hair loss. These treatments may be required for a long period of time. Hair transplant may be considered in patients who have lost a significant amount of hair.

# DISCOID LUPUS (SEE CHAPTER 1, SCALP DERMATITIS, DLE)

# TRACTION ALOPECIA

**Sonal Muzumdar and Andrew Kelsey**

## Clinical Features

- Traction alopecia is caused by hairstyles that pull on the hair, such as tight braids, buns, or ponytails. The use of chemical relaxants on hair may also contribute to the disease because chemically treated hair may be more susceptible to breakage with traction. Women of African or Caribbean descent are more commonly affected.
- Patients typically present with nonscarring alopecia in areas of high scalp tension. The frontal and temporoparietal scalp are most commonly involved, but other areas of the scalp may also demonstrate alopecia, depending on the patient's hairstyle. Classically, patients may retain a fringe of hair along the involved hairline, known as the "fringe sign."
- Affected patients may develop a secondary folliculitis (traction folliculitis) that presents with perifollicular erythema, papules, and pustules in involved regions of the scalp.

## Differential Diagnosis

The differential diagnosis for traction alopecia includes frontal fibrosing alopecia (FFA). The two conditions may be distinguished from one another in a few ways.

- FFA classically presents with scarring alopecia along the frontal hairline. Scarring is rarely seen with traction alopecia, especially early on in the disease course.
- FFA may involve hair loss at sites other than the scalp, such as the eyebrows and eyelashes. In traction alopecia, the scalp is almost always the only involved site of hair loss.

## Work-Up

- Traction alopecia may be diagnosed with a careful history and physical examination.
- Patients may report using tight hairstyles, such as braids or ponytails.
- On examination, patients may demonstrate nonscarring alopecia at areas of tension in the scalp. A fringe of smaller, fine hair may be present at the involved hairline. Erythematous papules or pustules may also be present in involved areas.
- Under dermoscopy, hair casts may be seen around the proximal hair follicles in involved regions.

## Warning Signs/Common Pitfalls

Early on in the disease course, traction alopecia may be reversible. Thus early detection is key because scarring may occur later in the disease as a result of permanent damage to the hair bulb from the recurrent or persistent traction.

## Management

- Patients should be counseled to avoid hairstyles that cause excess traction on their hair. They should also avoid thermal and chemical treatment of their hair.
- Patients with traction folliculitis (inflammatory papules and pustules) in involved scalp regions should

be given topical and/or oral antibiotics. Topical corticosteroids can occasionally be used as well to temporarily to decrease inflammation.

- Topical minoxidil has been demonstrated to benefit some patients with traction alopecia.
- Later in the disease course of traction alopecia, patients may develop scarring and permanent hair loss. Hair transplantation may be considered in these patients.

## Counseling

Your hair loss is caused by a condition called "traction alopecia." In this condition, patients lose hair because of a tight hairstyle pulling the hair from the scalp. Using heat or chemicals in your hair may make it more brittle and more susceptible to break from traction. In addition to hair loss, you may notice redness or bumps in the affected area.

This condition is typically reversible if caught early. The most important thing to do is loosen your hairstyle and style your hair in a way that does not pull on the scalp. You should also avoid using heat or chemicals in your hair. If you have redness or inflammation of your scalp, your healthcare provider may treat you with antibiotics and possibly topical steroids. Over-the-counter topical minoxidil (such as Rogaine) may also have some benefits in this condition. Reversing your traction alopecia early is important because your hair loss is still reversible. If you wait too long, you may develop scarring in the areas of hair loss, which can become permanent.

Tinea Capitis (See Chapter 1 Scalp Dermatitis)

# Nail Disease

# 15

# Conditions that Frequently Affect a Single Nail

## MELANONYCHIA

**Brett Sloan**

### Clinical Features

Melanonychia is dark brown or black pigmentation on the nail plate. There are numerous causes, the most concerning being melanoma of the nail unit.

Melanonychia can present as diffuse darkening of the nail plate or, more commonly, as a longitudinal line, which is known as "longitudinal melanonychia" (LM). Melanonychia is a misnomer because the nail pigmentation is not necessarily the result of melanin. The discoloration can be because of melanin, exogenous pigment, medications, fungi, or bacteria.

Evaluation of melanonychia is similar to the evaluation of any pigmented lesion. A commonly used acronym is ABCDEF.

**A** stands for age because the incidence of nail melanoma is higher in people in their 50s, 60s, or 70s.

**B** signifies borders and breadth. Well-defined, sharp borders and a diameter of less than 3 mm are good signs.

**C** is for change. It is important to assess whether the lesion has changed over time or been present without change for many years.

**D** is for digit. The thumb and the great toe are the most common sites of nail unit melanoma.

**E** is for extension onto the skin around the nail plate. This is called the Hutchinson sign, and it is extremely concerning for melanoma.

**F** is for family history. As with cutaneous melanoma, a family history of melanoma or dysplastic nevus syndrome is a risk factor for developing nail unit melanoma.

### Differential Diagnosis

The differential diagnosis of true melanonychia includes two broad categories: pigment because of an increased numbers of melanocytes (nail simple lentigines, nail melanocytic nevi, and melanoma) and pigment because of activation of normally quiescent melanocytes (melanocyte activation). The vast majority of

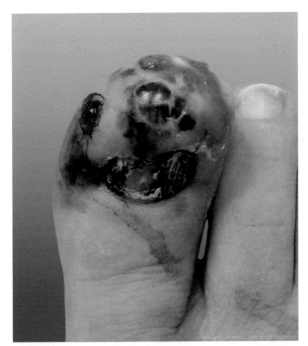

**Fig. 15.1** Acrolentiginous Melanoma. (From the University of Connecticut Department of Dermatology Grand Rounds Collection.)

melanocytes are found in the nail matrix and do not normally produce melanin. When activated, they produce pigment in the nail plate.

Causes of melanocyte hyperplasia include nail matrix nevi and melanomas (Fig. 15.1). Distinguishing between the two can be difficult and if there are any concerning features, a nail matrix biopsy is warranted. Nail matrix nevi are more common in children and are usually less than 3 mm in size, evenly pigmented, and do not involve any of the nail folds. Subungual melanomas are rare, accounting for between 0.7% to 3.5% of melanomas worldwide. It is the most common form of melanoma in Black people, Asians, and Hispanics.

There are numerous causes of melanocyte activation, all of which can produce melanonychia.

- Trauma from nail biting (onychophagia), nail picking (onychotillomania), ill-fitting shoes, or occupational/recreational hazards can be a cause.
- Physiologic causes are considered a normal variant in people with darkly pigmented skin and usually involve multiple nails.
- There are also numerous common medications that can cause melanocyte activation, including but not

limited to the cyclines, psoralens, zidovudine, phenytoin, fluoride, chemotherapeutics, antimalarials, ketoconazole, and ibuprofen.

- Another cause is postinflammatory hyperpigmentation after inflammation of the nail folds from eczema, contact dermatitis, psoriasis, or connective tissue disease.
- Systemic diseases, such as Addison disease, Cushing syndrome, acquired immunodeficiency syndrome, hyperthyroidism, porphyria, graft versus host disease, and malnutrition, can cause melanocyte activation.

## Differential Diagnosis

The differential diagnosis for melanonychia includes subungual hematomas, infectious etiologies, and exogenous pigments.

- Subungual hematomas usually present as a purple or black macule under the nail plate. It migrates distally with the growth of the nail plate.
- Infectious causes are usually fungal organisms or bacteria that produce pigment. There is a growing list of over 20 fungal species that produce subungual debris. If LM is present, it typically is wider distally and tapers proximally. *Pseudomonas aeruginosa* causes green nail syndrome. It produces pyocyanin and pyoverdine, blue and green pigments that can cause the nail to appear from yellow to green to black in color. It is most commonly seen in people who keep their hands submerged in water for extended periods (e.g., dishwashers, housekeepers, healthcare workers).
- Exogenous pigment found on the nail could include tobacco, dirt, tar, paint, or henna. Often, a supporting history can be elicited and these can be wiped off with an alcohol swab.

## Work-Up

- A thorough history should be completed with a focus on information about any potential trauma, any history of skin disease, and a full medication history (including over-the-counter medications and supplements).
- A review of systems should focus on potential systemic diseases that could cause melanonychia.
- A full-body skin examination, including the genitalia and oral mucosa, should be performed to look for other areas of hyperpigmentation or clues to systemic diseases that can cause nail hyperpigmentation.

Examination of all the nails is necessary. If the patient is wearing nail polish, this should be removed.

- If there is thickening of the nail plate or subungual debris, a nail clipping should be sent to the microbiology lab for culture or to the pathology lab for periodic acid–Schiff staining.
- If any of the features previously outlined as concerning for melanoma are present, the patient should be referred to a dermatologist experienced in performing nail matrix biopsies.

## Initial Steps in Management

Management of melanonychia should focus on ruling out malignancy.

The patient should immediately be referred to a dermatologist for evaluation for biopsy in a few instances:

- The pigmented band is new and greater than 3 mm wide.
- The pigmented band is new and changing in color or symmetry.
- There is a personal history of melanoma.
- There is any pigment on the skin around the nail (nail folds).

For solitary pigmented bands less than 3 mm in width and stable, it would be prudent to take a clinical image for the chart and follow up in 3 to 6 months to assess for interval change. Encourage patients to take a photograph of the affected nail with their personal cell phone for reference. This way, they can assess for any changes that may occur before the scheduled follow-up visit.

If there is any sign of skin disease on the finger that could be causing the inflammation and subsequent melanocyte activation, it should be treated with a mid-potency topical steroid, such as triamcinolone 0.1% ointment applied twice daily until resolution.

If there is thickening of the nail plate or subungual debris that has tested positive for nail fungus, treatment with an oral antifungal is warranted. Oral terbinafine 250 mg daily for 6 weeks for fingernails and 12 weeks for toenails is generally effective.

There is no medical reason to treat patients with multiple pigmented bands because there are no treatments available that will lighten the bands. The bands will fade and potentially disappear if they are secondary to melanocyte activation and the source of the activation is treated.

## Warning Signs/Common Pitfalls

The ABCDEs of pigmented bands should catch the warning signs of melanoma. Patient history is essential when it comes to changes in size or color of the band.

It also should be noted that melanomas can bleed and present as subungual hematomas. Thus all subungual hematomas should be evaluated and followed up on appropriately until resolution.

Likewise, onychomycosis is extremely common in the general population and can occur in conjunction with nail melanoma. If the onychomycosis is successfully treated and the pigment remains, the patient should be referred for a biopsy.

## Counseling

Pigmented bands and darkening of the nails is extremely common and the vast majority of causes are completely benign. Melanoma, although rare, can occur under the nail and this is the diagnosis we do not want to miss. A nail biopsy would be recommended if you have a history of melanoma, the band is solitary and new, the band is greater than 3 mm, the band has been changing in size or color, and/or there is pigmentation on the skin around the nail. These are all concerning signs for melanoma. Moles and lentigines (so-called "sun spots") can also occur under the nail, yet typically are smaller than 3 mm and are evenly pigmented and stable in size and color.

When multiple nails are involved, the causes are numerous and less concerning for malignancy. Oftentimes, these bands are because of your race because they are common normal findings in skin of color. They can also be the result of certain medications, trauma, and any skin disease that affects the skin around the nail.

# ERYTHRONYCHIA

**Brett Sloan**

## Clinical Features

Longitudinal erythronychia (LE) is a relatively common nail condition that presents with a longitudinal red or pink band extending from the lunula to the distal nail plate. The differential diagnosis of LE is broad but is generally divided into causes of solitary LE or LE involving multiple nails.

LE is often associated with nail plate changes. These can present as longitudinal ridges or grooves, distal

V-shaped nicks, chipping, splitting, and onycholysis (separation of the nail plate from the nail bed). It can also be associated with splinter hemorrhages and hyperkeratosis at the distal end of the LE.

## Differential Diagnosis

The differential diagnosis for solitary LE includes benign conditions, such as onychopapilloma, wart, glomus tumor, and scar. It also includes malignant conditions, such as Bowen disease (squamous cell carcinoma [SCC] in situ), SCC, and amelanotic melanoma.

- Onychopapillomas are the most common cause and are benign tumors that originate in the nail matrix. They are commonly associated with distal nail splinting and hyperkeratosis of the nail bed at the distal end of the LE.
- Warts rarely present as a solitary pink band. They are more commonly associated with cutaneous warts on the nail folds or under the nail plate.
- Glomus tumors are benign tumors of the glomus body, a temperature-sensitive organ in the nail bed that helps maintain digit circulation under cold conditions. They are typically painful when pressed or exposed to temperature change.
- Bowen disease and SCC present as evolving erythronychia and are often associated with nail dystrophy and nail bed hyperkeratosis. SCC is the most common malignancy of the nail bed.
- Amelanotic melanoma is a very rare form of melanoma. Although less than 7% of cutaneous melanomas are amelanotic, 20% to 30% of nail melanomas are amelanotic. Any evolving pink or red band should be referred for biopsy.

The potential causes of multiple nail involvement include lichen planus (LP), Darier disease, graft versus host disease, amyloidosis (Fig. 15.2), and hemiplegia. It is often idiopathic.

- LP can present with only involvement of the nails. This can present as multiple bands of LE. More commonly, it is associated with rough thin nail plates. Without treatment, this can progress to scarring manifested as dorsal pterygia (growth of the proximal nail fold onto the nail bed).
- Darier disease is a rare autosomal dominant skin disease that is associated with red and white nail bands with distal V-nicking of the nail plate (Fig. 15.3). Greasy, scaly papules on the head and chest in a seborrheic distribution and warty papules

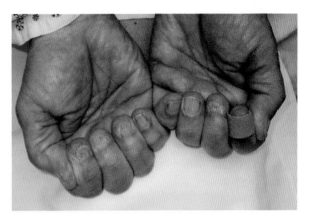

**Fig. 15.2** Nail Dystrophy in a Patient with Immunoglobulin Light Chain Amyloidosis. (From the University of Connecticut Department of Dermatology Grand Rounds Collection.)

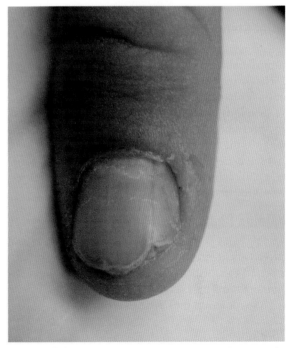

**Fig. 15.3** Erythronychia and V-Nicking in a Patient with Darier Disease. (From the University of Connecticut Department of Dermatology Grand Rounds Collection.)

on the dorsal hands are also manifestations of Darier disease.

- There is an ever-growing list of systemic conditions associated with multiple bands of erythronychia. For this reason, a thorough history, review of systems, and physical examination is essential.

## Work-Up

A thorough history should include any potential trauma and any history of skin disease or systemic disease. A review of systems should focus on potential systemic diseases that could cause LE.

A full-body skin examination, including the genitalia and oral mucosa, should be performed to look for cutaneous LP, Darier disease, or clues to systemic diseases that could be causing LE. Examination of all the nails is necessary. If the patient is wearing nail polish, this should be removed.

If pain is elicited with palpation or temperature changes and glomus tumor is suspected, imaging may be useful for diagnosis or preoperative planning. Both color-duplex ultrasonography and high-resolution magnetic resonance imaging (MRI) have been proven to be useful in establishing the diagnosis.

## Initial Steps in Management

Management of erythronychia should focus on ruling out malignancy.

The patient should immediately be referred for evaluation for biopsy if the band is new and changing; there is a subungual mass; there is tenderness upon palpation or with temperature changes; or there is associated dystrophy of the nail.

If the patient is unsure if the band is new or changing, a clinical image should be taken and followed up on every 3 to 6 months to assess for change.

## Warning Signs/Common Pitfalls

Warning signs revolve around missing a potential skin cancer. Patient history is extremely important, especially in regard to whether the band is new or changing or symptomatic. There should be a low threshold to refer for biopsy if any of the concerns are present.

## Counseling

Pink or red bands are not uncommon and the vast majority of causes are completely benign. Skin cancer, although rare, can occur under the nail and this is the diagnosis we do not want to miss. Evaluation for nail biopsy would be recommended if you have a history of skin cancer, the band is solitary and new, the band has been changing in size or color, there is an associated mass underneath the nail, there are textural changes to the nail plate, and/or there is tenderness or pain in nail.

When multiple nails are involved, the causes are numerous and less concerning for malignancy.

# HABIT TIC DEFORMITY

**Brett Sloan and Sonal Muzumdar**

## Clinical Features

- Habit tic deformity may affect any fingernail, but the thumbs are most commonly involved.
- Characteristic findings include a central, longitudinal depression in the nail and transverse, parallel ridging across the nail plate. The cuticle may be damaged or absent altogether.

## Differential Diagnosis

The differential diagnosis for habit tic deformity includes median canaliform dystrophy.

- Habit tic deformity can be differentiated from median canaliform dystrophy in terms of ridging and cuticles.
  - In median canaliform dystrophy, ridging is typically oblique, resembling a fir tree, rather than transverse, as in habit tic deformity.
  - In median canaliform dystrophy, cuticles are typically normal, whereas they may be atrophied or absent altogether in habit tic deformity.

## Work-Up

- Habit tic deformity may be diagnosed with a careful physical examination. Although any nail may be involved, the thumbnails are most frequently affected. Common nail findings include a central depression of the nail, transverse ridging across the nail bed, a hypertrophied lunula, and an absent cuticle.
- A history of picking or rubbing of the cuticle or nail, either from the patient or a relative, may be suggestive of habit tic deformity. Nevertheless, it is important to note that many patients are not conscious of this habit and may not report this in their history.

## Warning Signs/Common Pitfalls

In habit tic deformity, rubbing or picking at the cuticle and proximal nail is often not done consciously. As such, patients may not recall traumatizing their nails. Despite this, consider habit tic deformity if characteristic physical examination findings are present.

## Management

- Treatment focuses on discouraging manipulation of the nail. This may be achieved through the use of physical barriers (such as bandages or tapes) to cover the nail, cyanoacrylate adhesive between the proximal nail fold and the nail plate to allow for healing, and bland ointment applied proximally to distally over the nail to demonstrate improved symptoms.
- For persistent cases, cognitive behavioral may be used to teach patients not to pick at their nails.
  - Other options include N-acetylcysteine 600 mg taken orally daily or selective serotonin reuptake inhibitors (SSRIs) in those considered to have coexisting psychiatric disorders.

## Counseling

The changes in your nail are caused by a condition called habit tic deformity. In habit tic deformity, people pick or rub their cuticles and their nails. This is often done unconsciously and many people may not even realize that they are doing it. However, the picking or rubbing can cause damage to the nail and make it look abnormal.

The findings seen in your nail are reversible. Treatment is aimed at preventing you from picking or rubbing at your cuticles. You can try putting a bandage or tape over your nails to prevent you from picking at them. Putting a special instant glue on your cuticles may also help. For some people, putting an ointment on the nails also helps. In severe cases of habit tic deformity that do not respond to those treatments, we can try cognitive behavioral therapy to keep you from picking at your nails. A type of antidepressant medication called a "selective serotonin reuptake inhibitor," or "SSRI," may also help.

# 16

# Multiple Nails

## ONYCHOMYCOSIS

**Douglas Albreski**

### Clinical Features

A fungal infection of the nail, referred to as "onychomycosis" or "tinea unguium," is an infection of the nail in which the organism changes the structure and shape of the nail plate, leading to thickening, changes in appearance, and/or discoloration. Changes in appearance are dependent on the organism and site of infection.

- There are five common types of onychomycosis.
  - Distal dystrophic onychomycosis (distal subungual onychomycosis) is the most common type. It is caused by *Trichophyton rubrum,* which infects the distal nail unit, causing distal nail plate separation and subungual hyperkeratosis.

- White superficial onychomycosis is commonly caused by *T. mentagrophytes,* which grow on the surface of the nail plate and lead to further destruction of the nail plate if left untreated.
- Proximal subungual onychomycosis, which may also be caused by *T. rubum,* is the least common type and is associated with the organism entering through the disruption of the cuticle region. This type often causes nail loss and is associated with patients with untreated HIV.
- Candida onychomycosis involves a yeast infection along the proximal or lateral nail folds, with the most common type involving the hands. It is associated with patients who have increased water exposure to their hands.
- Total dystrophic onychomycosis is when the disease completely absorbs the nail plate and can lead to permanent damage, even after successful treatment.

## Differential Diagnosis

The differential for onychomycosis includes inflammatory nail dystrophy, bacterial nail infections, traumatic onychodystrophy, nail bed or osseous tumors, yellow nail syndrome, malignancies of the nail unit, and uncommon nail conditions like idiopathic onycholysis. Similar symptoms can sometimes also result from the use of certain drugs.

- Inflammatory nail dystrophy is the result of an inflammation of the nail unit, which includes the matrix and nail bed. These changes are associated with the location and degree of inflammation; common types are psoriatic nail dystrophy, lichen planus (LP) nail involvement, and contact dermatitis.
  - Psoriatic nail dystrophy is associated with the so-called "pitting" and classic "oil stain" signs; pain is associated with nail bed inflammation.
  - LP nail involvement is associated with nail plate splitting that has a winglike or so-called "pterygium" appearance (Fig. 16.1).
  - Contact dermatitis results from the inflammation of the nail folds after exposure to a sensitizing agent, such as acrylics (false nails) or topical nail preparations; if chronic exposure to the agent occurs, it can cause nail changes.
- Bacterial nail infections present with the causative organism usually infiltrating the borders of the nail unit and are associated with nail plate discoloration.
- Traumatic onychodystrophy results from injury of the nail unit; trauma can include direct traumatic injury or accumulation of repetitive microtrauma.

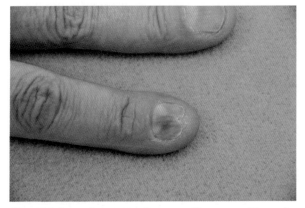

**Fig. 16.1** Pterygium, secondary to nail trauma. (From the UConn Department of Dermatology Grand Rounds Collection.)

Black-purple discoloration is common when there is a subungual hemorrhage.

- Nail bed or osseous tumors can cause structural changes to the nail unit, resulting in nail plate deformities.
- Yellow nail syndrome is a rare condition that results from increased lymphatic effusion, causing yellowing of the nail plate.
- Malignancies of the nail unit can cause structural changes, resulting in nail plate deformities. Black discoloration or a streak on the nail plate and/or unit may be an indicator of malignant melanoma.
- Uncommon nail conditions resembling onychomycosis include drug-induced nail dystrophy, pachyonychia congenita, and idiopathic onycholysis.
- Some drugs cause onycholysis (lifting of the nail plate from the nail bed) or photo-onycholysis via damage to the nail bed. The list of drugs known to cause these reactions includes psoralens, doxycycline, oral contraceptives, diuretics (thiazides), antibiotics (fluoroquinolone), nonsteroidal antiinflammatory drugs (NSAIDs), taxanes, captopril, retinoids, phenothiazines, clofazimine, and some anticonvulsants (sodium valproate).

## Work-Up

Onychomycosis requires disease confirmation by way of laboratory diagnosis because of the varying treatment options and differing lengths of therapies. Topical agents may require up to a year of therapy. Meanwhile, oral agents tend to be safe but can have various medical contraindications and potential drug interactions.

- Scraping subungual debris and placing it on a glass slide, staining it with potassium hydroxide (KOH), and then heating the slide results in an easy-to-perform slide preparation that can be examined in the clinic under a microscope to identify hyphae and quickly confirm the diagnosis.
- Diagnosis can be confirmed by culturing the nail plate and subungual debris. Culturing, unfortunately, is time consuming, often yields false-negative results, and may produce contaminants, all of which can delay therapy. Use of a dermatophyte test medium (DTM) provides results much more quickly, but the results are generalized; fortunately, most agents treat dermatophytes very well. A final diagnostic method is histologic examination; periodic acid–Schiff (PAS) staining

can confirm hyphae involvement, rule out contamination, and assist in ruling out inflammatory, non-mycotic nails.

## Initial Steps in Management

Treatment options vary; the two most common methods involve topical agents and oral antifungal medications. A decision on treatment course is determined by the patient's medical history, drug interactions, and patient compliance with the recommended course of treatment. Topical treatments are lengthy and less successful; oral medications have shorter therapeutic courses and higher success rates but carry a higher risk for an adverse medical outcome.

## Oral Antifungal Agents

The most common oral antifungal agents are terbinafine and itraconazole.
- Oral terbinafine 250 mg should be taken once daily for a total of 6 weeks for fingernails and 12 weeks for toenails.
- Oral itraconazole 200 mg should be twice daily for 1 week, then 3 weeks off; this cycle is repeated once more (for a total treatment time of 2 months) for fingernails and twice more (for a total treatment time of 3 months) for toenails.
- Oral antifungal agents have pediatric dosing recommendations based on weight and length of treatment, which is similar to adult dosing.

## Topical Antifungal Agents

Topical antifungal agents are commonly used when there is minimal disease, only a few nails are involved, and/or underlying medical concerns contraindicate the use of oral agents. Unlike oral antifungal agents, topicals have poorer penetration, resulting in lower effectiveness. Topical agents also have a higher incidence of contact dermatitis and skin irritation. On the other hand, topical agents can be used and are highly successful in the treatment of white superficial onychomycosis because of the excellent drug-to-fungal exposure. Nevertheless, many insurances will not cover the cost of these preparations and the patient will have to pay out of pocket. The most efficacious, and common, topical antifungal nail solutions available are efinaconazole, tavaborole, and ciclopirox.
- Efinaconazole 10% solution is applied to the affected nail daily for up to 48 weeks.

- Tavaborole 5% solution is applied to the nail surface and distal nail edge daily for up to 48 weeks.
- Ciclopirox 8% solution is applied to the nail and surrounding nails folds daily for up to 48 weeks. Ciclopirox also requires weekly removal of residual agent on the nail with alcohol.

## Surgical Treatment and/or Serial Debridement

Mechanical reduction is available as a final treatment option when the nail plate is totally dystrophic, which may lead to pain, ingrown nails, or injury to adjacent digits. Mechanical reduction is critical for the patient with diabetes and for high-risk patients who are neuropathic or have peripheral vascular disease.

## Other Treatment Options

Other treatment options are available, but they usually require out-of-pocket costs and have very limited peer review studies confirming their success rates. The two most notable options are laser treatment and photodynamic therapy.

## Warning Signs/Common Pitfalls

The most common concern when treating onychomycosis is the development of ingrown nails as regrowth and reattachment of the nail plate to nail bed occurs. Mycotic infections can cause onycholysis, which is the separation of the nail plate from the bed. During treatment, this separation resolves; the nail should thus not be debrided back too aggressively because this will eliminate the lytic edge of the plate, which is necessary to allow for proper nail regrowth over the folds and prevent an ingrown nail.

One common pitfall is an inadequate therapeutic course of treatment; if residual infection is present, reoccurrence will most likely occur over time.

Severe dystrophy and permanent nail lysis allows for easy reinfection because of the lack of nail plate reattachment and lack of the natural antifungal tissue barrier.

Finally, there are hereditary predispositions to fungal infections and onychomycosis; even after successful treatment, a reinfection may occur upon the next exposure.

## Counseling

Nail fungus, medically referred to as "onychomycosis," is an infection of the nails that can affect the toenails and fingernails. This condition, if left untreated, can spread to other nails and can cause skin fungal infections. Not all changes to the nails are caused by fungus, so your healthcare provider may perform sample testing to confirm a diagnosis. There are many treatment options, ranging from taking a pill (which tends to have a higher success rate and shorter treatment course but higher risk for an adverse medical outcome) to applying a topical agent to the nails (which tends to have a lower success rate and longer treatment course of up to a year but minimal side effects).

After successful treatment, it is necessary to prevent reexposure and reinfection. Daily inspections of the feet are required, looking for signs of redness and itchy and peeling skin. Self-care is important and nail instruments should be clean; avoid sharing your instrument. Using over-the-counter (OTC) antifungal foot sprays and powders may help prevent reinfection. Finally, general fungal prevention begins with wearing protective shoes and avoiding walking barefoot in highly infected areas, such as locker rooms, public pools, hotels, and other areas with high exposure rates.

Because the fungus can remain in your socks or shoes, we recommend you consider replacing your insoles or disinfecting your footwear with antifungal powder or sprays; washing your socks in hot water; and alternating shoes so that you do not wear the same pair 2 days in a row, thus allowing your shoes to dry out completely, which can help prevent a reinfection.

# NAIL SPLITTING

### Brett Sloan

## Clinical Features

Nail splitting, also known as "onychoschizia," is a common nail plate problem encountered by dermatologists. The nails plates are brittle, soft, and/or thin and develop lamellar (horizontal) splitting because of loss of intracellular adhesion.
- Onychoschizia is seen more frequently in women and in the elderly.
- Repeatedly wetting and drying of the hands is the most common cause of onychoschizia and is frequently found in nurses, custodians, and hairdressers.
  - It has also been attributed to nail cosmetics, nail procedures, and occupational exposure to various chemicals.
  - Repeated microtrauma to the nail from typing, picking things up with the nails, excessively buffering

them, and/or nail biting (onychophagia) can also contribute to onychoschizia.
- Dietary deficiencies in iron, selenium, and zinc can lead to nail changes that may result in onychoschizia.

## Work-Up

The cause of onychoschizia can usually be ascertained by obtaining a thorough medical history. Rarely do vitamin deficiencies or chronic medical problems cause onychoschizia. On the other hand, iron deficiency anemia, hypothyroidism, chronic pulmonary disease, and chronic renal disease have all been associated with nail splitting. Based on the review of systems, iron studies, a hemoglobin level, renal studies, and/or a thyroid panel may be warranted.

## Initial Steps in Management

The initial steps in management of onychoschizia are to avoid the offending behavior. This would include avoiding excessive hand washing; occupational exposure to cements, solvents, alkalis, acids, anilines, and thioglycolates; nail cosmetics (especially nail enamel removers and hardeners); nail procedures (such as the application of premixed acrylic nails, nail sculpting, or excessive use of manicure tools); and any repeated trauma to the nails.

There are small preliminary studies supporting the use of biotin 2.5 mg/day for up to 6 months. These studies demonstrated a modest increase in nail thickness and resolution of lamellar splitting. Most dermatologists, however, no longer recommend biotin routinely because biotin supplements can alter routine blood tests (e.g., thyroid function testing, troponins).

The use of moisturizers containing alpha-hydroxy acids, phospholipids, or lanolin after soaking the nails in water for 5 to 10 minutes has shown to be of some benefit.

## Warning Signs/Common Pitfalls

The vast majority of the time nail splitting is simply a cosmetic issue, and the cause can be accurately discovered based on history. Nevertheless, the healthcare provider should be vigilant to potential medical problems that could predispose the nail to split. A review of systems, as discussed in the work-up section, is essential.

Patients taking biotin should be counseled that this may lead to inaccurate blood tests, specifically for thyroid and cardiac troponin levels. It can cause falsely high levels of T3 and T4, falsely low levels of thyroid-stimulating hormone (TSH), and falsely low troponin levels.

## Counseling

Your nails, like your skin, are very susceptible to drying and are vulnerable to water, harsh chemicals, and nail cosmetics. When your nails get dry, they are predisposed to chipping and splitting. It is essential that you avoid excessive exposure to moisture and chemicals that can damage your nails. If exposure to water or chemicals is unavoidable, it is important that you wear gloves with cotton liners to limit the exposure. It is best to avoid all nail cosmetics and procedures to minimize stress on the nail plate. Like your skin, the consistent use of a moisturizer on the nail plate and skin around the nail after soaking your nail for 5 to 10 minutes in water or after bathing/showering will help strengthen the nail over time. The dietary supplement biotin has been shown to improve nail strength and decrease splitting. It is generally safe but has some potential side effects and can interfere with certain blood tests, so you should discuss its use with your healthcare provider before taking it.

# DRUG ERUPTIONS INVOLVING THE NAIL UNIT

**Brett Sloan**

## Clinical Features

Medications can affect the nails in different ways. They can affect the nail plate, the nail bed, or the skin around the nail. Because nails grow slowly, medication effects on the nail plate might not be readily apparent and may be delayed by several weeks or months.
- Numerous chemotherapeutics and targeted immunotherapeutic agents cause paronychia, which is an inflammation of the lateral and proximal nail folds.
  - These would include taxanes, methotrexate, epidermal growth factor (EGFR) inhibitors, tyrosine kinase inhibitors, vascular endothelia growth factor inhibitors, and CD20 antagonists.
  - Retinoids, cyclosporine, and certain HIV medications can also cause paronychia.
- Periungual pyogenic granulomas, which are a beefy and benign vascular tumor, are induced by retinoids, cyclosporine, indinavir, and EGFR inhibitors.

Beau's lines (Fig. 16.2) are horizontal depressions across the nail plate caused by a temporary arrest of the

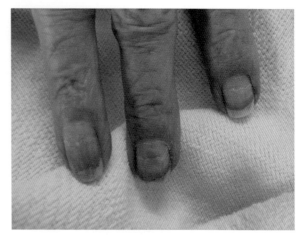

**Fig. 16.2** Beau's lines. (From the UConn Department of Dermatology Grand Rounds Collection.)

nail matrix. Onychomadesis, also known as "nail shedding," occurs when there is a more significant arrest in the nail matrix.
- These conditions are classically caused by chemotherapeutics. Nevertheless, retinoids, antiseizure medications, and certain antibiotics have also been reported to induce these changes.

Medications can affect the nail bed and interfere with how the nail plate adheres to the nail bed. Onycholysis occurs when the nail plate separates from the nail bed. Meanwhile, photo-onycholysis occurs when ultraviolet light triggers onycholysis.
- Photo-onycholysis can be seen with the use of doxycycline, NSAIDs, oral contraceptives, quinolone antibiotics, taxanes, thiazides, psoralens, and retinoids.

Nail plate pigmentation can be caused by activation of melanocytes in the nail matrix. This causes longitudinal brown lines to appear on the nail plates.
- It has been associated with chemotherapeutics, psoralens, hydroxyurea, and zidovudine and usually occurs 3 to 8 weeks after starting therapy.

Nail pigmentation can also be because of deposition of pigment in the nail bed.
- Minocycline can cause a bluish-gray discoloration, whereas antimalarials can cause a brown discoloration.
- Rarely do medications deposit pigment into the nail plate; however, tetracycline and gold salts can turn the nail plate yellow, and clofazimine can cause the plate to turn brown.

## Work-Up

A thorough medication history, including of OTC medications, should be taken. The medical history should also focus on other potential causes of nail changes.

- Recent surgery, stress, or trauma can cause Beau's lines.
- Onycholysis can be caused by occupational and household exposures to water and harsh chemicals; hypothyroidism and hyperthyroidism; psoriasis; onychomycosis; or connective tissue disease.
- If there is purulent discharge associated with paronychia, it should be cultured to help guide appropriate therapy.
- Nail pigmentation can be a normal variant based on the patient's race or could be because of endocrine diseases, connective tissue diseases, trauma, nail matrix nevi, nail matrix lentigines, or melanoma.

## Initial Steps in Management

The initial steps in management revolve around identifying the cause and then, if possible, discontinuing the offending medication. If the medication is vital and cannot be discontinued, management depends on the specific nail change and how distressing it is to the patient. Nail pigmentation is a cosmetic concern and not associated with symptoms; however, nail fold and bed abnormalities can cause significant distress.

Paronychia is best managed with warm soaks four times a day. If there is an accompanying cellulitis or if the patient is immunocompromised, has peripheral vascular disease, or has diabetes, a short course of systemic antibiotics that covers staphylococcus bacteria is indicated. If an abscess is present, it should be incised and drained. Pyogenic granulomas should be referred to a dermatologist for evaluation and treatment.

Drug-induced onycholysis is best treated by avoiding wet work, removing any nail plate that is not attached to the nail bed, and applying a mid-potency topical steroid twice daily.

## Warning Signs/Common Pitfalls

The most common pitfall is failure to recognize that nail changes could be secondary to either a prescription or OTC medication.

Any paronychia that is not resolving with conservative treatment should be referred to a dermatologist. A solitary pigmented or red band in the nail plate should also be referred to a dermatologist because this may represent a malignancy in the nail matrix.

## Counseling

Your nails, like your skin, are susceptible to developing side effects from medications. Medications can cause the skin around the nails to become red and tender, which can lead to infection. This is best treated with warm soaks, although some patients will also require antibiotics. Medications can also cause the nail plate to detach from the nail bed. This can make the nail susceptible to trauma and infections. To get the nail to reattach, it is best to stop taking the offending medication, if possible, cut away any nail that is not attached to the nail bed, and apply a mid-potency topical steroid to the nail bed. Nail discoloration can also occur from numerous medications and is usually reversible upon discontinuing the offending medication. There is no negative impact to your health from treatment medication–related discoloration; because it is not harmful, treatment for this pigmentation is not necessary.

# NAIL PSORIASIS

**Christian Gronbeck and Diane Whitaker-Worth**

## Clinical Features

Approximately 10% to 55% of patients (adults and children) with psoriasis have involvement of the nail bed or nail matrix. Nail psoriasis (Fig. 16.3) presents with a variety of findings, many of which are not specific to psoriasis. For example, nail psoriasis affects the fingernails more often than the toenails, but it can affect both.

Nail psoriasis almost always affects multiple nails and presents with one or more specific nail-related findings.

- Pitting involves small depressions in the nail plate surface that are caused by involvement of the proximal nail matrix.

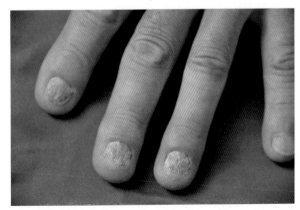

**Fig. 16.3** Nail psoriasis. (From the UConn Department of Dermatology Grand Rounds Collection.)

- Punctate (true) leukonychia involves white foci in the nail plate that do not go away when pressure is applied and that are caused by nail matrix involvement.
- Red spots in the lunula are less common than other findings and are caused by nail matrix involvement.
- Subungual hyperkeratosis is nail thickening with debris caused by increased keratinization of the distal nail bed.
- Splinter hemorrhages are typically on the distal nail bed because of capillary rupture in the dermis underlying the nail plate.
- Onycholysis is the separation of the nail plate from the nail bed and is caused by psoriasis of the nail bed.
- The so-called "oil drop sign" involves areas of yellow-orange discoloration that are visible through the nail plate.
- Nail plate crumbling is the disintegration of the nail plate because of the increased fragility of the nail.

Nail psoriasis occasionally occurs in the absence of typical cutaneous psoriasis in patients with psoriatic arthritis.

- Regardless of whether cutaneous psoriasis is present elsewhere, the presence of nail psoriasis increases the likelihood that a patient has or will develop psoriatic arthritis.

## Differential Diagnosis

The differential diagnosis for nail psoriasis most commonly includes LP, onychomycosis (fungal infection), and alopecia areata (AA). In general, nail psoriasis is easily differentiated from all of these entities, except for onychomycosis, by the presence of psoriasis elsewhere on the body. There are also a few additional signs that suggest a diagnosis of nail psoriasis.

- Psoriasis does not cause scarring of the nails (pterygium) or twenty-nail dystrophy (trachyonychia) like LP. In milder cases, nail LP can overlap with psoriasis; however, identification of the primary dermatosis elsewhere can distinguish between these two conditions.
- Patients with AA may develop trachyonychia (Fig. 16.4), which is not seen in nail psoriasis. Nail findings in AA can mimic those of psoriasis; however, identification of the primary dermatosis elsewhere can distinguish between these two conditions.
- Onychomycosis is the most difficult nail condition to distinguish from nail psoriasis because patients with known psoriasis/nail psoriasis can subsequently

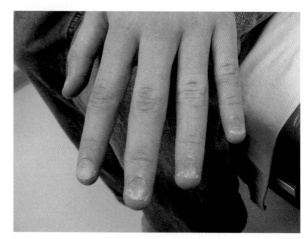

**Fig. 16.4** Trachyonychia in a patient with alopecia areata. (From the UConn Department of Dermatology Grand Rounds Collection.)

develop onychomycosis. Onychomycosis affects the toenails more often than the fingernails and when it affects the fingernails, it may only affect one hand (so-called "two foot, one hand" onychomycosis). In cases where there is diagnostic uncertainty and the patient desires treatment, a nail clipping (for culture and/or PAS) is recommended to differentiate between the two. This clipping should be performed from fingernails if they are what is bothersome because identification of onychomycosis of the toenails does not necessarily mean the patient's fingernail findings are also fungal in origin.

## Work-Up

The diagnosis of nail psoriasis is generally established through a total-body skin examination and patient history. Patients should receive a total-body skin examination because psoriatic plaques in other regions may support a diagnosis of psoriasis (if this diagnosis has not already been established). Specifically, this examination should be targeted toward the scalp and extensor surfaces, which are common sites for plaque psoriasis ( Chapter 3)

- Visualization of well-demarcated, inflamed plaques in characteristic skin regions (elbows, areas, scalp, knees) with significant scaling supports the diagnosis of plaque psoriasis.

As previously mentioned, it is frequently necessary to rule out onychomycosis in patients with known psoriasis that have dystrophic fingernails that are not responsive to psoriasis-directed management.

- A nail clipping of the fingernails (if affected) should be performed and sent for tissue culture and/or PAS stain to rule out onychomycosis.
  - Tissue culture is more sensitive for a diagnosis of onychomycosis; however, it takes weeks to return results.
  - PAS is much quicker than tissue culture; however, it is less sensitive and does not necessarily rule out a diagnosis of onychomycosis when negative.

Once a diagnosis of nail psoriasis has been made, it is imperative to evaluate for concomitant psoriatic arthritis because delaying the management of psoriatic arthritis by even 6 months can result in irreversible joint damage.

- Examination of the joints for active inflammation can be helpful, but it has poor sensitivity and absence of examination findings certainly does not rule out a diagnosis of psoriatic arthritis.
- Use of a standardized screening questionnaire, such as the Psoriasis Epidemiology Screening Tool (PEST), can be implemented easily; however, none of the available screening tools are more than 80% sensitive.
- In cases where there is suspicion for psoriatic arthritis (even in the absence of positive screening), it is best to refer the patient to a psoriatic arthritis specialist urgently to ensure prompt management.

## Initial Steps in Management

Many patients with nail psoriasis are not bothered by their nail disease; however, in cases of nail dystrophy and/or psoriatic arthritis, aggressive management is required.

Dystrophic nail disease is almost never responsive to topical therapy alone. Given its strong association with psoriatic arthritis, referral to a dermatologist or rheumatologist for initiation of systemic therapy is indicated.

Patients with mild disease or who decline referral for systemic therapy can be started on a high-potency topical corticosteroid (betamethasone 0.05% cream) twice daily, a topical vitamin D analog (calcipotriene 0.005% cream) twice daily, or a combination of both.

Importantly, the fingernails take 6 months to grow out and the toenails take 12 to 18 months. For this reason, even in cases where therapy is successful, treatment will take months before benefit is observed.

## Warning Signs/Common Pitfalls

It is recommended to screen patients with psoriasis for psoriatic arthritis at regular intervals and to refer patients to a psoriatic arthritis specialist (dermatologist or rheumatologist) if this is suspected.

In cases where patients with presumed dystrophic nail psoriasis fail to improve despite appropriate therapy, a nail clipping to evaluate for onychomycosis is recommended.

## Counseling

You have nail psoriasis. Nail psoriasis occurs in many individuals who have been diagnosed with skin psoriasis. In some cases, nail psoriasis can be so severe that it can be bothersome and can interfere with your daily activities. Additionally, having nail psoriasis may mean that you are at a higher risk for developing psoriatic arthritis, a type of destructive joint disease related to psoriasis.

Because you are at an increased risk for psoriatic arthritis, it is important that you tell your healthcare provider if you are having morning stiffness in your joints, including your lower back, that lasts more than 1 hour, and/or joint pain. Similarly, if you notice joints that are swollen or that become red-hot, it is important that you contact your healthcare provider immediately.

If you are bothered by your nail psoriasis or develop signs of psoriatic arthritis, you may need a pill or injection to manage your condition.

# Drug Reactions

# 17

# Drug Rashes

*Aziz Khan, Reid A. Waldman, and Jane M. Grant-Kels*

## CHAPTER OUTLINE

## MORBILLIFORM DRUG ERUPTION

### Clinical Features

Morbilliform drug eruption, also called "exanthematous" or "maculopapular drug eruption," is the most common form of cutaneous drug eruption, accounting for more than 80% of drug eruptions.

- The term "morbilliform" is often used to describe this condition because the morphology and distribution of the rash looks similar to those of viral exanthems (i.e., measles).

Morbilliform drug eruption is considered to be a type IVc hypersensitivity reaction and is caused by a wide variety of medications. Morbilliform drug eruption occurs in 1% to 5% of first-time drug users and is characterized by a widespread, maculopapular, symmetrically distrib-uted rash. The highest drug-specific incidence is reported among patients exposed to antibiotics (1%–8%), particularly beta-lactams.

Clinical manifestations usually appear about 3 to 14 days (typically within the first week) after initiation of the culprit drug; however, the rash can appear earlier if the person is already sensitized to the drug from previous exposure. Drugs commonly implicated in morbilliform drug eruption include antibiotics (e.g., beta-lactam antibiotics, sulfonamides, fluoroquinolones); allopurinol; anticonvulsants (e.g., lamotrigine, carbamazepine, phenytoin, phenobarbital); antivirals (e.g., nevirapine, abacavir); and oxicam nonsteroidal antiinflammatory drugs (NSAIDs).

Systemic symptoms include a fever, which is typically low grade (less than 100.4° F), and pruritis.

## Cutaneous Manifestations

- Skin lesions usually present as erythematous macules and/or papules, mainly on the trunk and extremities. The lesions can coalesce to form patches or plaques.
- Rarely, pustules, bullae, or purpuric lesions may develop, particularly on the dependent areas of the lower extremities.
- Typically, there is no mucosal involvement.
- Symmetric drug-related intertriginous and flexural exanthem (SDRIFE; previously known as "baboon syndrome") is an uncommon variant of morbilliform drug eruption, which typically presents as symmetric, sharply defined erythema of the gluteal, intertriginous, and flexural areas. Systemic symptoms are usually absent. It is most often seen in male patients exposed to aminopenicillins. Rarely, SDRIFE is a manifestation of systemic contact dermatitis to nickel or mercury. Systemic contact dermatitis is a condition in which a person who is already sensitized to a substance through skin contact gets exposed to it via a systemic route, resulting in a cutaneous eruption.

## Differential Diagnosis

The differential diagnoses for a maculopapular rash are broad and include viral exanthems, bacterial exanthems, autoimmune disease, and drug eruptions. A temporal relationship between rash onset and exposure to the offending drug helps differentiate drug exanthems from other exanthems.

- The evolution, distribution, and morphology of the rash and the absence of symptoms typically associated with viral, bacterial infections (e.g., fever, sore throat, lymphadenopathy) can help distinguish viral/bacterial exanthems from drug eruptions.
- Viral exanthems (measles, rubella) are typically seen in unimmunized children or young adults. Serologic tests supplement history and physical findings to help differentiate viral exanthems from other causes of maculopapular rash.
- Infectious mononucleosis can cause a maculopapular rash in adults, usually after administration of ampicillin.
- Acute retroviral syndrome caused by human immunodeficiency virus (HIV) infection usually presents with a transient maculopapular rash. Accompanying symptoms include fever, malaise, sore throat, and lymphadenopathy. HIV testing should be performed in patients at risk for HIV infection who present with a maculopapular rash.

- Autoimmune antibody testing should be obtained if a cutaneous autoimmune disease like SLE is suspected.

It is essential to distinguish morbilliform drug eruption from other forms of severe cutaneous drug reactions, including DRESS and SJS/TEN. Morbilliform drug eruptions lack the mucosal findings associated with the aforementioned conditions. These conditions can be further differentiated based on skin biopsy findings.

- SJS/TEN usually presents within 4 weeks of drug exposure and is characterized by severe, generalized mucosal involvement and a high-grade fever.
- DRESS syndrome is characterized by a high-grade fever, systemic/visceral involvement, and limited mucosal involvement.
- Acute generalized exanthematous pustulosis (AGEP) presents within 48 hours of drug exposure (typically to beta-lactam antibiotics) and is characterized by multiple pinpoint pustules distributed over the whole body with limited mucosal involvement.

## Work-Up

The diagnosis of morbilliform drug eruption is suspected when a patient presents with a new-onset maculopapular rash and a recent drug exposure.

A careful review of the complete medication list, including prescription, over-the-counter (OTC), and herbal medications, should be done. The timeline of drug exposure and symptoms onset should be documented to assess for drug causality. History of previous and recent exposure to topical medications should also be obtained. Travel history, sick contacts, recent febrile illness, and exposure to any ticks should be obtained to assess for an infectious etiology.

Careful examination of the skin and all mucosal surfaces should be performed because a morbilliform drug eruption can sometimes be the heralding sign of a more severe cutaneous drug eruption. The presence of mucosal involvement, skin tenderness, or a high-grade fever (greater than 100.4° F) should raise suspicion for a severe evolving cutaneous drug reaction, including a drug reaction with eosinophilia and systemic symptoms (DRESS) and/or Stevens-Johnson syndrome/toxic epidermal necrolysis (SJS/TEN).

Laboratory investigations are generally not routinely performed if the diagnosis and drug causality is certain. Nevertheless, in uncertain cases, the following tests should be obtained to confirm the diagnosis and exclude other conditions that mimic morbilliform drug eruption.

- A complete blood count (CBC) with differential and peripheral blood smear should be done to look for the eosinophilia that occurs in patients with DRESS.
- Liver function tests and renal function tests are often abnormal in patients with DRESS or SJS/TEN.
- Viral serologies can be completed, as guided by clinical presentation and history.
- Autoimmune antibody testing should be obtained if a cutaneous autoimmune disease like systemic lupus erythematosus (SLE) is suspected.

A skin biopsy to diagnose morbilliform drug eruption is not routinely performed; however, a skin biopsy for histopathologic examination and direct immunofluorescence (DIF) should be obtained if the diagnosis is uncertain and/or to exclude severe cutaneous drug eruptions like DRESS and SJS/TEN. Typical histopathological features include vacuolar interface dermatitis with a superficial perivascular and interstitial inflammatory infiltrate composed mostly of lymphocytes but often with some neutrophils and eosinophils.

## Initial Steps in Management

Identification and prompt withdrawal of the culprit drug remains the mainstay of treatment. Morbilliform drug eruption is a self-limiting disease, and withdrawal of the offending agent usually results in the resolution of cutaneous manifestations in about 5 to 14 days. Postinflammatory hyperpigmentation can occur, especially in patients with darker skin.

For symptomatic relief of pruritus, topical steroids and oral antihistamines are used. Either first-generation oral antihistamines (e.g., diphenhydramine, hydroxyzine) or second-generation oral antihistamines (e.g., cetirizine, loratadine) can be used. Second-generation antihistamines are generally less sedative and are preferred over first-generation drugs. These are usually continued until the pruritus subsides.

High-potency topical steroids are preferred over systemic steroids.

- Clobetasol dipropionate 0.05% cream (or a similar strength topical steroid) can be taken twice daily for 1 week or until symptoms resolve. It should not be used on the face.
- For the face, patients can use hydrocortisone 2.5% cream twice daily (or a similar strength topical steroid) until resolution.

It is essential to avoid reexposure to the same or structurally similar medications. Desensitization can be considered if the culprit drug is of essential therapeutic importance with no other alternative therapeutic options (e.g., antibiotics in cystic fibrosis). These patients should be closely monitored.

## Warning Signs/Common Pitfalls

Morbilliform drug eruption can sometimes be the foreshadowing sign of a more severe cutaneous drug eruption. Hence it is vital to closely monitor patients for signs typically associated with DRESS and SJS/TEN. The presence of fever, mucosal involvement, skin tenderness, or abnormal laboratory findings should warrant further workup for DRESS and SJS/TEN.

SDRIFE should be differentiated from malignant intertrigo, a condition characterized by painful, erythematous skin patches in the intertriginous areas. Malignant intertrigo occurs 2 to 3 weeks after exposure to chemotherapeutic agents.

Patients should be counseled about strict avoidance of the causative drug and chemically related medications.

## Counseling

Morbilliform drug eruption is a relatively common side effect of a medication that affects the skin. It causes red, itchy spots to appear on the skin. Many medications can potentially cause morbilliform drug eruption; a list will be provided to you.

In addition to drugs, other viral and bacterial infections can present with similar spots. Nevertheless, in contrast to a rash caused by infections, fever and sore throat are typically absent in morbilliform drug eruption. If the etiology of the outbreak is uncertain, however, the doctor will perform specific laboratory tests to help differentiate a drug rash from a rash caused by an infection.

In your case, the offending drug should be stopped, and it is recommended that you strictly avoid this drug in the future. Structurally similar drugs can also cause the same reaction, and it is recommended that you talk with your healthcare provider before starting any new medications. You should learn the names of the medications you should avoid and keep a written record on your person. Your pharmacy should also make a note that you have had a drug reaction and should have a list of medications you should avoid. Consider wearing a medical alert bracelet to let people know which medications to avoid.

You should alert your healthcare provider or go to the emergency room immediately if you develop any fever, blistering of the skin, or mouth sores. You should also regularly follow up with your primary healthcare provider.

# URTICARIAL DRUG ERUPTION

## Clinical Features

Urticarial drug eruption is the second most common form of cutaneous drug eruption.

- Urticaria occurs in approximately 20% of individuals at some point in life.
- It is caused by numerous triggers, including drugs, foods, infections, insect bites, latex, blood product transfusions, systemic diseases, and physical stimuli.
- Urticaria is characterized by transient, evanescent, intensely pruritic wheals that individually resolve without scarring in hours.
  - Urticaria is divided into acute (less than 6 weeks) and chronic urticaria (greater than 6 weeks) based on the duration of recurring symptoms.
  - Angioedema may occur in association with urticaria in about 40% of patients.
    - Urticaria involves edema in inflammation in the superficial layers of skin and mucosa, whereas angioedema involves the deeper layers of skin and mucosa.
  - Urticaria may be limited to the skin or may occur as a part of systemic allergic reactions like anaphylaxis.

Drug-induced urticaria is triggered by both immunologic and nonimmunologic mechanisms and is mediated by mast cells in the superficial dermis. Basophils also play a role in the pathogenesis. Angioedema occurs through similar mechanisms and is characterized by histamine release in the dermis and subcutaneous tissue.

- Immunologic urticaria occurs because of an allergic reaction to a medication (i.e., an immunoglobulin E [IgE]–mediated type 1 hypersensitivity reaction).
- Nonimmunologic urticaria occurs because of direct histamine release from mast cells (opiates, vancomycin) and leukotriene formation/histamine release (NSAIDs).
  - Note that NSAIDs can cause urticaria through both immunologic and nonimmunologic mechanisms.
  - Angiotensin-converting enzyme (ACE) inhibitors cause angioedema without urticaria through decreased bradykinin breakdown.

- Medication-induced serum sickness can also present with urticaria.

Drug-induced immunologic urticaria is characterized by the development of a rash within minutes to hours after exposure to the culprit drug.

Drugs commonly implicated in drug-induced immunologic urticaria include antibiotics (such as beta-lactam antibiotics or sulfonamides, but virtually any category of antibiotics can cause immunologic urticaria); NSAIDs; and latex.

Drugs commonly implicated in drug-induced nonimmunologic urticaria include narcotics, anesthetic muscle relaxants, vancomycin (which causes red man syndrome), radiocontrast agents, and NSAIDs.

## Systemic Symptoms

- Fever is typically absent in drug-induced urticaria.
- Lesions are intensely pruritic and painless.
- Difficulty breathing, wheezing, and/or shock can occur when associated with anaphylaxis or angioedema.

## Cutaneous Manifestations

- Skin lesions are characterized by episodic, transient, swollen, pale pink or erythematous plaques.
- It can involve any area of the skin or mucosa.
- Lesions often occur with associated central pallor and blanch with pressure.
- Lesions may or may not be associated with surrounding skin erythema.
- The lesions vary in size from few millimeters to centimeters (Fig. 17.1).
- Lesions may be oval, round, or serpiginous in shape.
- Lesions are intensely pruritic, particularly at night.
- The lesions typically disappear within 24 hours, leaving normal skin with no scarring or hyperpigmentation.
- A urticarial drug eruption may be associated with angioedema and/or anaphylaxis.
- Urticarial vasculitis should be suspected if lesions are painful, last longer than 24 hours, and leave residual ecchymosis or hyperpigmentation.

## Differential Diagnosis

The differential diagnoses for urticaria are broad, and possible triggers include drugs, foods, infections, insect bites, latex, blood product transfusions, systemic conditions, and physical stimuli. The diagnosis of drug-induced urticaria is made clinically. Through a detailed history and examination, other etiologies of urticaria should be ruled

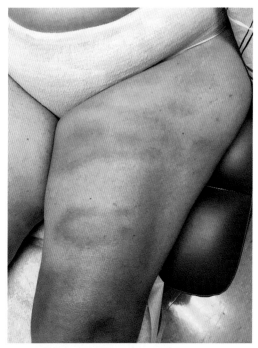

**Fig. 17.1 Drug-Induced Urticaria Multiforme Secondary to Nivolumab.** These large urticarial plaques are called "urticaria multiforme" because they clinically mimic erythema multiforme.

out. A temporal relationship between rash onset and exposure to the offending drug helps differentiate drug-induced urticaria from other forms of urticaria.

Certain pruritic conditions, such as atopic dermatitis (AD) and contact dermatitis, although pruritic, are not usually confused with urticaria. AD presents with a pruritic rash but the lesions appear eczematous, last for days or weeks, and leave postinflammatory hyperpigmentation upon resolution. In contrast, an urticarial rash resolves within 24 hours, leaving normal skin. Contact dermatitis is characterized by an eczematous rash or vesicular, erythematous papules in the areas of direct skin contact with the precipitating contactant.

Other forms of drug eruptions, such as morbilliform drug eruption, may also be associated with pruritus. Unlike urticaria, however, the lesions are characterized by small macules/papules, which last for days.

## Work-Up

A diagnosis of drug-induced urticaria is suspected when a patient presents with new-onset hives and recent drug exposure.

A careful review of the complete medication list, including prescription, OTC, and herbal medications, should be performed. The timeline of drug exposure and symptoms onset should be documented to assess for drug causality. History of previous and recent exposure to topical medications should also be obtained. Travel history, sick contacts, recent febrile illness, and exposure to any ticks should be obtained to assess for an infectious etiology. In addition to drugs, urticaria can be triggered by numerous other conditions, as previously discussed.

History and physical examination should be focused on ruling out other etiologies of urticaria (e.g., foods, infections, insect bites, latex, blood product transfusions, systemic conditions, and physical stimuli), identifying any associated angioedema, and identifying any systemic allergic reaction (such as anaphylaxis).

Careful examination of the skin and all mucosal surfaces should be performed because urticarial drug eruption can be associated with angioedema and anaphylaxis. If the lesions have resolved by the time of evaluation, patients should be shown photographs of urticaria and asked if their lesions appeared similar. Patients should be asked to take pictures of the lesions in the future because the lesions might disappear by the time a healthcare provider evaluates them.

Laboratory investigations are generally not routinely performed if the diagnosis and drug causality is certain. In uncertain cases, however, certain tests should be obtained to confirm the diagnosis and exclude other conditions that cause an urticarial eruption. These tests include a CBC with differential and peripheral blood smear; liver function tests and renal function tests; viral serologies, as guided by clinical presentation and history; a urinalysis; erythrocyte sedimentation rate (ESR); autoimmune antibody testing and skin biopsy if urticarial vasculitis is suspected; and allergen testing.

A skin biopsy is not routinely performed to diagnose drug-induced urticaria. Skin allergen testing is not routinely performed in patients with drug-induced urticaria because of the high prevalence of false-positive results. Nevertheless, skin prick tests may help in the diagnosis of drug-induced urticaria from antibiotics.

## Initial Steps in Management

Identification and prompt withdrawal of the culprit drug remains the mainstay of treatment. Drug-induced urticaria is often self-limiting, and withdrawal of the offending agent results in the resolution of cutaneous manifestations. Typical lesions of acute urticaria last for less than 24 hours; however, patients might develop recurrent new transient lesions until the culprit drug is cleared out of the system.

For symptomatic relief of pruritus, oral antihistamines are used. Either first-generation oral antihistamines (e.g., diphenhydramine, hydroxyzine) or second-generation oral antihistamines (e.g., cetirizine, loratadine) can be used. Second-generation antihistamines are less sedative and are the preferred agents in both adults and children. These are usually continued until pruritus subsides.

- For adults and children older than 12 years, cetirizine 10 mg may be taken orally daily and increased to twice daily if needed.
- For children aged 6 to 12 years, cetirizine 5 mg oral daily may be taken, and the dose can be increased to 10 mg per day.
- For children aged 2 to 5 years, cetirizine 5 mg oral daily is recommended.
- For children aged 6 months to 2 years, cetirizine 2.5 mg oral daily is recommended.

Systemic glucocorticoids are not routinely used for isolated drug-induced urticaria. Nevertheless, systemic steroids should be used in addition to antihistamines if angioedema or anaphylaxis is suspected.

It is essential to avoid reexposure to the same or structurally similar medications because reexposure may lead to potentially catastrophic anaphylaxis or angioedema.

## Warning Signs/Common Pitfalls

It is essential to look for angioedema or signs of anaphylaxis when evaluating a patient with drug-induced urticaria. Patients with features of angioedema or anaphylaxis should be closely monitored.

Patients with immunogenic drug-induced urticaria should be referred to an allergist or dermatologist; these patients need to be prescribed and educated about the use of epinephrine (Epi-Pen) for self-injections if needed.

Patients should be counseled about strict avoidance of the causative drug and chemically related medications.

## Counseling

Drug-induced urticaria is a relatively common side effect of a medication that affects the skin. It causes raised, light pink to red lesions or swelling (hives) to appear on the skin. These lesions are typically very itchy. Some people who get hives can also develop angioedema (a condition in which the lips, eyelids, and face become swollen and puffy) and anaphylaxis (characterized by trouble breathing, wheezing, passing out, and low blood pressure). Drug-induced urticaria in itself is self-limiting; however, angioedema and anaphylaxis are potentially severe drug reactions. Many medications can potentially cause an urticarial drug eruption; a list will be provided to you.

In addition to drug allergies, an allergy to many other things can cause hives. These include foods, plants, insect bites, latex, and infections.

In your case, the offending drug should be stopped, and it is recommended that you strictly avoid this drug in the future. Structurally similar drugs can also cause the same or potentially a worse reaction, and it is recommended that you talk with your healthcare provider before starting any new medications. You should learn the names of the medications you should avoid and keep a written record with yourself. Your pharmacy should also make a note that you had a drug reaction and should have a list of medications you should avoid. Consider wearing a medical alert bracelet to let people know which medications to avoid.

You should go to the emergency room immediately or call for an ambulance (call 911) if you develop difficulty breathing; swelling of the lips, face, eyelids, or hands; wheezing; abdominal pain, nausea, or vomiting; loss of consciousness or syncope; or dizziness.

You should regularly follow up with your primary healthcare provider.

## LICHENOID DRUG ERUPTION

### Clinical Features

Lichenoid drug eruption, also known as "drug-induced lichen planus," is a rare form of cutaneous drug eruption.

- It is characterized by the development of papules resembling lichen planus (LP) and occurs months to years after drug exposure.
  - The period between drug exposure and the appearance of the rash depends on the type of drug, host immune response, and previous exposure to the drug.

- On average, the latent period is about 2 to 3 months. For penicillamine, however, a latent period of up to 3 years has been reported.

The immunologic mechanism of lichenoid drug eruption remains unclear. Cytotoxic CD8 T cells and dendritic cells are thought to play an essential role in the pathogenesis of the disease. A wide variety of medications can cause lichenoid drug eruption.

Drugs commonly implicated in lichenoid drug eruption include antibiotics (e.g., tetracyclines, ethambutol, isoniazid, streptomycin); antifungals (e.g., ketoconazole, griseofulvin); allopurinol (which typically involves the oral mucosa); antihypertensives (e.g., ACE inhibitors, thiazide diuretics, beta-blockers, nifedipine); gold salts; penicillamine; antimalarials (e.g., chloroquine, hydroxychloroquine, quinine); NSAIDS; and tumor necrosis factor–alpha antagonists (e.g., infliximab, etanercept, adalimumab).

In terms of systemic symptoms, fever is absent and pruritis is a common symptom.

## Cutaneous Manifestations

- Skin lesions usually present as symmetric, flat-topped, erythematous, or violaceous papules, mainly on the trunk and extremities.
- The lesions are often polygonal and confluent.
- A photosensitive lichenoid reaction (Figs. 17.2 and 17.3) has been reported with a variety of drugs; the lesions in these patients are often photodistributed.
- In contrast to LP, the lesions are larger and potentially more eczematous or psoriasiform. Wickham

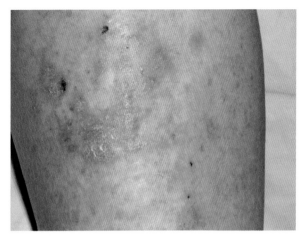

**Fig. 17.3** Drug-induced lichen planus on the shin (close-up).

striae are typically absent. Nails and mucous membranes are uncommon.
- Rarely, nails demonstrate ridging and brittleness as part of the hypersensitivity reaction.
- The lesions are typically pruritic, but some patients are asymptomatic.
- When lesions resolve, postinflammatory hyperpigmentation is noted, particularly in patients with darker skin.

## Mucosal Manifestations

- Mucosal involvement in lichenoid drug eruption is rare. If present, however, it typically involves the oral mucosa.
- The lesions generally are identical to those of oral LP.
- An erosive oral lichenoid eruption presents with pain and burning.
- A reticular oral lichenoid eruption is usually asymptomatic.

## Work-Up

The diagnosis of lichenoid drug eruption is suspected when a patient presents with an LP-type rash and a drug exposure known to cause lichenoid eruptions. It is also suspected in cases where a lichenoid rash is biopsied and the biopsy shows the presence of eosinophils and/or parakeratosis. A careful review of the complete medication list, including prescription, OTC, and herbal medications, should be performed.
- The timeline of drug exposure and symptoms onset should be documented to assess for drug causality.

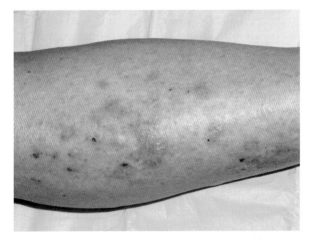

**Fig. 17.2** Drug-induced lichen planus on the shin.

- This type of drug eruption can occur immediately after initiating a new medication or not present for several months or even a year or more, making identification of the culprit drug challenging.
- History of previous and recent exposure to topical medications should also be obtained.
- A careful examination of the skin and all mucosal surfaces should be performed.

Laboratory investigations are not routinely performed if the diagnosis and drug causality is certain. Nevertheless, in some cases, autoimmune antibody testing can be obtained to exclude other conditions that mimic lichenoid drug eruption (e.g., SLE).

A skin biopsy for histopathologic examination and DIF should be obtained to confirm the diagnosis and exclude mimics. Typical histopathologic features include interface dermatitis with basal vacuolar alteration and colloid bodies. There is a dense, dermal band like infiltrate of lymphocytes that obscures the dermoepidermal junction. Histologically, it is often challenging to differentiate a lichenoid drug eruption from other forms of lichenoid eruptions. Features that may favor lichenoid drug eruption over other lichenoid eruptions include focal parakeratosis, eosinophils within the inflammatory infiltrate, spongiosis, and extension of the inflammatory infiltrate deeper into the dermis around the superficial and deeper dermal blood vessels.

## Initial Steps in Management

Identification and prompt withdrawal of the culprit drug remains the mainstay of treatment. The lesions generally resolve over weeks to months after discontinuing the culprit drug. Postinflammatory hyperpigmentation can occur, especially in patients with darker skin.

Treatment options for symptomatic patients (pruritus, pain) include topical steroids, systemic steroids, and oral antihistamines. There are no randomized clinical trials comparing the relative efficacy of these agents, and their use is mainly based on clinical experience.

For patients with limited skin involvement, topical steroids are preferred over systemic steroids and oral retinoids. Generally, high-potency topical steroids are preferred.

- Clobetasol dipropionate 0.05% cream (or a similar strength topical steroid) can be used twice daily for 2 to 4 weeks or until symptoms resolve. High-potency topical steroids should not be used on the face.

- For the face, use a hydrocortisone 2.5% cream twice daily (or a similar strength topical steroid) until resolution.

For symptomatic patients with extensive skin involvement, systemic steroids should be used. Oral antihistamines to treat pruritus can also be helpful, such as prednisone 30 to 60 mg per day for 2 to 6 weeks, followed by a 2 to 6 weeks taper.

Rarely, oral retinoids, such as acitretin 25 to 35 mg per day for 6 to 12 weeks, have been used in recalcitrant patients or in those for whom systemic steroids are contraindicated.

For patients with symptomatic oral involvement (erosive oral lichenoid eruption), high-potency topical steroids are the preferred agents. If patients fail topical therapy, then oral prednisone can be used at a similar dose as previously mentioned.

It is essential to avoid reexposure to the same or structurally similar medications. Nevertheless, sometimes the culprit drug is of essential therapeutic importance and cannot be discontinued. In these cases, possible options include decreasing the dose of the culprit drug, concomitantly treating the patient with topical steroids, and concomitantly treating the patient with oral steroids (especially in patients with extensive, symptomatic disease).

## Warning Signs/Common Pitfalls

Lichenoid drug eruption should be differentiated from LP. The morphology of skin lesions of both conditions is similar. In contrast to LP, however, lichenoid drug eruption lesions are larger and can present with a more eczematous or psoriasiform appearance. Wickham striae are typically absent. Nails and mucous membranes are often spared. Lichenoid drug eruption lesions typically involve the trunk and extensor surfaces of extremities. In contrast, LP lesions tend to involve flexural areas and are symmetrically distributed over the extremities. Oral involvement is more common in LP. A temporal relationship between rash onset and exposure to the offending drug further helps to differentiate these conditions.

## Counseling

Lichenoid drug eruption is an uncommon side effect of a medication that affects the skin and, rarely, the oral mucosa. It causes small, red or purple bumps to appear on the skin. The lesions can be itchy and bothersome.

Rarely, it can cause similar lesions to appear in the mouth, which can be painful. There are many medications that can potentially cause lichenoid drug eruption; a list will be provided to you. Once you have this type of drug reaction, you are at an increased risk for developing similar reactions in the future.

In your case, the offending drug should be stopped, and it is recommended that you strictly avoid this drug in the future. Structurally similar drugs can also cause the same reaction, and it is recommended that you talk with your healthcare provider before starting any new medications. You should learn the names of the medications you should avoid and keep a written record on your person. Your pharmacy should also make a note that you had a drug reaction and should have a list of medications you should avoid. Consider wearing a medical alert bracelet to let people know which medications to avoid.

You should go to the emergency immediately or call for an ambulance (call 911) if you develop any fever, blistering of the skin, or mouth sores. You should also regularly follow up with your primary healthcare provider.

# 18

# Drug Reactions With Systemic Symptoms

*Aziz Khan, Reid A. Waldman, and Jane M. Grant-Kels*

## ACUTE GENERALIZED EXANTHEMATOUS PUSTULOSIS

### Clinical Features

Acute generalized exanthematous pustulosis (AGEP) is an uncommon, severe cutaneous eruption that is attributed to drugs in more than 90% of cases (Fig. 18.1). It is characterized by the rapid development of numerous superficial sterile pustules on an erythematous base. It has an estimated incidence of 1 to 5 cases per million per year. AGEP commonly affects adults and shows a slight female predominance.

AGEP is considered to be a T cell–mediated, sterile, neutrophilic, type IVd hypersensitivity reaction. The

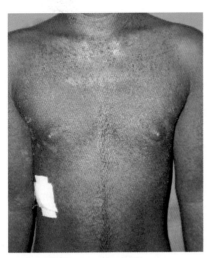

**Fig. 18.1** Drug Reaction with Eosinophilia and Systemic Symptoms Syndrome. Notice the diffuse, exfoliative dermatitis. Patient initially presented with a morbilliform eruption. (Courtesy Preeti Jhorar, MD.)

rash usually develops within hours to days of drug exposure, with a typical latency of 24 to 48 hours.

Drugs commonly implicated in AGEP include a large number of medications, such as antibiotics (particularly ampicillin/amoxicillin, macrolides, sulfonamides, and quinolones), antifungals (e.g., terbinafine, ketoconazole, fluconazole), hydroxychloroquine, diltiazem, and drugs with weaker association (such as omeprazole, corticosteroids, oxicam nonsteroidal antiinflammatory drugs [NSAIDs], and antiepileptic drugs).

Infections commonly implicated in AGEP are *Mycoplasma pneumoniae* infection, *Chlamydia pneumoniae*, *Escherichia coli*, cytomegalovirus, coxsackie B4, and parvovirus B19.

In terms of systemic symptoms, a fever of at least 100.4° F is almost always present.

## Cutaneous Manifestations

- AGEP involves numerous pinhead-sized, nonfollicular, sterile pustules on an erythematous, edematous base.
- The rash typically begins on the flexural areas and progresses to the trunk and extremities within hours. Many patients are near erythrodermic.
- The lesions generally are pruritic and sometimes are associated with a burning sensation.
- Mucosal involvement is reported in about 20% of cases and is typically confined to a single site, especially the mouth or lips.

## Common Laboratory Findings

- Neutrophilic leukocytosis and elevated C-reactive protein (CRP) levels are common.
- Eosinophilia is seen in 30% of cases.
- Hypocalcemia is seen in 75% of cases.
- Another common laboratory finding is a negative Gram stain and culture of the pustules.
- Systemic involvement is reported in 17% of cases and typically include elevated creatinine (kidney injury) and transaminitis (liver injury) levels.

## Differential Diagnosis

It is essential to distinguish AGEP from other forms of drug reactions, including drug reaction with eosinophilia and systemic symptoms (DRESS), Stevens-Johnson syndrome/toxic epidermal necrolysis (SJS/TEN), and exanthematous drug eruptions.

- SJS usually presents within 4 weeks of drug exposure and is characterized by severe, generalized mucosal involvement. In contrast, AGEP presents within 48 hours of drug exposure (typically beta-lactam antibiotics) and is characterized by multiple pinpoint pustules distributed over the whole body. Mucosal involvement in AGEP is usually limited to one site (mostly the mouth) without any erosions. These conditions can be further differentiated based on skin biopsy findings.
- Generalized acute pustular psoriasis may be difficult to distinguish from AGEP. Acute generalized pustular psoriasis most commonly occurs in individuals with known psoriasis who have either recently received a course of systemic corticosteroids or have been exposed to another psoriasis exacerbator. History of psoriasis, absence of drug exposure, longer symptom duration, and papillary dilated or tortuous blood vessels, as well as psoriasiform epidermal hyperplasia on histopathology, favor the diagnosis of psoriasis. Drugs can also trigger acute pustular psoriasis; however, the spectrum of inciting drugs differ between these two conditions.
- Bullous impetigo is another differential to consider that generally affects children. It clinically manifests as small vesicles or pustules on the face and/or flexural areas. The pustules usually rupture, leaving erosions with a honey-colored crust. In contrast to AGEP, Gram stain and culture of the pustule grows *Staphylococcus aureus.*
- Other pustular eruptions from bacterial or fungal infections can be excluded by clinical picture,

history, histopathologic, and smears or cultures of the lesions.

## Work-Up

The diagnosis of AGEP is suspected when a patient presents with fever, rapid development of a pustular rash, and recent drug exposure or febrile illness.

A careful review of the patient's complete medication list, including prescription, over-the-counter (OTC), and herbal medications, should be performed. The timeline of drug exposure and symptoms onset should be documented to assess for drug causality. Travel history and exposure to any ticks should be obtained to evaluate for an infectious etiology.

Tests that should be obtained as a part of the work-up to confirm the diagnosis and exclude other conditions that mimic AGEP include a complete blood count (CBC) with differential and peripheral blood smear, liver function tests, renal function tests, bacterial and fungal cultures from blood, a Gram stain and culture of the pustules, and imaging studies (guided by clinical presentation).

A skin biopsy for histopathologic examination should be performed to support the diagnosis and exclude AGEP mimics. The histologic findings include subcorneal or intraepidermal spongiform pustules, which are associated with dermal edema and a superficial and midperivascular (as well as interstitial) inflammatory infiltrate that contains neutrophils and eosinophils. In contrast to pustular psoriasis, papillary dilated and tortuous blood vessels and psoriasiform epidermal hyperplasia are absent.

In the case of polypharmacy, a patch test can be performed to identify the causative agent.

## Initial Steps in Management

Identification and prompt withdrawal of the offending agent is the mainstay of treatment. AGEP is a self-limiting disease, and withdrawal of the offending agent results in the resolution of cutaneous manifestations in about 2 weeks. Those with a more generalized skin involvement or older patients may require admission for fluid/electrolyte replacement and nutritional support.

Symptomatic patients (those with pruritus, pain, and/or burning) are generally treated with medium-potency topical steroids.

- Fluocinolone acetonide 0.025% ointment (or a similar strength topical steroid) can be applied twice daily for 1 week or until symptoms resolve. It should not be used on the face.
- For the face, patients should use hydrocortisone 2.5% cream twice daily (or a similar strength topical steroid) for 1 week or until symptoms resolve.

## Counseling

Acute generalized exanthematous pustulosis (AGEP) is a rare side effect of a medication that affects the skin. The rash appears suddenly after drug exposure and is characterized by multiple small pus-filled spots and skin edema. AGEP is triggered by medications in more than 90% of cases. There was no way to determine that you would get AGEP from the medication that caused your rash before starting that medication. AGEP is caused by a wide variety of drugs, most commonly antibiotics. The list of medications that can potentially cause AGEP will be provided to you. Rarely, AGEP is caused by a viral or bacterial infection.

AGEP is a self-limiting disease and usually resolves without any complications after the causative drug is discontinued. AGEP can happen again after the reintroduction of the causative drug.

In your case, the offending drug should be stopped, and it is recommended that you strictly avoid this drug in the future. Structurally similar drugs can also cause the same reaction, and it is recommended that you discuss with your healthcare provider before starting any new medications. You should learn the names of the medicines you should avoid and keep a written record on your person. Your pharmacy should also make a note that you had a drug reaction and should have a list of medications you should avoid. Consider wearing a medical alert bracelet to let people know which medications to avoid.

# DRUG REACTION WITH EOSINOPHILIA AND SYSTEMIC SYMPTOMS

## Clinical Features

Drug reaction with eosinophilia and systemic symptoms (DRESS) is a rare, potentially life-threatening adverse drug reaction with a long latency period.

- It was initially described after the introduction of phenytoin and thus was historically called "phenytoin hypersensitivity syndrome."
  - Many other medications have since been implicated and numerous names have been used, including

"anticonvulsant hypersensitivity syndrome" and "drug-induced hypersensitivity syndrome."
  • The term DRESS was coined in the late 1990s and is currently the most accepted terminology.
• Clinical manifestations typically appear anywhere from 2 to 8 weeks (with a mean of 3 weeks) after initiation of the culprit drug.
  • They include fever, malaise, skin eruption, hematologic abnormalities, lymphadenopathy, and visceral involvement.
• DRESS is associated with a 10% mortality rate.
The etiology of DRESS is complex and likely involves three factors: a genetic predisposition that alters immune response, a trigger that may involve a viral infection, and a drug to which the patient may have a defect in drug metabolism.
DRESS is fortunately rare, with an incidence ranging from 1 in 1000 to 1 in 10,000 drug exposures.
• The frequency varies depending on the drug type and appears to be higher in patients taking anticonvulsants, particularly lamotrigine.
Common drugs implicated in DRESS include anticonvulsants (such as phenytoin, carbamazepine, phenobarbitone, and lamotrigine); antibiotics (e.g., minocycline, dapsone [especially in patients with HLA-B*13:01 haplotype], sulfonamides, beta-lactam antibiotics), antivirals (including nevirapine, telaprevir, raltegravir, and abacavir [HLA-B*5701 haplotype]), allopurinol (especially in patients with HLA-B*58:01 haplotype), and chemotherapeutic/immunotherapeutic agents (such as imatinib, sorafenib, and vemurafenib).
Systemic symptoms include fever, malaise, lymphadenopathy, and symptoms of visceral involvement.

## Cutaneous Manifestations

• DRESS starts as a morbilliform eruption that rapidly progresses to a diffuse, confluent skin erythema. Some patients complain of pruritus. In about one-fourth of patients, the erythema progresses to exfoliative dermatitis (Fig. 18.1).
• It initially involves the face and upper part of the trunk and upper extremities with eventual extension to the lower extremities.
• It involves more than 50% of the body surface area (BSA).
• Symmetric, persistent, facial edema with erythema is present in more than 50% of cases (Fig. 18.2).
• Erythema and tenderness of mucous membranes without erosions are seen in more than half of the cases.

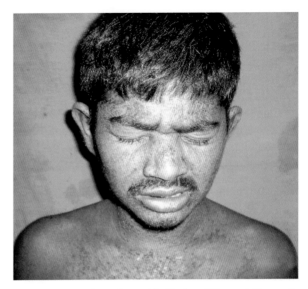

**Fig. 18.2** Drug Reaction with Eosinophilia and Systemic Symptoms Syndrome. *Notice the characteristic facial edema.* (Courtesy Preeti Jhorar, MD.)

• Other less commonly reported features include the development of vesicles, bullae, pustules, target lesions, and purpura.
In terms of systemic involvement, the frequency of organ involvement depends on the inciting agent (e.g., allopurinol-induced DRESS usually causes kidney injury).

## Hematologic Involvement

• With hematologic involvement, leukocytosis with eosinophilia is usually present.
• Thrombocytopenia and anemia is rare but sometimes reported.

## Liver Involvement

• When the liver is involved, asymptomatic hepatitis (either hepatocellular or cholestatic damage) is more common (70% patients), but patients may also present with hepatomegaly and jaundice.
• In severe cases, fulminant hepatic failure may develop and is responsible for most of the mortality associated with DRESS syndrome.

## Kidney Involvement

• Acute kidney injury (tubulointerstitial nephritis) develops in about 11% of patients, especially in patients on allopurinol.

- It is manifested by a rise in blood urea nitrogen (BUN) and creatinine levels.
- Other features include low-grade proteinuria and abnormal urinary sediment with eosinophils.

### Lung Involvement

- Lung involvement may include interstitial pneumonitis with nonspecific symptoms of cough and difficulty breathing.
- Hypoxemia is also sometimes present.

### Other Organ Involvement

Several other organs can also be involved in DRESS, including the heart (myocarditis, pericarditis), pancreas (pancreatitis), thyroid (thyroiditis), and eyes (uveitis).

- Thyroid involvement is unique in that it may present months after acute DRESS has resolved.

## Differential Diagnosis

It is essential to rule out an infectious etiology before starting any immunosuppressive therapy. Other severe cutaneous drug eruptions, infectious agents, and autoimmune conditions can mimic DRESS and should be carefully investigated.

- SJS usually presents within 4 weeks of drug exposure and is characterized by severe, generalized erosive mucosal involvement. In contrast, mucosal involvement in DRESS is generally limited to one site (mostly mouth or pharynx) without any erosions. These two conditions can be further differentiated based on skin biopsy findings.
- Another significant differential to consider is AGEP, which, unlike DRESS, presents within 3 days of drug exposure and is characterized by multiple pinpoint pustules distributed over the whole body.
- Acute cutaneous lupus erythematosus can present similarly to DRESS and can be differentiated by the presence of specific autoantibodies and interface dermatitis on skin biopsy.
- Sézary syndrome and angioimmunoblastic T cell lymphoma are other relevant differentials to consider. These can be differentiated from DRESS based on specific histologic findings.

## Work-Up

A diagnosis of DRESS is suspected when a patient presents with skin eruption and systemic symptoms after exposure to a new drug. Often, the initial dilemma is to rule out an infectious etiology. Exposure to a high-risk medication in the previous 2 to 8 weeks of symptoms onset supports the clinical suspicion of DRESS.

A careful review of the complete medication list (including prescription, OTC and herbal medications) should be performed.

- The timeline of drug exposure and symptoms onset should be documented to assess for drug causality.
  - It is unlikely for a drug to be the cause of DRESS if initiated within 2 weeks of symptoms onset or taken for more than 3 months before symptoms onset.
- Travel history and exposure to ticks should be obtained to assess for an infectious etiology.
- A careful examination of the skin should be performed, focusing on the clinical manifestations of DRESS.

Blood tests that should be obtained as a part of the work-up to confirm the diagnosis and exclude other conditions that mimic DRESS include a CBC with differential and peripheral blood smear (look for eosinophilia and leukocytosis), liver function tests, and renal function tests.

- Blood cultures should be obtained.
- Testing for viral hepatitis, Epstein-Barr virus, cytomegalovirus, human herpesvirus (HHV) 6 and 7, and human immunodeficiency virus (HIV) should be performed.

Imaging studies, guided by clinical presentation, are recommended.

A skin biopsy for histopathologic examination and direct immunofluorescence (DIF) will help support the diagnosis and exclude DRESS mimics. The histologic findings are usually nonspecific and include mild spongiosis, acanthosis, and interface vacuolar alteration. There is a predominantly perivascular, lymphocytic infiltrate in the superficial dermis, with eosinophils and dermal edema.

## Initial Steps in Management

Identification and prompt withdrawal of the offending agent remains the mainstay of treatment. These patients should be admitted to the hospital and carefully monitored for fluid status, electrolyte abnormalities, and other complications of DRESS.

Patients without severe systemic involvement can be treated symptomatically. For skin inflammation, high- or super high–potency topical steroids are preferred over systemic steroids.

- Patients can use clobetasol dipropionate 0.05% cream (or a similar strength topical steroid) twice daily until symptoms resolve. It should not be used on the face.

- For the face, patients can use hydrocortisone 2.5% cream twice daily (or a similar strength topical steroid) until resolution.

### Patients with Severe Liver Involvement

- Patients with severe liver involvement should be closely monitored in the hospital with a hepatologist consultation. Liver injury can evolve into acute liver failure, necessitating consideration for liver transplantation.
- Systemic steroids are not shown to improve hepatic involvement (although they are used for other manifestations of DRESS).

### Patients with Lung or Kidney Involvement

- Patients with lung or kidney involvement are treated with moderate to high-dose systemic steroids.
- The starting dose is 0.5 to 2 mg/kg per day of prednisone or prednisone until there is clinical and laboratory improvement. This is followed by a prolonged taper over 8 to 12 weeks.
- Oral cyclosporine can be used as a second-line agent for patients who do not respond to systemic steroids or if steroids are contraindicated.

The skin and systemic manifestations gradually resolve after the withdrawal of the offending agent. The average recovery time ranges from 6 to 9 weeks. Nevertheless, in some patients, the disease might persist for several months with periods of remissions and relapses. The severity of liver involvement is associated with a prolonged clinical course.

### Warning Signs/Common Pitfalls

Patients should be counseled about strict avoidance of the causative drug and chemically related medications. Family members should also be advised to avoid the causative drug.

### Counseling

Drug reaction with eosinophilia and systemic symptoms (DRESS) is a rare side effect of a medication that affects the skin and internal organs. It causes the skin to turn red, involving more than half of the body's surface area. Swelling of the face is commonly seen. This drug hypersensitivity reaction can also involve the mucosal surfaces (typically mouth or pharynx) and internal organs, including the liver, kidneys, and lungs. Many medications can potentially cause DRESS, and a list will be provided to you.

In your case, the offending drug should be stopped, and it is recommended that you strictly avoid this drug in the future. Structurally similar drugs can also cause the same or potentially a worse reaction, and it is recommended that you talk with your healthcare provider before starting any new medications. You should learn the names of the medications you should avoid and keep a written record on your person. Your pharmacy should also make a note that you had a severe drug reaction and should have a list of medications you should avoid. Consider wearing a medical alert bracelet to let people know which medications to avoid.

You should go to the emergency room immediately or call for an ambulance (call 911) if you develop any fever, difficulty breathing, trouble swallowing, abdominal pain, yellowish skin or eyes, decreased urine amount, or change in color of urine.

You should regularly follow up with your healthcare provider, who will periodically check your blood counts, liver, and renal function. Topical creams and possibly some pills will be prescribed to alleviate your symptoms. Please use or take them as prescribed.

## STEVENS-JOHNSON SYNDROME AND TOXIC EPIDERMAL NECROLYSIS

### Clinical Features

SJS (Fig. 18.3) and TEN (Fig. 18.4) are rare, life-threatening hypersensitivity reactions that involve the skin and

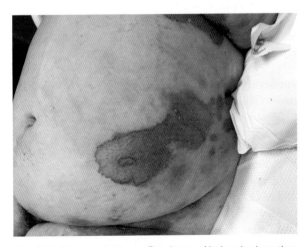

**Fig. 18.3 Stevens-Johnson Syndrome.** Notice the less than 10% body surface area involvement. (From the University of Connecticut Grand Rounds Collection.)

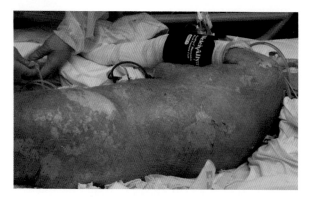

**Fig. 18.4** Toxic Epidermal Necrolysis. Notice the greater than 80% body surface area involvement. (Courtesy Justin Finch, MD.)

mucous membranes. They are more commonly triggered by medications and rarely by an infection.

SJS, SJS/TEN overlap, and TEN occur along a continuum of disease and are distinguished based on the degree of skin detachment. SJS is defined as skin detachment of less than 10%, TEN is defined as skin detachment of greater than 30%, and SJS/TEN overlap shows 10% to 30% skin detachment. In all three conditions, mucous membranes are involved in greater than 90% of cases, typically at two or more different sites. We will use the term SJS/TEN to collectively refer to SJS, TEN, and SJS/TEN overlap syndrome.

SJS/TEN is fortunately very rare, with a reported incidence of 1 to 2 cases per million person years. It can affect individuals of any age and is more common in those with an active malignancy or an HIV infection. SJS/TEN is a medical emergency with a mortality rate ranging from 5% for SJS to 30% for TEN.

SJS/TEN is considered to be a delayed type of hypersensitivity reaction, commonly triggered by medications. Clinical manifestations typically appear about 4 to 28 days (with an average of 14 days) after initiation of the culprit drug. The most vulnerable period seems to be the first 8 weeks after the initiation of a new medication. The risk decreases after 8 weeks, and drugs used for a more extended period are unlikely to be the cause of SJS/TEN.

Medications commonly implicated in SJS/TEN include allopurinol (especially for patients with the HLA-B*58:01 haplotype), anticonvulsants (such as lamotrigine, carbamazepine, phenytoin, and phenobarbital), antibiotics (e.g., sulfonamides, beta-lactam antibiotics,

fluoroquinolones), antivirals (including nevirapine), oxicam NSAIDs, and chemotherapeutic/immunotherapeutic agents (such as thalidomide, capecitabine, afatinib, vemurafenib, tamoxifen, and immune checkpoint inhibitors).

Infections commonly implicated in SJS/TEN include *Mycoplasma pneumoniae* infection and Herpes simplex virus (HSV) infection.

Systemic symptoms and severe mucocutaneous involvement characterize the acute phase of SJS/TEN. Once the precipitating cause is identified and the medication is discontinued or the infection is treated, SJS/TEN lasts for approximately 1 to 2 weeks, followed by a gradual reepithelialization over 2 to 4 or more weeks.

Systemic symptoms may precede mucocutaneous lesions by 1 to 3 days and may include a fever (typically exceeding 102.2° F), malaise, myalgia, arthralgia, dysphagia, stinging eyes, photophobia, runny nose, and decreased appetite.

### Cutaneous Manifestations

- Skin lesions usually begin as erythematous or violaceous macules/patches with purpuric centers.
- Atypical targetoid lesions with darker centers may be present.
- As the disease progresses, the lesions evolve into bullae and erosions and the skin begins to peel away.
- Skin is tender to the touch, often out of proportion to the skin changes.
- The lesions typically start on the face and trunk. As the disease progresses, the lesions spread to other areas, sparing the scalp. Palms and soles are rarely involved.
- The Nikolsky sign (in which slight rubbing of apparently uninvolved skin results in sloughing of skin) is typically positive.
- The Asboe-Hansen sign or "bulla spread sign" (extension of bullae to an adjacent unblistered skin surface when pressure is applied on top of bullae) may also be present.

### Mucosal Manifestations

- Involvement of mucosa occurs in more than 90% of cases and is characterized by erythema, hemorrhagic erosions, and painful crusts.
- Oral mucosa is almost invariably involved and can lead to dehydration secondary to impaired oral intake.

- Pharyngeal mucosa is involved in nearly all patients.
- Ocular involvement is reported in about 80% of cases and the most common findings are severe conjunctivitis, pseudomembrane formation, purulent eye discharge, corneal ulceration, anterior uveitis, and late sequelae (including development of scarring and synechiae between the eyelids and conjunctiva).
- The genitourinary tract is affected in up to 60% of cases; typical findings are urethritis leading to urinary retention, genital erosions, ulcerative vaginitis, and vaginal synechiae.
- The lower respiratory tract, esophagus, and intestines are less frequently affected.

## Complications and Sequelae

The risk and severity of acute complications with SJS/TEN are proportional to the degree of skin detachment. Extensive denuded skin results in excessive fluid losses, electrolyte imbalance, renal failure, increased infections, and multiorgan failure. Septic shock from *S. aureus* and *Pseudomonas aeruginosa* is the leading cause of mortality in these patients. Pneumonia is a frequent complication and can lead to acute respiratory distress syndrome, requiring mechanical ventilation in about 25% of patients.

### Long-Term Sequelae

- Cutaneous sequelae may include postinflammatory hypopigmentation or hyperpigmentation, scarring, and nail dystrophies.
- Patients may also have severe dry eyes, ingrown eyelashes, corneal scarring (leading to visual impairment), dry mouth, caries, periodontal disease, urinary retention, vaginal dryness, introital stenosis, chronic bronchitis, and bronchiectasis.
- Some patients may suffer from depression and decreased quality of life.

## Differential Diagnosis

It is vital to distinguish SJS/TEN from other forms of drug reactions, including DRESS and exanthematous drug eruptions. These conditions can be further differentiated based on skin biopsy findings. SJS/TEN usually presents within 4 weeks (average of 2 weeks) of drug exposure and is characterized by severe, generalized mucosal involvement.

In contrast, mucosal involvement in DRESS is generally limited to one site (mostly mouth or pharynx) without any erosions.

Exanthematous drug eruptions lack the mucosal findings associated with SJS/TEN.

Another important differential to consider is AGEP, which typically presents within 3 days of drug exposure (usually to beta-lactam antibiotics) and is characterized by multiple, pinpoint pustules distributed over the whole body.

Erythema multiform (Figs. 18.5 and 18.6) usually presents with typical target lesions and involves less than 10% BSA. Bullae formation and mucosal involvement is limited. It is most commonly (in 90% of cases) associated with HSV infection.

SJS/TEN should also be differentiated from staphylococcal scalded skin syndrome (SSSS), which is characterized by generalized erythema followed by the rapid

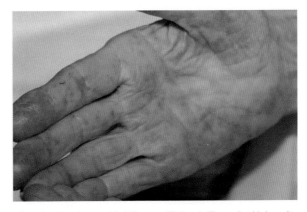

**Fig. 18.5** Erythema Multiforme (Palms). (From the University of Connecticut Grand Rounds Collection.)

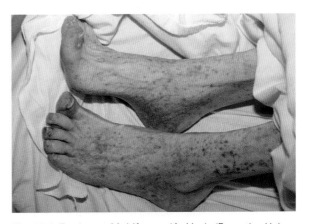

**Fig. 18.6** Erythema Multiforme (Ankles). (From the University of Connecticut Grand Rounds Collection.)

development of skin sloughing. SSSS does not involve the mucosa, and histologically only the upper layers of the epidermis are affected, compared with the full-thickness epidermal necrosis seen with SJS/TEN.

### Work-Up

The diagnosis of SJS/TEN is suspected when a patient presents with a fever, rapidly progressive rash, and a recent drug exposure or febrile illness.

A careful review of the complete medication list, including prescription, OTC, and herbal medications, should be performed. The timeline of drug exposure and symptoms onset should be documented to assess for drug causality. It is unlikely for a medication to be the cause of SJS/TEN if taken for more than 8 weeks before symptoms onset. Travel history and exposure to any ticks should be obtained to assess for an infectious etiology. Careful examination of the skin and all mucosal surfaces should be performed. Nikolsky sign and/or Asboe-Hansen sign should be elicited if clinically warranted.

Tests that should be obtained as a part of the work-up to confirm the diagnosis and exclude other conditions that can mimic SJS/TEN include a CBC with differential and peripheral blood smear, liver function tests, renal function tests, bacterial and fungal cultures from blood, and imaging studies (guided by clinical presentation).

A skin biopsy for histopathologic examination and DIF should be obtained to help support the diagnosis and exclude SJS/TEN mimics. A punch biopsy (equal to or greater than 4 mm) or deep shave biopsy is typically preferred. The histologic findings include necrotic keratinocytes scattered in the basal layer of the epidermis with interface and a superficial perivascular inflammatory infiltrate. Subepidermal bullae and full-thickness epidermal necrosis is seen in later stages of the disease. DIF is always negative.

## Initial Steps in Management

Identification and apt withdrawal of the culprit drug is of paramount importance. Early withdrawal of the causative drug has been shown to decrease mortality. Any patient suspected to have SJS/TEN should be admitted to the hospital and closely monitored for complications. It is essential to assess the severity of the disease on admission for appropriate triage. The SCORTEN (SCORe of Toxic Epidermal Necrosis) scale generates a validated prognostication score based on seven independent clinical and laboratory variables. These include age equal to or greater than 40 years, malignancy, at least 10% BSA detached, heart rate of at least 120 beats/min, serum urea greater than 10 mmol/L, serum glucose greater than 14 mmol/L, and serum bicarbonate less than 20 mmol/L. Patients with a SCORTEN score of 2 or more or skin detachment of more than 30% BSA should be admitted to an intensive care unit (ICU) or a burn unit, if available.

Supportive care is an integral part of the therapeutic approach and includes wound care, fluid/electrolyte management, nutritional support, prevention and treatment of superinfections, and pain control.

### Wound Care

- The degree of skin detachment should be assessed daily and documented as a percentage of total BSA.
- There is no consensus regarding optimal wound care. Some centers prefer debridement of the necrotic skin, whereas other centers prefer to leave the separated skin in place, working as a biologic dressing.
- There are no randomized clinical trials to compare the relative efficacy of silver-containing nonadherent nanocrystalline gauze dressing over petrolatum-impregnated gauze. Nevertheless, the nanocrystalline bandage may be preferred because it can be left in place for a week, minimizing the need for painful dressing changes.

### Fluid and Nutrition

- Renal function and electrolytes should be closely monitored.
- A crystalloid solution to maintain an adequate urine output of 0.5 to 1 mL/kg/h should be administered intravenously.
- The room temperature should be set between 86°F and 89.6°F to prevent excessive fluid loss and calorie expenditure.

### Pain Control

- Skin detachment in these patients predisposes them to severe pain and is further exacerbated by the need for frequent wound care procedures. Adequate pain control with narcotic or nonnarcotic analgesics should be attained.

### Superinfections

- Prophylactic antibiotics are not recommended to prevent superinfections.

- Infection control precautions, including sterile handling, proper hand hygiene, and antiseptic solutions for disinfection, should be employed.
- Skin should be closely monitored for any signs of superinfection.
- Blood cultures, skin cultures, and catheter cultures should be obtained every 48 hours.
- Any suspected or confirmed infection should be treated promptly.

### Other Complications

- Ophthalmology consultation should be sought on admission to get a baseline eye examination. Any eye involvement should be closely monitored and immediately treated in consultation with an ophthalmologist.
- A urology/gynecology team should be consulted for patients with a suspected genitourinary involvement.

### Specific Systemic Therapy

There are no randomized trials to support a particular systemic therapy for SJS/TEN. The immunosuppressive therapies used for the treatment of SJS/TEN are based on clinical experience and local guidelines. There is increasing evidence from case series that cyclosporine may help slow the progression of SJS/TEN.

### Systemic Steroids

- The use of steroids remains controversial and its effectiveness is not well studied in clinical trials.
- Although some observational studies indicated a potential benefit of a short-course systemic steroid therapy (prednisone 1–2 mg/kg/day for 3–5 days), other studies have shown an increased frequency of complications and mortality.
- Steroid therapy is not recommended, especially in those with extensively denuded skin, because it increases the risk for infection and protein catabolism.

### Intravenous Immune Globulin

Although intravenous immune globulin (IVIG) is a frequently used, consensus-approved therapy for SJS/TEN, the data regarding its efficacy are conflicting. Several case series, meta-analyses, and systemic reviews have failed to show any survival benefit with IVIG use.

### Cyclosporine

There are no randomized trials that assess the efficacy of cyclosporine in SJS/TEN; however, there is growing evidence from case series and systemic reviews that cyclosporine may slow the disease progression. The recommended dose is 3 to 5 mg/kg per day.

### Thalidomide

Thalidomide has been shown to increase mortality in patients with TEN, and its use is contraindicated.

### Tumor Necrosis Factor Inhibitors

A few case reports and a small unblinded clinical trial have demonstrated that tumor necrosis factor (TNF) inhibitors, such as etanercept and infliximab, may halt the progression of skin detachment and potentially improve survival. These early studies are promising; however, additional studies are needed to assess efficacy and determine the optimal dose and duration of therapy.

### Other Therapies

- Combination therapy with IVIG and systemic steroids have shown equivocal results.
- A potential benefit of plasmapheresis was demonstrated in early case series; however, recent studies have not demonstrated any clinically significant improvement in mortality, length of stay, or time to reepithelization.

## Warning Signs/Common Pitfalls

Patients should be counseled about strict avoidance of the causative drug and chemically related medications.

## Counseling

Stevens-Johnson syndrome (SJS) is a rare side effect of a medication that affects the skin and mucosal surfaces (inner lining of mouth, eyes, genitals, airways, and digestive tract). It causes the skin to turn red and peel away from the body. A more severe form of SJS is called "toxic epidermal necrolysis" or "TEN." Both SJS and TEN are most commonly triggered by medications that cannot be predicted. There are many medications that can potentially cause SJS/TEN, and a list will be provided to you.

Fever is often the first symptom, followed by sore throat, difficulty swallowing, dry eyes, and body aches. This is followed by skin rash, blister formation, and peeling away of the skin surface.

In your case, the offending drug should be stopped, and it is recommended that you strictly avoid this drug in the future. Structurally similar drugs can also cause the same reaction, and it is recommended that you talk with your healthcare provider before starting any new medications. You should learn the names of the medications you should avoid and keep a written record on your person. Your pharmacy should also make a note that you had a drug reaction and should have a list of medications you should avoid. Consider wearing a medical alert bracelet to let people know which medications to avoid.

You should go to the emergency room immediately or call for an ambulance (call 911) if you develop any symptoms of SJS/TEN.

You should regularly follow up with your primary healthcare provider, who will periodically check your blood counts, liver, and renal function.

## DRUG-INDUCED BULLOUS PEMPHIGOID (SEE CHAPTER 3, BODY DERMATITIS)

## DRUG-INDUCED PEMPHIGUS (SEE CHAPTER 3, BODY DERMATITIS)

# Children and Pregnant Women

# 19

# Dermatoses of Pregnancy

*Jeff Shornick*

## CHAPTER OUTLINE

## INTRODUCTION

There are four accepted entities included in the dermatoses of pregnancy. They are pemphigoid gestationis (PG; also known as "herpes gestationis" or "gestational pemphigoid"); polymorphic eruption of pregnancy (PEP; also known as "pruritic urticarial papules and plaques of pregnancy" or "PUPPP"); atopic eruption of pregnancy (AEP); and intrahepatic cholestasis of pregnancy (ICP; also known as "obstetric cholestasis" or "jaundice of pregnancy").

Nomenclature in this group is somewhat confusing because names and nomenclature have changed as understanding has evolved. Disagreement persists as to whether additional entities should be added (e.g., pustular psoriasis associated with pregnancy) or whether a given entity should be carved out as distinctive (e.g., whether or not pruritic folliculitis of pregnancy should be lumped into AEP). The best way to think about

dermatoses of pregnancy is that PG, PEP, and cholestasis are all sufficiently defined to be clearly recognizable (although PEP awaits a defining biomarker), and AEP stands for everything else.

Such a classification admittedly leaves room for improvement, but that will not happen until we have a clearer understanding of mechanisms.

It is more likely that an itchy pregnant woman has something unrelated to pregnancy, such as scabies, than a specific dermatosis of pregnancy. Therefore the first differential step is always to decide whether the pregnancy is causative or coincidental.

Nearly all articles on the specific dermatoses of pregnancy include ICP, which is not really a dermatosis. ICP presents with pruritus and excoriations, but it is not really a specific dermatosis. ICP is included in the dermatoses of pregnancy because patients present with pruritus and a rash, but to the dermatologist's eye, the rash is entirely secondary.

Some skin diseases may be worse during pregnancy (such as psoriasis and eczema herpeticum), but these are not considered among the dermatoses of pregnancy. Preexisting diseases that can be made better or worse by pregnancy are also not considered to be dermatoses of pregnancy.

# PEMPHIGOID GESTATIONIS

## Clinical Features

PG is the most clinically distinct and histopathologically defined of the dermatoses of pregnancy. For patients with rash, PG is the diagnosis to exclude.

- PG is rare, occurring in approximately 1 out of every 50,000 pregnancies.
- It is mediated by an immunoglobulin (Ig)G with specificity for the 16th domain of the extracellular component of type XVII collagen (NC16A), also known as "BP180."
  - The antigen is demonstrable by direct immuno-fluorescence (DIF) in 100% of patients and by enzyme-linked immunosorbent assay (ELISA) to the NC16A antigen in over 90% of patients.
  - It is thought that aberrant expression of this antigen in the placenta induces an immune response, and that the antibody then crossreacts with the skin.
  - There are distinctive human leukocyte antigen associations in PG, strongly suggesting a genetic predisposition.
- PG typically develops during the second or third trimester, although explosive onset during the immediate postpartum period can occur in up to 25% of patients.
- First onset in the periumbilical area occurs in 50% of patients, but onset may also be on the palms, soles, or extremities.
  - Facial involvement is uncommon and mucosal involvement is rare.
- The primary lesion ranges from intensely pruritic urticarial papules and plaques to tense, grouped (so-called "herpetiform") blisters.
  - Urticarial lesions without blisters can occur but are seen in fewer than 10% of cases.
- PG not infrequently improves or clears as the pregnancy progresses, but 75% of patients flare with delivery or during the immediate postpartum period, often dramatically so.
- Recurrence during use of oral contraceptives has been reported and recurrence during subsequent gestations is the rule, although skip pregnancies may occur.
- There is no increased maternal risk in PG.
  - There is, however, an increased risk for premature delivery (32% before 38 weeks and 16% before 36 weeks) and a slightly increased risk for small-for-gestational-age births.
  - Transient involvement in the newborn may be seen in up to 10% of cases.
- PG tends to improve over the weeks to months after delivery.
  - Flares with menstruation or during use of oral contraceptives have been reported.
- Disease typically recurs during subsequent gestations, often with first onset earlier in pregnancy; however, skip pregnancies have been reported in up to 10% of cases.

## Work-Up

Referral to a dermatologist should be considered for work-up and treatment. A skin biopsy should be done for routine pathology and DIF.

- Histopathology usually shows an increase in eosinophils, often lined up along the dermoepidermal junction.
- DIF shows complement along the epidermal fragment of the basement membrane zone, with or without IgG. This finding is quite similar to that seen in bullous pemphigoid and is unique to the pregnancy rashes. It remains the defining characteristic of PG, occurring in 100% of cases.

Indirect immunofluorescence (IIF) is less reliable; however, ELISA for NC16A (BP180) is detectable in over 90% of cases, offering a reliable alternative to biopsy. Antibody titers do not correlate with the degree of skin involvement.

Antithyroid antibodies are increased, although their clinical relevance is unclear. Most patients are clinically euthyroid. On the other hand, the risk for subsequent autoimmune thyroid disease, especially Graves disease, is clearly increased in those with a history of PG, affecting about 10% of patients.

## Differential Diagnosis

The primary differential in PG is between PEP and a wide variety of diseases unrelated to pregnancy. Immunofluorescence or ELISA is the key to differentiating

PG. Most typically, the relentless progression of unbearable itch associated with urticarial lesions, rapidly progressing to clustered, tense blisters, is characteristic of PG.

## Initial Steps in Management

PG is rare; treatment guidelines are driven by expert opinion.

Because PG is not associated with significant maternal or fetal risk and because it tends to remit spontaneously postpartum, it is imperative not to create disproportionate risk from therapy.

- Topical steroids and antihistamines are rarely of benefit.
- Systemic steroids (prednisolone 0.25–0.5 mg/kg/d or prednisone 0.5–1 mg/kg/d) remain the treatment of choice.
- Many patients improve during the latter part of pregnancy, only to flare at the time of delivery. Because profound flares at delivery are common, one should be prepared to initiate or increase steroids during the immediate postpartum period.

Close collaboration with the obstetrician and hospital neonatologist are recommended.

## Warning Signs/Common Pitfalls

PG may recur during use of oral contraceptives. Recurrence, often with earlier onset during subsequent gestation(s), is the rule. Subsequent pregnancies are not contraindicated but are likely to be unpleasant because of the disease, treatment, or both.

Patients with a history of PG are at increased risk for autoimmune thyroid disease (10% risk).

## Counseling

You have a disease called "pemphigoid gestationis" (PG). "Gestationis" refers to pregnancy; thus the name means "pemphigoid occurring during pregnancy." It is very rare and also very unpleasant, but it is not dangerous to you or your baby.

Pemphigoid is caused by an antibody against a normal component of skin; in other words, it is as if you have developed an allergy to yourself. We do not know why this happens, but there is evidence to suggest it develops in the placenta and that the responsible antibody then crossreacts with normal skin.

PG is unpredictable. Untreated, it often (but not always) improves as pregnancy progresses, only to flare at the time of delivery, sometimes dramatically so. In

about one-quarter of patients, it only develops in the immediate postpartum period. It tends to burn itself out over a period of months after delivery. It sometimes recurs with the use of oral contraceptives and it almost always comes back during subsequent pregnancies.

PG poses no threat to your well-being. There is no significant threat to your baby either, except that there is a slight risk for premature delivery or a small-for-gestational-age birth. About 10% of babies have transient skin involvement, similar to your own, but it typically resolves quickly, without treatment.

Treatment usually starts with antihistamines and creams. Unfortunately, they are not terribly effective. Thus oral steroids are the treatment of choice (especially prednisone). Prednisone usually works quickly and because it is not uncommon for PG to improve on its own, its use is often temporary. It is important to remember that PG tends to flare at the time of delivery, so even if you are happy with creams for the time being, oral steroids may be needed later.

People who have had PG are at a higher risk for developing low thyroid over time (about a 10% risk). There are no other long-term problems known to be associated with PG.

# POLYMORPHIC ERUPTION OF PREGNANCY

## Clinical Features

PEP is the most common name for this group, although the term PUPPP is preferentially used in the United States and Australia.

PEP is the most common specific dermatosis of pregnancy, occurring in 1 out of every 120 to 300 pregnancies.

- The cause of PEP is unknown.
  - An increase in activated T cells within dermal infiltrates has led to speculation that PEP may be a consequence of a delayed T-cell hypersensitivity to skin antigens.
- PEP most commonly presents during the third trimester in primiparous women.
- Patients most typically develop urticarial papules, plaques, or excoriations, which classically begin on (or are even confined to) the abdominal striae during the last trimester or immediate postpartum period.
  - Rapid spread to the trunk or extremities is characteristic.

- Targetoid or dyshidrotic lesions may be seen (which led to the change in nomenclature from PUPPP to PEP).
- The large, tense blisters of PG are absent, but microblisters have been described.
- Facial involvement is uncommon (less than 12% of cases).
- Mucosal involvement is not seen.
- Most cases (around 75% to 85%) occur in primiparous women, but first onset after multiple pregnancies has been reported.
- PEP rarely recurs during subsequent gestations.
- No maternal risks or complication(s) are noted, except for an increased incidence of excessive weight gain and fetal twinning.
- Because there is no definitive test for PEP, the diagnosis remains a clinical one.

## Differential Diagnosis

The differential includes early PG or PG without blisters, toxic drug eruption, viral exanthems, and urticaria.

## Work-Up

Although patients can be frantic with itch, PEP is a benign, self-limited problem. Spontaneous resolution within 4 to 6 weeks of delivery is typical. Nevertheless, referral to a dermatologist should be considered for the work-up and treatment.

Skin biopsy should be done for routine pathology and DIF.

- Histopathology is typically nonspecific, with or without eosinophils.
- DIF is negative.
- IIF is negative. Serum tests for BP180 are negative.
- Serum levels of bile salts and transaminases are normal.

## Initial Steps in Management

Management is symptomatic. Potent topical steroids and antihistamines may provide symptomatic support. Systemic steroids are quite helpful but not always necessary.

## Counseling

You have a skin condition with two common names, "polymorphic eruption of pregnancy" (abbreviated to "PEP") and "pruritic urticarial papules and plaques of pregnancy" (also known as "PUPPP"). The two terms are interchangeable. PEP is of unknown cause. It is more common in women with excessive weight gain or who are carrying twins for reasons we do not know. It most typically starts on the belly, often in stretch marks, then rapidly spreads to the trunk and extremities. It rarely goes to the face. It usually goes away by itself within weeks of delivery and rarely recurs during subsequent pregnancies. Except for the discomfort it causes, it poses no risk to you or your baby. Treatment is symptomatic, usually with creams and antihistamines. Oral prednisone can be very effective but is usually reserved for severe symptoms.

# ATOPIC ERUPTION OF PREGNANCY

## Clinical Features

AEP warehouses several entities (such as pruritic folliculitis of pregnancy), which may or may not be distinct. Until such time as there is a unique identifier for this (or any subgroup of this), confusion will remain. The unifying feature of AEP is that there is no diagnostic clarity, only a similar clinical pattern (Fig. 19.1).

- AEP is less common than PEP, estimated at around 1 in 300 to 450 pregnancies, and is by far the most confusing of the dermatoses of pregnancy.
- AEP usually presents with pruritic papules, patches, or pustules on extensors, typically during the second or third trimester of otherwise uncomplicated pregnancies.
  - Truncal involvement is not uncommon.
  - The striae are usually spared, helping to differentiate this group from PEP.

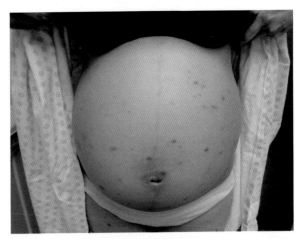

**Fig. 19.1 Atopic Eruption of Pregnancy.** Notice the excoriations from pruritus. (From the UConn Department of Dermatology Grand Rounds Collection.)

- There is a personal or family history of atopy in up to 50% of patients.
- For many, however, AEP appears to be their first manifestation of disease.
- Pruritus is intense and excoriations are the rule. There may be pustules but not blisters.
- Resolution is spontaneous and typically rapid after delivery, but duration up to 3 months has been reported.
- There are no maternal or fetal risks associated with AEP.
- Recurrence during subsequent pregnancies is variable.

## Work-Up
- Histopathology is nonspecific.
- DIF and IIF are negative.
- Serum IgE may or may not be elevated. Serum bile acids and liver function tests are (by definition) normal.

## Initial Steps in Management
Treatment is symptomatic with topical or systemic corticosteroids depending on disease severity.

## Counseling
Atopic eruption of pregnancy is an itchy rash that appears during pregnancy. As miserable as it is, it is not dangerous and poses no risk to you or your baby.

At least half of women with your condition have a personal or family history of atopy (such as eczema, asthma, or hay fever). Although half of the women do not have a personal or family history of atopy, we think pregnancy somehow triggers the atopic tendency in this group. All tests for other rashes associated with pregnancy are normal, labor and delivery are normal, and there are no ill effects for your baby.

Treatment is symptomatic, usually with bland creams, topical steroids, or antihistamines. Oral treatment is rarely required, and the rash usually goes away by itself over weeks to months after delivery. It may or may not recur if you get pregnant again.

## CHOLESTASIS OF PREGNANCY

### Clinical Features
ICP is characterized by impaired transport of bile acids from hepatic cells into the gallbladder.
- Increased intracellular bile acids lead to hepatic injury and leakage of bile acids into the blood.

- There is a broad spectrum of clinical presentations, but the primary feature is pruritus associated with cholestasis; there is no primary dermatologic lesion.
- Patients present with pruritus plus elevated serum bile acids, typically 3 to 100 times the normal level, and (usually) abnormal lever function tests, all in the absence of an alternative explanation.
  - Pruritus can precede identifiable serum anomalies. Symptoms are usually worse on the palms and soles, are worse at night, and may wax and wane without apparent correlation to serum levels of bile salts or liver enzymes.
- ICP typically presents during the last trimester of otherwise uneventful pregnancies.
  - Nevertheless, onset as early as 7 weeks has been reported.
- The incidence of ICP varies in different racial groups. It seems to be highest in Chile-Bolivia (6%–27%), China (2.3–6%), and Sweden (1%–1.5%), and lowest among Black Americans.
- ICP occurs in approximately 1 out of every 1000 pregnancies in the United States.
  - It is more common in those with preexisting hepatitis C, a history of gallstones, multiparous women, and those using assisted reproduction.
  - There is an increased risk for ICP in first-degree relatives of those with a confirmed diagnosis, suggesting a genetic predisposition.
- Around 10% to 50% of patients develop signs of hepatitis, such as dark urine, light-colored stools, or jaundice, usually within 4 weeks of presentation.
- Failure of pruritus to stop within days of delivery or the persistence of elevated liver function tests suggests underlying hepatic or primary biliary disease.
- Recurrence during subsequent gestations occurs in 45% to 70% of cases. Recurrences may also occur with use of oral contraceptives.
- If ICP lasts for weeks, vitamin K absorption may be impaired, leading to a prolonged prothrombin time.
  - Without exogenous vitamin K, fetal prothrombin activity may lead to an increased incidence of intracranial hemorrhage.
  - The prothrombin time should be monitored and intramuscular vitamin K administered as necessary.
    - Vitamin K anomalies are, however, rare.
- Meconium staining and premature labor occurs in 20% to 60% of cases. An increase in fetal distress is

clear. Whether and by how much fetal mortality is increased is disputed.

## Work-Up

Elevated bile acids, with or without elevated transaminases, defines the disease. Increased bile acids are typically 3 to 100 times the normal level. In those without jaundice, elevated bile acids may be the only identifiable laboratory abnormality. Conjugated (direct) bilirubin is increased but rarely above 2 to 5 mg/dL. Alkaline phosphatase, gamma–glutamyl transferase, and cholesterol are unreliable during pregnancy and aspartate aminotransferase typically remains below four times normal, even in those with ICP. ICP is associated with an increased frequency of mutations in biliary transport enzymes.

- Hepatic ultrasonography is normal. Liver biopsy is not indicated.
- Serum bilirubin is increased in 10% of patients. Patients may develop jaundice, malabsorption of fats (steatorrhea), or reduced absorption of vitamin K (rare).
- The cause of pruritus remains unclear. There is no correlation between serum levels of bile salts and itch.
- A maternal serum bile acid level greater than 40 micromoles per liter is associated with increased preterm delivery, meconium staining of the amniotic fluid, fetal hypoxia, and stillbirth.
- Fetal development can appear normal up to the time of spontaneous abortion, suggesting a vascular or cardiac (arrhythmic) event.

## Initial Steps in Management

Ursodeoxycholic acid (UDCA; 500–2000 mg/day) is the treatment of choice. It improves pruritus, normalizes liver enzymes, decreases the risk for premature birth, improves fetal outcome, and reduces utilization of the neonatal intensive care unit.

- Antihistamines and bland topicals are helpful to reduce pruritus.
- There is consensus (but not clear evidence) to support delivery at 36 to 38 weeks.

## Warning Signs/Common Pitfalls

The primary cutaneous finding is excoriations, which results in a risk for secondary infection.

ICP is associated with an increased risk for gestational diabetes, dyslipidemia, large babies, and preeclampsia.

Patients with a history of ICP have an increased long-term risk for diabetes mellitus, thyroid dysfunction, psoriasis, inflammatory polyarthritis, Crohn's disease, and cardiovascular disease. Patients with a history of ICP may also suffer a long-term increased risk for cholelithiasis and cancer of the liver or biliary tree.

## Counseling

You have a condition called "cholestasis of pregnancy." It is caused by a hormonally induced defect in moving chemicals called "bile salts" out of the liver. Some of those chemicals leak into your bloodstream, causing you to itch. We do not know why this happens. Because it is more common in some countries than others and because it is more common in siblings of those who already have it, we think there is a genetic predisposition. It is, by definition, a pregnancy-related problem; when the pregnancy goes away, the problem goes away, but it sometimes recurs with the use of birth control pills and it comes back during subsequent pregnancies somewhere between 45% and 75% of the time.

There are some risks associated with cholestasis, but most patients have nothing more than itch.

For the mother, mild jaundice (yellowing of the eyes, dark urine, light-colored stools) occurs up to half of the time. With significant disease, there is an increased risk for fetal distress. These risks are both dramatically lowered by treatment. Still, for these reasons, your doctor is likely to recommend delivery at 36 to 38 weeks. Regardless of treatment, all symptoms tend to resolve quickly after delivery.

For the baby, cholestasis is associated with meconium staining (leakage of bowel contents into the fluid surrounding the baby). That, in turn, can cause respiratory problems. There is also a small risk for spontaneous abortion associated with cholestasis. Both of these risks are lowered by treatment, but they are another reason your doctor is likely to recommend delivery before full term.

There is a simple, highly effective treatment for cholestasis called "UDCA" (ursodeoxycholic acid), which is a pill that helps the liver get rid of the bile salts that back up in the liver. It usually works quickly and well and can be stopped once your hormones return to normal. UDCA reduces the itch and reduces the likelihood of both meconium staining and premature delivery.

Having cholestasis does not mean you should never have another baby. Cholestasis is likely, however, to recur if you get pregnant again, something that needs to be factored into your thinking.

# Miscellaneous Skin Conditions

# Ulcers

*Ayman Grada and Tania Phillips*

## DIABETIC ULCERS

Diabetic wounds are multifactorial in etiology. Patients with long-standing diabetes develop polyneuropathy, which creates sensory, motor, and proprioceptive abnormalities and can lead to insensate skin and foot deformities. Combined with vascular disease and immunosuppression, patients have a high risk for trauma, subsequent ulceration, and infection. Most diabetic foot ulcers (DFUs) result from peripheral neuropathy (60%–70%), peripheral vascular disease (15%–20%), or a combination of both (15%–20%). Approximately

2% to 3% of all patients with diabetes will develop a DFU in a given year, and 10% to 25% of all patients with diabetes will develop at least one DFU in their lifetime. Approximately 50% to 60% of patients with a DFU have clinical signs of infection at the time of hospital admission. DFU accounts for nearly two-thirds of all nontraumatic amputations performed in the United States.

## Clinical Features

### Symptoms

- Sensory neuropathy results in the loss of protective sensation (as evidenced by an abnormal 10-point monofilament examination). Patients frequently complain of skin burning, numbness, itching, needle-like pain, and paresthesia.
- Autonomic neuropathy results in reduced sweating and dry, scaly feet.
- DFUs are often painless.

### Location

- The majority of DFUs originate at sites of pressure, including plantar metatarsal phalangeal joint prominences and the plantar surface of the heel (Fig. 20.1). They can also originate within the toe web spaces.

### Clinical Findings

- Motor neuropathy leads to difficulty in activating certain extensor muscles, resulting in inadequate pressure distribution and altered foot anatomy, such as hammer toes, claw toes, or a high or flattened arch (Charcot foot).
- The wound often appears punched out with a thick rim of callus.

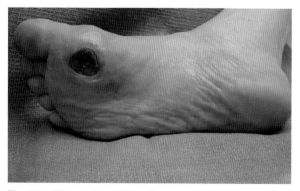

**Fig. 20.1 Diabetic Foot Ulcer.** Note the classic location. (Courtesy Tania Philips, MD.)

- Peripheral pulses may be diminished or absent if there is coexisting arterial disease.
- Patients with neuropathy may have altered sensation to light touch, pinpricks, or joint position sense.

## Differential Diagnosis

The differential includes nondiabetic neuropathic ulcers, arterial ulcers, pressure ulcers, calciphylaxis, venous ulcers, and drug-induced cutaneous necrosis.

## Work-Up

- Diagnosis is based mainly on history and physical examination. Location and physical characteristics are key.
- A patient with diabetes who has foot calluses should be checked for neuropathy (using nylon monofilament, testing vibration sense, and proprioception).
- Ulcer depth should be assessed by probing for bone with a metal instrument. If the ulcer can be probed to bone, there is a high correlation with osteomyelitis.
- There is a high risk for wound infection in patients with diabetes and classic signs can often be masked. Therefore there should be a lower threshold in putting patients with diabetes on antibiotics if infection is suspected.
- The ankle brachial index (ABI)/toe brachial index (TBI) should be calculated.
  - Note that the ABI can be unreliable in DFU because of noncompressible (or partly compressible) arteries.
  - If the ABI is high or arterial disease is suspected, the TBI should be measured in the vascular lab.
- Hemoglobin A1c (HbA1c) levels should also be tested.
  - Good diabetic control is needed to facilitate healing.

## Initial Steps in Management

- A comprehensive assessment and physical examination of both the patient and wound is critical.
- Tight control of blood glucose levels and lifestyle modifications is often necessary. It is also important to manage other contributing systemic factors, such as hypertension and peripheral arterial disease.

### Infection Control

Treatment of tinea pedis and onychomycosis will prevent the development of skin cracks and bacterial entry (which can lead to cellulitis). If present, treat concomitant cellulitis or osteomyelitis with the appropriate antibiotics.

## Surgical Debridement

Surgical (sharp) debridement at frequent intervals has been shown to heal neuropathic wounds more rapidly. Necrotic and callus tissue should be debrided to a healthy bleeding base. This allows for a more thorough examination of the wound and activation of platelets and allows the proliferative phase of healing to begin.

## Avoiding Repetitive Trauma

Patients can avoid repetitive trauma by using mechanical off-loading and pressure relief techniques. These may include adhering to bed rest; using crutches, a walker, or a wheelchair; and wearing therapeutic shoes or sandals (matching the shoe gear to the anatomic alterations). Total contact casting can be a useful first step in managing Charcot foot. Foams and padding can also be used to off-load pressure.

## Prevention

Patients should be tested regularly with a 10 g monofilament on the feet. Loss of this sensation increases the risk for undetected injuries, which can lead to amputations.

Prevention is important and involves daily foot inspections, meticulous hygiene, and properly fitting shoes. Advise smoking cessation if applicable because smoking increases the risk for ulcer formation.

Wound dressings are selected based on ulcer appearance and other wound characteristics (e.g., dry, exudative, infected). Ulcer beds should be kept clean and moist (not wet).

## Advanced/Adjunctive Options

- In complicated or recalcitrant cases where there is no evidence of ulcer healing, a few different treatment modalities can be tried. These may include hyperbaric oxygen therapy, skin-equivalent dressings, negative-pressure dressings (e.g., vacuum-assisted closure or VAC dressings), or surgical interventions.
  - In terms of skin-equivalent dressings, bilayered skin constructs (such as Apligraf) and bioabsorbable membrane with human fibroblasts (such as Dermagraft) are bioengineered products that act as delivery systems for growth factors and extracellular matrix. Both have been approved by the U.S. Food and Drug Administration (FDA) and are indicated for recalcitrant diabetic foot ulcers that have no exposed muscle, bone, or tendon; are not infected; and have had aggressive debridement.

- Surgical interventions should be made on an individual basis and may involve revascularization to restore arterial perfusion and reduce the risk for amputation; foot/joint revision; wound closure; or coverage by plastic surgery.

## Warning Signs/Common Pitfalls

- Good patient care should take a multiprofessional approach, involving primary care, endocrinology, podiatry, and orthopedic and vascular surgery specialists.
- The insensate foot is generally poorly understood by patients; therefore patient education and continuous reinforcement is crucial.
- Liberal moisturizers with emollients, such as unscented petroleum jelly, are recommended to prevent cracking and fissuring of the skin.
- Patients should not attempt to trim calluses or cut their nails on their own, especially if they have impaired vision.
- Patients should never walk barefoot.
- Patients should always check the insides of their shoes before putting them on. Many patients cannot detect a foreign body in their shoe if they have insensate feet.
- Patients should test water temperature with their elbow before taking a bath.
- Exposed bone generally indicates osteomyelitis. Ulcers can become deep, and underlying osteomyelitis should be considered when ulcers do not heal with off-loading therapies.
- Vascular imaging may be helpful, including duplex ultrasonography, computed tomography angiography, or magnetic resonance angiography. Vascular surgical intervention can salvage a limb in many cases.
- Imaging may be helpful, especially if there is a concern for osteomyelitis.
- ABI is unreliable in patients with diabetes and should not be used in these patients to exclude the presence of arterial diseases. ABI can often be falsely elevated because of vessel calcification. In these cases, toe brachial index is helpful because the small toe vessels do not become calcified.
- Biopsy should be done if there is a concern for malignancy.

## Counseling

Your healthcare provider has diagnosed you with a diabetic foot ulcer, which is caused by sensory nerve damage resulting from high blood sugar levels. Because of the nerve damage, patients may lose their ability to sense pain and hence are at an increased risk for injuring the feet; even a minor injury can become serious quickly if it goes unnoticed. Nerve damage can also weaken certain foot muscles and contribute to foot deformities. It is crucial that you do whatever you can to control your blood sugar levels. It is also advisable that you eat a well-balanced, healthy diet and stop smoking.

There are several things you can do to reduce your chances of developing foot problems. In addition to managing your blood sugar, practice good foot care habits and check your feet daily to prevent complications.

- Avoid walking barefoot or wearing shoes without socks because you could step on something without realizing it and because there is significantly more pressure on bare feet. Test bath water with your fingers instead of stepping into it.
- Be careful when trimming your nails. Trim your toenails straight across and avoid cutting them too short. You can remove any sharp edges using a nail file. Never cut your cuticles or allow anyone else (e.g., a manicurist) to do so. See a foot care provider (such as a podiatrist) if you need treatment for an ingrown toenail or callus.
- Wash and check your feet daily. Use lukewarm water and mild soap to clean your feet. Thoroughly dry your feet, especially between the toes, by gently patting them with a clean, absorbent towel. Apply a moisturizing cream or lotion.
- Choose socks and shoes carefully. An orthotics consultation is recommended.
- Be sure to get regular foot examinations. If you have lost sensation in your feet, you should inspect your feet nightly for injury.

Your healthcare provider will recommend some wound dressings and may alter your medications to try to achieve better control of any underlying conditions that you might have that are contributing to this disease.

# PRESSURE ULCERS

Pressure ulcers are areas of localized damage to the skin and underlying soft tissue caused by unrelieved pressure to soft tissue that is compressed between a bony prominence and an external surface for a prolonged period of time. Risk factors include an age of 65 or older, impaired circulation and tissue perfusion, immobilization, undernutrition, decreased sensation, and incontinence. Especially in the elderly, hip fracture and hospitalization are major risk factors for pressure ulcers.

## Clinical Features

- A pressure injury is typically identified by its characteristic appearance and by its location over a bony prominence (including the medial and lateral metatarsal heads). The sacrum is the most common location (resulting in bedsores or decubitus ulcers), followed by the heels.
- Pressure ulcers present clinically as large areas of undermining, which extend circumferentially; have fibrotic tissue (including necrotic eschar); often present with deep probing to the level of bone and undermining of skin edges; and have surrounding periwound erythema.

## Differential Diagnosis

The differential includes neuropathic/diabetic ulcers, arterial ulcers, and venous ulcers.

## Work-Up

- The most widely used system for clinical staging comes from the National Pressure Injury Advisory Panel (NPIAP), which classifies pressure injuries into four stages based on the extent of soft-tissue damage.
  - Stage 1 indicates intact skin or nonblanching erythema.
  - Stage 2 involves partial-thickness skin loss with loss of the epidermis and some of the dermis.
  - Stage 3 involves full-thickness loss of skin with the epidermis and dermis gone and damage to or necrosis of subcutaneous tissues.
  - Stage 4 indicates full-thickness skin loss with extensive destruction; tissue necrosis; and damage to the underlying muscle, tendon, bone, or other exposed supporting structures.
  - If an injury is unstageable, that indicates obscured full-thickness skin and tissue loss.
  - A deep-tissue pressure injury presents as persistent, nonblanchable, deep red, maroon, or purple discoloration.
- Recommended tests include hematocrit, transferrin, prealbumin, albumin, and total and CD4 lymphocyte counts.

## Initial Steps in Management

- Pressure redistribution is the mainstay of pressure ulcer prevention.
- Reduce pressure through frequent repositioning and by using protective padding and support surfaces.
- Maintain and improve tissue tolerance to pressure to prevent injury.
  - Moisturize to protect skin from drying, avoid massaging over bony prominences, protect the skin from incontinence, and provide adequate hydration/nutrition.

### Local Wound Care

- Local wound care involves cleansing, debridement (mechanical, sharp, enzymatic, or autolytic), and addressing moisture (to keep the area from becoming macerated or eroded).
- Cleanse the wound with normal saline and an irrigation pressure of 4 to 15 psi (with a 35 mL syringe and 19-gauge angiocatheter).
- Wound dressing should be based on the characteristics (wet, dry, or infected).

### Warning Signs/Common Pitfalls

- A nutritional assessment is recommended in patients with pressure injury, particularly those with stage 3 or 4 pressure ulcers.
- The undermined edges of pressure ulcers should be removed surgically because they often provide an ideal pocket for infection.

### Counseling

Your healthcare provider has diagnosed you with a pressure ulcer. This usually means you have remained in the same position for too long and have put undue pressure on the skin overlying a bony prominence. Reposition yourself often, use protective padding, lubricate your skin, and make sure to eat a well-balanced diet.

## VASCULITIS ULCERS

- Vasculitis ulcers result from the pathologic process of inflammation and destruction of blood vessels. A total of 50% of them are idiopathic.
- Cutaneous signs of vasculitis include palpable purpura, skin ulcerations, and Raynaud phenomenon.

## Clinical Features

- Clinical presentation can be widely variable.
- They are most often bilateral and commonly occur below the knee.
- Palpable purpura can cause a burning or stinging sensation. Plaques and ulcers can be very painful (Fig. 20.2).
- They are associated with many disease states.
- Their classification is based on the size of the vessel involved.

### Leukocytoclastic Vasculitis

Leukocytoclastic vasculitis is a form of vasculitis ulcer that starts with the deposition of circulating immune complexes. These activate the classic and alternative complement pathways (C3, C4, C5) and inflammatory cells.

Leukocytoclastic vasculitis results from a heterogeneous group of underlying medical issues, including infection, chemical, or drug exposure; connective tissue disease; Henoch-Schönlein syndrome; mixed essential cryoglobulinemia; malignancy; Churg-Strauss; and Wegener granulomatosis.

### Clinical Features

Painfully palpable purpura is the most common finding, consisting of nonblanching, 1- to 3-mm, violaceous, round, regular papules, characteristically involving the lower extremities (Fig. 20.3). In severe cases, ulcers on the ankles and legs can appear.

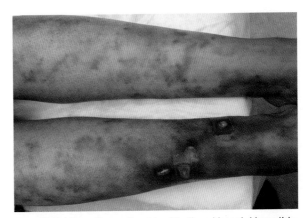

**Fig. 20.2 Ulcer Secondary to Medium-Vessel Vasculitis.** (From the UConn Grand Rounds Collection.)

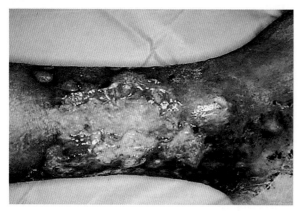

**Fig. 20.3** Leukocytoclastic Vasculitis. (Courtesy Vincent Falanga, MD.)

## Differential Diagnosis

The differential includes drug-induced lupus erythematosus, polyarteritis nodosa, cryofibrinogenemia, cryoglobulinemia, cholesterol emboli, and infection.

## Work-Up

- Skin biopsy is required to confirm cutaneous vasculitis. The optimal time for biopsy is less than 24 hours after the onset of a lesion.
- A careful drug history should be taken.
- To rule out other rheumatologic or infectious causes, lab tests may be required, such as an antinuclear antibody (ANA) test, antineutrophil cytoplasmic antibody (ANCA) test, rheumatoid factor, complement levels, anti-Ro, anti-La, and antiphospholipid antibody test.

## Initial Steps in Management

- Treat any underlying trigger, such as medications or infection.
- Recommend leg elevation and compression for lower extremity lesions, nonsteroidal antiinflammatory drugs (NSAIDs) for pain control, and antihistamines for pruritis.
- For some forms of leukocytoclastic vasculitis, colchicine (0.6 mg by mouth every 8–12 hours) or dapsone (100–150 mg by mouth every 24 hours) have been used.
- Although systemic steroids can be helpful, the chronic use of systemic steroids is not advised because it is associated with innumerable serious systemic side effects.

## Warning Signs/Common Pitfalls

Cannabis has been associated with vascular disease, but that finding may be confounded by the frequent presence of a smoking history.

## Counseling

Your healthcare provider has diagnosed you with an ulcer because of inflammation and damage to some of the blood vessels in your skin. This can arise spontaneously without a known underlying cause or may be associated with an underlying disease process. Your healthcare provider will likely perform a skin biopsy and order some blood tests. If the lesions are on your legs, keep them elevated at rest. Depending on the underlying etiology, the healthcare provider may prescribe some medications to reduce the inflammation.

# VENOUS ULCERS

Chronic venous insufficiency (because of dilated veins, incompetent venous valves, or poor calf muscle pump function) causes persistent inflammation, edema, prominent veins (varicosities), venous dermatitis, and venous leg ulcers (VLUs). VLUs are the most common form of leg ulcers, with an increasing incidence among the elderly of up to 3% to 4%.

## Clinical Features

- VLUs are most commonly found on the lower legs in the gaiter area, between the lower calf and ankle. The medial aspect is affected most frequently (Fig. 20.4).

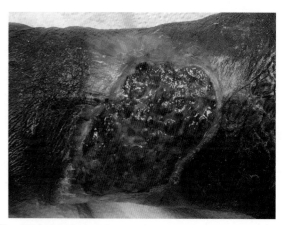

**Fig. 20.4** Venous Leg Ulcer. Note the classic location. (From the UConn Grand Rounds Collection.)

- Pain is usually mild.
- The typically shallow ulcer may have irregular sloping edges and moderate to heavy exudate.
- Surrounding skin may exhibit eczematous changes, erythema, scaling, weeping, induration, and crusting. Hemosiderin deposits (brown pigmentary skin changes) and lipodermatosclerosis are common findings. "Lipodermatosclerosis" refers to subcutaneous fibrosis and skin hardening caused by chronic inflammation and is associated with chronic venous insufficiency.
- The presence of exposed tendons or black eschar within the wound rules out venous etiology.

## Differential Diagnosis

The differential includes arterial ulcers, diabetic ulcers, pyoderma gangrenosum (PG), sickle-cell disease, livedoid vasculopathy, infection, and malignancy.

- Arterial ulcers are typically very painful; have a punched-out appearance; are located anteriorly or laterally on the lower extremity; and present with weak or absent distal pulses, cool feet, and loss of hair on the legs.
- Diabetic ulcers are usually painless. Look for punched-out ulcers, usually within a thick callus, that are typically located in pressure sites on the feet. These ulcers are associated with peripheral neuropathy and an elevated HbA1c.
- PG involves rapidly enlarging, often very painful ulcers that have a violaceous, undermined, border. These can occur anywhere and are tender to palpation.
- Sickle-cell disease is very painful and has a well-demarcated, punched out appearance. It is also resistant to treatment, with a high recurrence rate. Bilateral involvement is common and uncontrolled ulcers may become circumferential.
- Livedoid vasculopathy involves painful, recurrent, stellate, shallow ulcerations that are slow to heal, with depressed, white, atrophic, stellate scars with telangiectasia called "atrophie blanche."
- Infections that resemble venous ulcers include methicillin-resistant *Staphylococcus aureus* (MRSA) infection, atypical mycobacterial infections, deep fungal infections, and leishmaniasis.
- Primary cutaneous neoplasms, such as squamous cell carcinoma (SCC) or basal cell carcinoma (BCC), can ulcerate. Chronic ulcers can also undergo malignant transformation. They typically present as ulcers that are enlarging or failing to heal despite treatment, usually with exophytic or irregular wound edges. A Marjolin ulcer is an aggressive, ulcerating SCC that arises from a chronic wound.

## Work-Up

- A comprehensive history and physical examination are essential in the evaluation of chronic venous insufficiency and ulceration. Pulses are usually normal unless there is concomitant arterial disease.
- A venous duplex ultrasound scan can help to confirm the diagnosis.
  - Assess perfusion in the affected extremities.
  - Check foot temperature and pulses.
  - The ABI is a noninvasive tool used to diagnose peripheral arterial disease (PAD) and measure the systolic blood pressures in the ankle and the arm using a Doppler probe and a blood pressure (BP) cuff. ABI is calculated by dividing the BP in an artery of the ankle by the BP in an artery of the arm.
    - A normal ABI value is greater than 0.9 and less than 1.3.
    - In a noncompressible calcified vessel, the ABI value is greater than 1.3.
    - In positive peripheral arterial disease, the ABI value is less than 0.9.
- Skin biopsy (a deep wedge containing the wound margin and the wound bed) should be done if the diagnosis is in doubt or if there is a deterioration or no healing progress despite good wound care. A rule of thumb for performing a biopsy is 3 months of nonhealing.

## Initial Steps in Management

- Leg elevation and compression are the mainstays of treatment for venous ulcers. Compression can be provided with bandage systems (such as multilayer compression wraps or Unna boots), stockings/hosiery, or intermittent compression devices. For venous ulcers, 30 to 40 mm Hg pressure is recommended.
- Wound debridement accelerates healing by removing dead necrotic tissue, foreign material, and biofilms. In addition to enzymatic and traditional surgical methods, hydrosurgery is another good modality to remove nonviable tissue.
- Routinely cleanse the wound gently with saline or tap water.

- The dressing should be chosen based on the level of exudate.
  - For very moist wounds, absorptive dressings like alginates and hydrofibers should be used.
  - Dry wounds necessitate hydrogels and moderate drainage indicates hydrocolloids or foams.
- Once a dressing becomes saturated, it should be replaced. If clinical infection is suspected, antimicrobial dressings containing silver, iodine, honey, polyhexamethylene biguanide, or a combination of methylene blue and crystal violet can be used.
- Venous eczema may require mid- to high-potency topical corticosteroids applied twice daily around but not in the wound.
- Pentoxyfylline 400-800 mg three times daily have proven to be effective in the treatment of venous ulcers.
- Optimize the patient's nutrition with appropriate dietary supplementation.

### Warning Signs/Common Pitfalls

- Vascular surgery should be consulted if the ABI is equal to or less than 0.8.
- Surgical therapy should be considered after medical treatment options have been exhausted. Surgical options include punch grafts, split-thickness grafts, epidermal or dermal engineered grafts, and saphenous vein surgery. Endovenous ablation may also have a role in treatment.
- Contact dermatitis is a frequent complication of therapy, usually because of the use of topicals with neomycin, bacitracin, lanolin, or paraben preservatives.
- The differentiation between contact dermatitis and cellulitis of the leg is often difficult. It is often necessary to get a dermatology consult or to empirically treat with systemic antibiotics.
- Compressive leg stockings are a necessary long-term measure after healing. Patients should be warned to remove the garments if they notice any side effects of numbness, pain, tingling, or dusky toes.

### Counseling

You have been diagnosed with an ulcer on your legs because of leg veins that can no longer return blood back toward your heart the way they used to.

You should wear support hose, keep your legs elevated when sitting or at rest, and try to walk to exercise the muscles in your legs. Your healthcare provider will prescribe creams to use on your legs and may refer you to a vascular surgeon or specialist dermatologist to help you deal with this issue if it progresses despite treatment.

## PYODERMA GANGRENOSUM

PG is a poorly understood ulcerative skin disease. It is a neutrophilic dermatosis and is often associated with systemic inflammatory conditions, such as inflammatory bowel disease (IBD), rheumatoid arthritis, hematologic diseases (e.g., acute and chronic myelogenous leukemia, hairy cell leukemia, myelodysplasia, and immunoglobulin [Ig]A monoclonal gammopathy), or other immune diseases. PG is a diagnosis of exclusion.

### Clinical Features

- PG involves rapidly enlarging (in days), painful, exudating ulcers. They may start as pustules, which then develops an overlying necrotic bulla that ulcerates with purulent drainage. Edges of ulcers are elevated and undermined with violaceous borders and may have tiny pustules along the periwound. Lesions heal with irregular cribriform scarring (Fig. 20.5).
- The most common site is on the lower legs, but it may be seen at other sites.
- PG exhibits pathergy, which means that enlargement of the lesion may be exacerbated with minimal trauma; additionally, spontaneously occurring lesions can occur at the site of trauma.

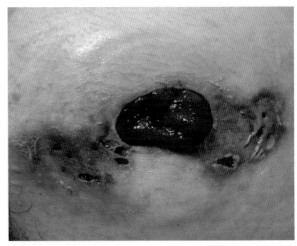

**Fig. 20.5 Peristomal Pyoderma Gangrenosum.** Note the cribriform scarring.

- Postsurgical PG may masquerade as wound dehiscence or infection.
- There are 4 main subtypes of PG: ulcerative, pustular, bullous, and vegetative.
  - Ulcerative is the most common form. It involves a painful ulcer with a purulent base and erythematous undermined border. The lower extremities and trunk are the most common sites of involvement.
  - Pustular PG involves discrete pustules with surrounding erythema, which usually occur in patients with IBD.
  - Bullous (also known as "atypical PG") is less common. It involves rapidly evolving vesicles that coalesce into bullae on an erythematous base. Lesions can evolve rapidly and there can be central necrosis. This subtype is most commonly seen in patients with an associated hematologic disease.
  - In vegetative PG, the head and neck are the most common sites. These are superficial ulcerations without a purulent base or undermined borders. A verrucous quality is often present.

## Differential Diagnosis

The differential for PG includes primary infections (such as MRSA infection, atypical mycobacterial infections, deep fungal infections, and leishmaniasis), venous ulcers, antiphospholipid antibody syndrome, calciphylaxis, vasculitis, malignancy (e.g., nonmelanoma skin cancer such as SCC or BCC), arthropod bite reactions, brown recluse spider bites, and trauma.

- Venous ulcers can be easily diagnosed by ordering a duplex ultrasound scan.
- Antiphospholipid antibodies are lupus anticoagulant and anticardiolipin antibodies.
- Calciphylaxis presents with eschars, is rapidly progressive, and is associated with renal disease.
- In vasculitis, Wegener is the most common cause of PG-like ulcers. Check the ANCA levels. Other conditions that may mimic PG include cutaneous polyarteritis nodosa, microscopic polyangiitis, granulomatous vasculitides, autoimmune connective tissue disease, and Behçet disease.
- Trauma resembling PG include factitial ulcers (Fig. 20.6).

## Work-Up

Skin biopsy and microbial work-up should be performed to rule out infectious etiologies. Lab tests that

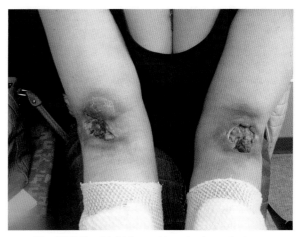

**Fig. 20.6 Factitial Ulcers.** Note the jagged edges.

may be ordered to rule out systemic disease include a complete blood count with or without a peripheral blood smear; serum electrolytes; liver function tests; urinalysis, ANCA; ANA; antiphospholipid antibody; rheumatoid factor; and serum and urine protein electrophoresis.

## Initial Steps in Management

- Referral to a dermatologist is recommended.
- The main goals of treatment are to control the inflammation and optimize wound care.
- Wounds should be cleansed gently with tepid sterile saline or a mild antiseptic before dressing changes. Wound dressings that promote a moist wound environment and do not adhere to the wound base are preferred because they may be beneficial for healing.
- Inflammation can be controlled by using superpotent topical steroids (such as clobetasol); intralesional injections with triamcinolone acetonide (10 mg/mL); and systemic dapsone with or without prednisone (start with 1 mg/kg per day). If no response is seen in a week, a second immunosuppressive agent, such as cyclosporine (4-10 mg/kg/day), should be added. Biologic agents that interfere with the action of tumor necrosis factor-alpha have emerged as powerful agents for the treatment of inflammatory conditions, including PG.
- In superficial or limited lesions, consider dapsone 100 to 200 mg daily, minocycline 100 to 200 mg daily, colchicine 100 mg twice daily, or clofazimine 100 mg twice daily.

## Warning Signs/Common Pitfalls

- Unnecessary traumatic insults to the wound, such as surgical debridement or the use of wet to dry dressings, and the application of caustic substances (e.g., silver nitrate) should be avoided. Because of the risk for pathergy, surgical intervention is controversial but usually contraindicated.
- PG tends to recur and persists without treatment. Recurrence occurs in approximately 30% of patients. Lesions may last from months to years.
- Patients should be monitored for clinical signs of wound infection (e.g., fever, warmth, swelling, malodor, lymphangitic streaks, increased drainage, pain) and should be treated appropriately with antibiotics if infection occurs.

## Counseling

You have been diagnosed with a poorly understood inflammatory disease that can cause painful ulcers in the skin. This disease often is associated with an underlying disease process, such as an autoimmune disease (e.g., ulcerative colitis, Crohn disease, arthritis). Please try not to traumatize your skin because this can make the ulcer worse or create new lesions. Your healthcare provider will take a thorough history, order some tests, and may inject the ulcers with steroids. Referral to a dermatologist is recommended.

# SURGICAL SITE WOUND INFECTION

Infection can delay wound healing. A wound infection indicates the presence of an organism with clinical signs and symptoms of illness. Colonization indicates the presence of an organism without symptoms of illness. All wounds are colonized with microbes; however, not all wounds are infected. Although colonization of a wound is not indicative of invasive infection, the presence of endogenous and/or exogenous organisms in biofilms increases the risk.

The Centers for Disease Control and Prevention (CDC) defines surgical site infection (SSI) as an infection related to an operative procedure that occurs at or near the surgical incision within 30 days of the procedure or within 90 days if prosthetic material is implanted at surgery. An infection involving a surgical bed may be superficial, involving the skin, or can be deeper, involving subcutaneous tissues and underlying structures. Risk factors include smoking, uncontrolled diabetes, obesity, malnutrition, immunosuppression, cardiovascular disease, prior incision, and irradiation at the surgical site. Surgical technique also plays a role, as does the proper application of skin antiseptic solutions.

*Staphylococcus sp.* is most commonly associated with surgical-site wound infections.

## Clinical Features

The surgeon generally makes the diagnosis of infection. Clinical criteria for defining SSI include a purulent exudate draining from a surgical site; a positive fluid culture obtained from a surgical site that was closed primarily; and/or a surgical site that is reopened in the setting of at least one clinical sign of infection (pain, swelling, erythema, warmth) and is culture positive or not cultured.

## Differential Diagnosis

The differential includes surgical dehiscence, or the opening of a previously closed wound. This may be related to infection, surgical technique, or extra pressure from the pulmonary toilet (coughing) and/or ileus.

## Work-Up

Diagnosis is clinical. Culture of purulent material, if present, can be helpful.

## Initial Steps in Management

- Mild topical antiseptics are frequently used to cleanse wounds. Nevertheless, antiseptics cannot be used for a prolonged period of time because of their ability to cause cytotoxicity.
- Iodine and silver-based dressings are commonly used as antimicrobial dressings in the management of wounds that are at risk for infection.
- Topical mupirocin ointment is an alternative topical therapy after cleansing the wound twice a day.
- Systemic signs, such as fever and leukocytosis, are indicators of progression to bacteremia or septicemia. In such cases, systemic antibiotics are warranted.

## Counseling

Your healthcare provider has noted that your surgical wound has become infected. Topical care will be recommended and prescribed. Please alert your healthcare provider if you develop a fever because oral antibiotics may then be needed as well.

Page numbers followed by "*f*" indicate figures, "*t*" indicate tables.